Practical Pharmacology for the
SURGICAL TECHNOLOGIST

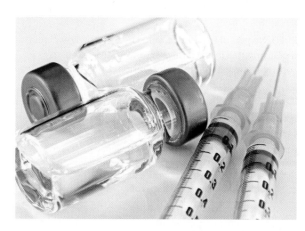

Practical Pharmacology for the
SURGICAL TECHNOLOGIST

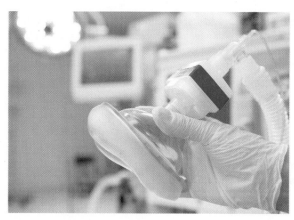

Teri Junge
MEd, CSFA, CST, FAST

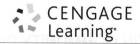

CENGAGE
Learning·

Australia • Brazil • Mexico • Singapore • United Kingdom • United States

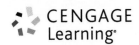

Practical Pharmacology for the Surgical Technologist
Teri Junge

SVP, GM Skills & Global Product Management: Dawn Gerrain

Product Director: Matthew Seeley

Product Manager: Stephen Smith

Senior Director, Development: Marah Bellegarde

Product Development Manager: Juliet Steiner

Senior Content Developer: Patricia Gaworecki

Product Assistant: Mark Turner

Vice President, Marketing Services: Jennifer Ann Baker

Senior Marketing Manager: Erica Glisson

Senior Production Director: Wendy Troeger

Production Director: Andrew Crouth

Content Project Management and Art Direction: Lumina Datamatics

Cover image(s): Voyagerix/Dreamstime; areeya_ann/Shutterstock; Pavel L Photo and Video/Shutterstock; Firma V/Shutterstock

Library of Congress Control Number: 2015954710

ISBN: 978-1-435-46980-8

Cengage Learning
20 Channel Center Street
Boston, MA 02210
USA

Cengage Learning is a leading provider of customized learning solutions with employees residing in nearly 40 different countries and sales in more than 125 countries around the world. Find your local representative at **www.cengage.com**.

Cengage Learning products are represented in Canada by Nelson Education, Ltd.

To learn more about Cengage Learning, visit **www.cengage.com**

Purchase any of our products at your local college store or at our preferred online store **www.cengagebrain.com**

Notice to the Reader

Publisher does not warrant or guarantee any of the products described herein or perform any independent analysis in connection with any of the product information contained herein. Publisher does not assume, and expressly disclaims, any obligation to obtain and include information other than that provided to it by the manufacturer. The reader is expressly warned to consider and adopt all safety precautions that might be indicated by the activities described herein and to avoid all potential hazards. By following the instructions contained herein, the reader willingly assumes all risks in connection with such instructions. The publisher makes no representations or warranties of any kind, including but not limited to, the warranties of fitness for particular purpose or merchantability, nor are any such representations implied with respect to the material set forth herein, and the publisher takes no responsibility with respect to such material. The publisher shall not be liable for any special, consequential, or exemplary damages resulting, in whole or part, from the readers' use of, or reliance upon, this material.

Printed in the United States of America
Print Number: 01   Print Year: 2

Dedication
This book is dedicated to my parents who urged me to begin a career in the medical field following my high school graduation, to Cousin Ruth who inspired me to pursue a career as a surgical technologist, Mary for mentoring me when I began teaching surgical technology, Bev for encouraging me to continue my education, my colleagues for supporting this textbook project by continually suggesting improvements and through answering endless questions, and to my close friends and family for surviving the challenges related to my working on an undertaking of this magnitude.
Additionally, this book is dedicated to surgical technology educators and surgical technology students who strive to ensure that their patients receive optimal care.

CONTENTS

REVIEWERS

Audrey Gabel, CST, AAS
Surgical Technology Program Director/Clinical
Coordinator/Instructor
Las Positas College
Livermore, CA

Douglas J. Hughes, MAE-CI, CSFA, CSA, CST, CRCST
Professor and Director of Surgical Technology
Columbia Basin College
Pasco, WA

Patricia Siefkas, AS, CST
Surgical Technology Program Director
San Joaquin Valley College
Bakersfield, CA

Shannon Valenzuela, CST
Surgical Technology Program Director/Instructor
South Plains College
Lubbock, Texas

PREFACE

Practical Pharmacology for the Surgical Technologist addresses the topic of pharmacology as it relates to the practice of surgical technology. The textbook is appropriate for use in accredited surgical technology education programs because it is compliant with the *Core Curriculum for Surgical Technology* (6th edition) (Core Curriculum) and meets the accreditation requirements for surgical technology education programs set forth by the Commission on Accreditation of Allied Health Education Programs (CAAHEP). The textbook focuses on the theory and skills that lead to safe medication practices in the surgical environment, containing introductory information for the surgical technology student as well as review materials for the experienced surgical technologist. Additionally, the textbook is a valuable resource to surgical technologists preparing to take the Certified Surgical Technologist (CST) examination administered by the National Board of Surgical Technology and Surgical Assisting (NBSTSA).

ROLE OF THE SURGICAL TECHNOLOGIST

Surgical technologists are allied healthcare professionals who are educated in theories and skilled in techniques specific to practice in the operating room. Surgical technologists are part of a team of specialists that care for the surgical patient preoperatively, intraoperatively, and postoperatively primarily in hospital and outpatient settings. Surgical technologists are responsible for many aspects of surgical case management and delivery of quality patient care in the operating room and must carry out those responsibilities at a high level of integrity and with concern for the patient's well-being while functioning as part of a team (Association of Surgical Technologists [AST], 2005).

Safe medication practices are a vital function of the surgical technologist during all three phases of surgical case management. A medication error can present life-threatening circumstances for the patient; therefore, all surgical team members must work together to ensure that safe medication practices are implemented.

SURGICAL TECHNOLOGY EDUCATION

Over 450 CAAHEP accredited surgical technology education programs are in existence in the United States today (Commission on Accreditation of Allied Health Education Programs [CAAHEP], 2014). And the Accrediting Bureau of Health Education Schools (ABHES) lists an additional 60 accredited surgical technology education programs (Accrediting Bureau of Health Education Schools [ABHES], 2014b). The length of a surgical technology education program varies from 9 to 24 months and graduates attain a diploma, a certificate of completion, or an associate degree (ABHES, 2014a; Accreditation Review Council on Education in Surgical Technology and Surgical Assisting [ARC/STSA], 2011a). According to CAAHEP (2009a), graduates of nearly half of the accredited programs earn an associate degree. The associate degree is the preferred minimum education for entry-level surgical technologists because the practicing surgical technologist must be intellectually and technically prepared to meet the demands of the profession (AST, 1993).

Accreditation

Accreditation is a process that provides assurance to potential students that an institution or a program within that institution complies with established standards of quality. Accrediting agencies are private national or regional associations that develop assessment criteria and determine whether an institution or program meets the required standards (United States Department of Education, 2011). In the United States, accrediting bodies are recognized as authentic by the United States Department of Education and/or the Council for Higher Education Accreditation. Standards used for evaluation address adequacy of the facility, availability of student support services (learning resources, financial aid, etc.), faculty qualifications, curriculum content, and student outcomes. The accreditation process typically consists of a self-study of compliance with the assessment criteria, which is followed by a site visit by a panel of experts to ensure compliance with the set standards. Information from the self-study and the recommendations of the review committee are forwarded to the accrediting body to determine accreditation status. In order to maintain accreditation, an institution or program may be required to submit annual updates and undergo periodic on-site review (Council for Higher Education Accreditation, 2010).

CAAHEP Accreditation

Most surgical technology education programs are accredited by CAAHEP in collaboration with the Accreditation Review Council on Education in Surgical Technology and Surgical Assisting (ARC/STSA). The goal of CAAHEP is to ensure that graduates of the allied health education programs that are accredited by their organization have the theoretical background and necessary skills that will allow the individual to function successfully in the chosen healthcare profession (CAAHEP, 2009a). "CAAHEP is the largest programmatic accreditor in the health sciences field … and is recognized by the Council for Higher Education Accreditation" (CAAHEP, 2009b).

In order to achieve initial CAAHEP accreditation and to maintain ongoing accreditation, surgical technology education programs must be in full compliance with the latest edition of the *Standards and Guidelines for the Accreditation of Educational Programs in Surgical Technology* (Standards). The Standards have been established by CAAHEP in cooperation with the American College of Surgeons (ACS) and the Association of Surgical Technologists (AST) (ARC/STSA, 2011a). To enhance understanding of and compliance with the Standards, ARC/STSA has developed the *Surgical Technology Standards Interpretive Guide* (SIG) that contains explanations and detailed examples of ways that a program may demonstrate compliance with the Standards (ARC/STSA, 2011b). Standard III (Resources) C (Curriculum) states that the surgical technology "program must demonstrate by comparison that the curriculum offered meets or exceeds the content demands of the latest edition of the *Core Curriculum for Surgical Technology*" (CAAHEP, 2004, p. 5).

ABHES Accreditation

The United States Department of Education also recognizes ABHES as an accreditor. A few surgical technology education programs are accredited by ABHES, which is a small regional agency that grants institutional and programmatic accreditation to private and public postsecondary institutions that offer one of three health education programs including surgical technology (ABHES, n.d.). Accreditation of a surgical technology education program through ABHES requires compliance with the *Accreditation Manual*, which includes adherence to the current edition of the Core Curriculum (ABHES, 2014a).

Core Curriculum

The Core Curriculum was developed by a committee of surgical technology educators and practicing surgical technologists appointed by the AST Board of Directors. As the professional organization for surgical technologists, one of AST's primary responsibilities is to "ensure that surgical technologists and surgical assistants have the knowledge and skills to administer patient care of the highest quality" (AST, 2011). The Core Curriculum establishes minimum educational standards to guide the teaching of surgical technology students and serves as an outcomes indicator for national programmatic accreditation and eligibility for national individual certification as a surgical technologist (Hughes & Junge, 2011).

The Core Curriculum is presented in an outline format and six pages of the current document are dedicated to pharmacology concepts and skills (Graft, et al., 2011). Several new topics were added to the pharmacology portion of the sixth edition of the Core Curriculums that were not included in previous editions. New content includes the following:

- The Joint Commission National Patient Safety Goals
- Terminology related to medication orders (stat, prn)
- Commonly confused drug names
- Use of alternative medications (herbal medicine, nutritional supplements)
- Drugs packaged in sterile packets
- Additional information concerning drug labeling and package inserts
- Drug handling supplies (control syringes, ear syringes, Toomey syringes, catheter tip syringes, intrathecal pumps)
- Labeling of drugs in containers on the sterile field
- Methods of transfer of drugs
- Blood replacement concepts
- Categories of drugs commonly used for surgical patients (nasal sprays, stains, miotics, respiratory inhalers) (Graft, et al., 2011).

Surgical technology education programs seeking initial or ongoing CAAHEP accreditation must demonstrate full compliance with the latest edition of the *Standards and Guidelines for the Accreditation of Educational Programs in Surgical Technology* (ARC/STSA, 2011a). Standard III C states that the surgical technology "program must demonstrate by comparison that the curriculum offered meets or exceeds the content demands of the latest edition of the *Core Curriculum for Surgical Technology*" (CAAHEP, 2004, p. 5). Table 1 consists of a correlation chart lists all requisite components of the pharmacology portion of the Core Curriculum and identifies the location of the relevant textbook content as it pertains to each component of the Core Curriculum.

TABLE 1 Core Curriculum Comparison Chart

Core Curriculum Component	Surgical Technologist's Guide to Pharmacology Chapter Location
1. Medication measurements	2
a. Conversion and equivalent tables	2
i. Metric system (terminology and conversions)	2
ii. Household system (terminology and conversions)	2
iii. Temperature conversion (Fahrenheit to Celsius/ Celsius to Fahrenheit)	2
iv. Units of Measure	2
1. oz	2
2. mL or ml	2
3. L	2
4. Gtt	2
5. Kg	2
6. Mg	2
b. Basic mathematics	2
i. Fractions	2
ii. Decimals	2
iii. Ratios	2
iv. Proportions	2
v. Percentages	2
c. Dosage calculations	2
i. Calculating unit per milliliter dosages	2
ii. Calculating amount/dosage delivered	2
d. Mixing Medications	2
i. Combining	2
ii. Reconstituting	2
iii. Diluting	2
2. Terminology	1, 7, 8
a. General definitions	1, 7, 8
i. Pharmacology	1
ii. Pharmacokinetics	7
1. Absorption	7
2. Distribution	7
3. Metabolism	7
4. Excretion	7
iii. Pharmacodynamics	8
1. Onset	8
2. Peak effect	8
3. Duration of action	8
b. Types of medication actions and effects	8
i. Actions	8
1. Synergist	8
2. Agonist	8
3. Antagonist	8
4. Additive	8
ii. Therapeutic actions	8
1. Indications	8
2. Contraindications	8
iii. Effects	8
1. Side effects	8
2. Adverse effects	8
3. Medications	1, 3, 4, 5, 6
a. Medication nomenclature	3
i. Chemical name	3
ii. Generic name	3
iii. Trade or brand name	3

6.	Lubricants	10
7.	Miotics	10
8.	Mydriatics	10
9.	Viscoelastics	10
xxvi.	Sedative-hypnotic agents	10
xxvii.	Staining agents	10
xxviii.	Tranquilizers	10
xxix.	Alternative medications	3
1.	Herbal medicine	3
2.	Nutritional supplements	3

Note. Adapted from the Table of Contents of the *Core Curriculum for Surgical Technology* (6th ed.) by Graft, et al. Copyright 2011 by the Association of Surgical Technologists.

Credentialing of the Surgical Technologist

Credentialing is a method of demonstrating that an individual meets an established minimum knowledge base in a given profession and is entitled to certain privileges because they have earned a credential (Credentialing, n.d.). The credential that is available to surgical technologists is certification. Certification is "recognition by an appropriate body that an individual has met a predetermined standard" (Frey, et al., 2008, p. 39). Two credentialing bodies offer certification for surgical technologists.

NBSTSA

The National Board of Surgical Technology and Surgical Assisting (NBSTSA) is the primary certifying agency for surgical technologists and offers the Certified Surgical Technologist (CST) credential. Currently, an individual may establish eligibility to test with the NBSTSA by currently or previously earning the CST credential or by graduating from a CAAHEP or ABHES accredited surgical technology education program. In 2012, a new option became available for military trained personnel (National Board of Surgical Technology and Surgical Assisting [NBSTSA], 2011b). The NBSTSA is accredited by the National Commission for Certifying Agencies (NCCA), which gives reliability and validity to the credential (NBSTSA, 2011a). According to the NBSTSA (2011d) Surgical Technologist Certifying Examination Outline, 20% of the questions in the basic science section relate to surgical pharmacology. The CST credential is renewed every four years through continuing education (60 continuing education credits required within a four year renewal cycle) or by reexamination (NBSTSA, 2011c).

NCCT

The National Center for Competency Testing (NCCT) is an independent secondary certifying agency that offers the Tech in Surgery-Certified (TS-C) credential. An individual with a high school diploma or the equivalent may establish eligibility to test with NCCT by also (National Center for Competency Testing [NCCT], n.d.b) graduating from a formal surgical technology education program and having one year of qualifying experience; or having seven years of qualifying experience; or by being licensed as a medical doctor (MD), registered nurse (RN), licensed practical nurse (LPN), or licensed vocational nurse (LVN) and having extensive experience in the role of a surgical technologist. The NCCT does not claim "allegiance to any specific professional organization or accreditor" (NCCT, n.d.b). The credential is not recognized in Tennessee and South Carolina (NCCT, n.d.b). The TS-C credential is renewed every four years through continuing education (14 clock hours per year required within a five year renewal cycle) (NCCT, n.d.a).

ORGANIZATION

The textbook consists of a table of contents, 10 chapters, an extensive glossary, a detailed index, and a substantial directory of drugs commonly used in the surgical environment. Each chapter begins with identification of the student learning outcomes (SLOs), followed by a listing of key terms contained within the chapter. Students will use the key terms to enhance understanding of the chapter content as each term is defined contextually (within the chapter) as well as in the glossary. Chapter content is presented in small segments using a typical manuscript format that is frequently supported visually with tables and other graphics (photographs, drawings, etc.). Sequencing of the chapters follows a logical progression with introductory and foundational information contained within the early chapters and more complex information that builds upon the preliminary information appears later in the textbook. Each chapter ends with a summary in an outline format and series of review questions that require the use of critical thinking skills; answers to the review questions are found at the end of the textbook.

The textbook content is compliant with the latest edition of the Core Curriculum; therefore, it is suitable for use in all CAAHEP and ABHES accredited surgical technology education programs. The focus is on the theory and skills that lead to safe medication practices in the surgical environment, and contains introductory information for the surgical technology student as well as review materials for the experienced surgical technologist. The textbook could be a valuable resource to surgical technologists preparing for the national certification examination.

TEACHING AND LEARNING PACKAGE

Student Resources

The following resources were developed to help students learn and practice the information essential to becoming certified as a skilled surgical technologist

MindTap for Practical Pharmacology for the Surgical Technologist

ISBN: 978-1-305-51117-0 (electronic access code) / 978-1-305-51118-7 (printed access card)

MindTap is a fully online, interactive learning experience built upon authoritative Cengage Learning content. By combining readings, multimedia, activities, and assessments into a single learning path, MindTap elevates learning by providing real-world application to better engage students and improve student outcomes. MindTap is device agnostic, meaning that it will work with any platform or learning management system and will be accessible anytime, anywhere: on desktops, laptops, tablets, mobile phones, and other Internet-enabled devices.

MindTap for Practical Pharmacology for the Surgical Technologist includes:

- An interactive e-book with highlighting, note-taking (integrated with Evernote), ReadSpeaker, and more.
- Flashcards for glossary terms and images
- Computer-graded activities and exercises:
  - Self-check and integration activities
  - Case studies
  - Certification style review exams

Instructor Resources

Instructor Companion Website to Accompany Practical Pharmacology for the Surgical Technologist

The Instructor Companion web site allows you to spend less time planning and more time teaching. The site can be accessed by going to Cengage.com/login to create a unique user log-in. Once your instructor account has been activated, you will have access to a comprehensive selection of digital support materials, including:

- The *Instructor's Manual to Accompany Practical Pharmacology for the Surgical Technologist*, with instructor support, course outlines and syllabi, and answers to end-of-chapter critical thinking review questions.
- PowerPoint presentations for each chapter highlighting the key concepts.
- Cognero test bank.

REFERENCES

Accreditation Review Council on Education in Surgical Technology and Surgical Assisting. (2011a). *Information on ARC/STSA*. Retrieved from http://arcst.org/about_arcst.htm

Accreditation Review Council on Education in Surgical Technology and Surgical Assisting. (2011b). *Surgical technology standards interpretive guide*. Retrieved from http://www.arcstsa.org/wp-content/uploads/2012/02/SIG-ST-0212-FINAL2.pdf

Accrediting Bureau of Health Education Schools. (2014a). *Accreditation manual* (17th ed.). Retrieved from http://www.abhes.org/assets/uploads/files/17th_Edition_Accreditation_Manual_2-11-2014.pdf

Accrediting Bureau of Health Education Schools. (2014b). *Directory of institutions and programs*. Retrieved from https://ams.abhes.org/ams/onlineDirectory/pages/directory.aspx

Accrediting Bureau of Health Education Schools. (n.d.). *Recognition*. Retrieved from http://www.abhes.org/recognition

Association of Surgical Technologists. (1993). *Associate degree concept resolution*. Retrieved from http://www.ast.org/pdf/Standards_of_Practice/Resolution_Associate_Degree.pdf

Association of Surgical Technologists. (2005). *Surgical technology: A growing career*. Retrieved from http://www.ast.org/pdf/GrowingCareer.pdf

Association of Surgical Technologists. (2011). *About AST*. Retrieved from http://www.ast.org/aboutus/about_ast.aspx

Commission on Accreditation of Allied Health Education Programs. (2004). *Standards and guidelines for the accreditation of educational programs in surgical technology*. Retrieved from http://www .caahep.org/documents/SurgTechStandardsFinal-May2004(1).pdf

Commission on Accreditation of Allied Health Education Programs. (2009a). *What is accreditation and why is it important?* Retrieved from http://caahep .org/Content.aspx?ID=1

Commission on Accreditation of Allied Health Education Programs. (2009b). *What is CAAHEP?* Retrieved from http://www.caahep.org

Commission on Accreditation of Allied Health Education Programs. (2014). *CAAHEP accredited program search*. Retrieved from http://www.caahep .org/Find-An-Accredited-Program

Council for Higher Education Accreditation. (2010). *The value of accreditation*. Retrieved from http://www .acpe-accredit.org/pdf/ValueofAccreditation.pdf

Credentialing. (n.d.). *Dictionary.com unabridged*. Retrieved from http://dictionary.reference.com/browse/ credentialing

Frey, K., et al. (2008). *Surgical technology for the surgical technologist: A positive care approach* (3rd ed.). Clifton Park, NY: Delmar Cengage Learning.

Graft, D., Bell, C., Bradley, B., Bidwell, J., Burton, A., Campbell, L., … Watts, E. (2011). *Core curriculum for surgical technology* (6th ed.). Littleton, CO: Association of Surgical Technologists.

Hughes, D. & Junge, T. (2011). *Surgical technology teaching improvement project*. Project for Dr. Pamela Lane-Garon's CI 285 course.

National Board of Surgical Technology and Surgical Assisting. (2011a). *About NBSTSA*. Retrieved from http://nbstsa.org/about/index.html

National Board of Surgical Technology and Surgical Assisting. (2011b). *CST examinations: Establishing eligibility to test*. Retrieved from https://nbstsa.org/ examinations-cst.html

National Board of Surgical Technology and Surgical Assisting. (2011c). *Renewal options*. Retrieved from http://nbstsa.org/renewal/index.html

National Board of Surgical Technology and Surgical Assisting. (2011d). *Surgical technologist certifying examination outline*. Retrieved from https://nbstsa .org/downloads/2011/2011_CST-outline.pdf

National Center for Competency Testing. (n.d.a). *Recertification/CE*. Retrieved on September 15, 2011, from http://www.ncctinc.com/CE

National Center for Competency Testing. (n.d.b). *Tech in surgery – certified (NCCT)*. Retrieved from http://www.ncctinc.com/documents/tech%20in%20 surgery%20-%20certified%20(ncct)%20brochure .pdf

United States Department of Education. (2011). *Accreditation in the United States*. Retrieved from http:// www2.ed.gov/admins/finaid/accred/index.html

ACKNOWLEDGEMENT

The author would like to acknowledge Mr. Michael Perry, CEO of San Joaquin Valley College, as well as the director of the Fresno Campus, Dr. John Swiger, for permitting use of the surgical technology simulation lab to obtain many of the photos used in this textbook. Additionally, the author would like to thank Jennifer Nyswonger, BS, CSFA, CST and Annalise Minks, AS, CST, for demonstrating the skills featured in the photos.

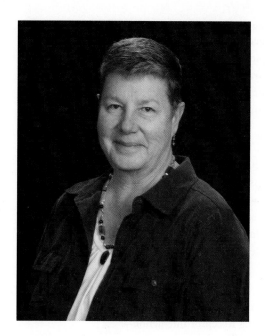

TERI JUNGE started her career in the operating room in 1974 and became a Certified Surgical Technologist (CST) in 1984 and a Certified Surgical First Assistant in 1992. She has been involved in surgical technology education since 1996 and is currently the surgical technology program coordinator at Triton College in River Grove, Illinois. She holds degrees in Surgical Technology (Associate of Applied Science), Health Services Administration (Bachelor of Science), and a Master of Arts in Education degree with an emphasis in Curriculum and Instruction. According to the CAAHEP Standards, "The Program Director must be responsible for all aspects of the program, including the organization, administration, continuous review, planning, development, and general effectiveness of the program" (CAAHEP, 2004, p. 3). Evaluation and selection of course materials, including textbooks, as well as planning curricular content are some of the responsibilities of the program director. When developing the pharmacology unit for classroom use, she examined the available resources for teaching the pharmacology portion of the program and found them to be limited. She identified a critical need for an additional resource and resolved to create a textbook designed to fill a perceived void in pharmacologic information currently available that is specifically relevant to the practice of surgical technology and to meet the necessary programmatic accreditation requirements. Ms. Junge has written numerous articles for *The Surgical Technologist*, participated on the Core Curriculum revision committee (5th edition), served in several capacities (such as author and editor) on several editions of *Surgical Technology for the Surgical Technologist: A Positive Care Approach*, and helped develop many educational products (such as the *Study Guide, Instructor's Manual*, and the video series) to accompany the textbook.

FIGURES

TABLES

Chapter ONE

INTRODUCTION TO PHARMACOLOGY

Student Learning Outcomes

After studying this chapter, the reader should be able to:

- Define the term *pharmacology*.
- Determine a time line of the events leading up to modern pharmacologic practice.
- List and describe federal and state drug regulations.
- Provide the rationale for the five narcotic classifications.
- Differentiate the roles of the Drug Enforcement Administration and the Food and Drug Administration.
- Explain the importance of The Joint Commission National Patient Safety Goals and identify the goals that relate to medication handling the surgical environment.
- Recognize the potential consequences to the patient should a medication violation occur.

Key Terms

Anatomy
Anesthesia
Antineoplastic
Apothecary
Circa
Drug Enforcement
  Administration (DEA)
Effects
Efficacy
Electuary

Food and Drug
  Administration (FDA)
Formulary
Indigenous
Mitigate
Monograph
Off-label use
Patent
Pathology
Pathophysiology

Pharmacist
Pharmacodynamics
Pharmacokinetics
Pharmacologist
Pharmacology
Pharmacopeia
Pharmacy
Physiology
Policy
Procedure

Properties
Prophylaxis
Protocol
Synthesize
Trademark
Uniform Resource Locator
  (URL)

DEFINITION OF THE TERM *PHARMACOLOGY*

The word *pharmacology* is derived from the Greek root word *farmakon* meaning drug and the suffix *logy* meaning to study. The term *pharmacology* is defined as the study of drugs. The study of drugs pertains to the composition, **properties**, and uses of the drug—especially those that make it medically effective, and the **effects** or characteristics of the drug. Sometimes the effects of the drug are called the actions of the drug.

A drug is described as a substance that is used to diagnose, treat, cure, **mitigate** (to make less severe), or prevent a disease or condition. *Prophylaxis* is the term used to describe preventive measures.

The term *pharmacologist* is used to describe one who has knowledge of drugs (origin, composition, action, uses, toxic effects, etc.) and the science of drug preparation. A pharmacologist usually works in a research setting. A **pharmacist** is a licensed health care professional educated to prepare and dispense drugs. A pharmacist usually works in a hospital or retail **pharmacy**. A pharmacy is a place where drugs are prepared and dispensed. The term *pharmacy* may also be used to describe the practice of drug preparation and dispensation as well as other services such as providing the consumer with information concerning prescribed medication(s) and other clinical services.

BRIEF HISTORY (TIME LINE) OF PHARMACOLOGY

Although there is no formal record of ancient history, it is believed that the people of the time used animal, mineral, and plant elements in a rudimentary fashion for medicinal properties. Whether by instinct or by trial and error, the benefit of each crude treatment was recognized and that knowledge was passed (verbally and through the use of demonstration) from one generation to the next to benefit others.

Medical texts written on clay tablets found in Mesopotamia that date back to approximately 2600 B.C.E. (before the Christian/common era) describe **apothecary** practitioners as a pharmacist, physician, and priest. The tablets describe the signs and symptoms of an illness, the prescribed treatment along with instructions for preparing the treatment, and a prayer to the gods. This concept is thought to be the basis for the current practice of combining spiritual care and traditional health care to promote healing.

Shen Nung, thought to be a Chinese Emperor (**circa** 2000 B.C.E.), is recognized for investigating the therapeutic qualities of hundreds of herbs by testing them on himself and writing about them in the *Pen Tsao*, which is loosely translated to *The Divine Farmer's Herb-Root Classic*. The *Pen Tsao* contains information about the medicinal properties of 365 healing compounds made from plant (barks, herbs, roots), mineral, and animal sources. Nung's documented experiments are credited with being the beginning of traditional Chinese herbal techniques still in use today.

The Egyptian goddess of knowledge, Thoth, is credited with providing a 42-volume work (*The Medical Book of Thoth*) prescribing methods for Egyptians to live healthy lives (circa 1600 B.C.E.). One volume in particular lists combinations of plant and animal mixtures as cures for many human complaints. The *Ebers Papyrus* (1552 B.C.E.) is thought to be an extension of *The Medical Book of Thoth* and possibly a combination of several ancient writings. The *Ebers Papyrus* consists of a scroll that measures over 66 feet in length and nearly 12 inches in width that contains roughly 700 formulas, remedies, and incantations designed to treat physical and mental illnesses. Other topics covered in the *Ebers Papyrus* include contraception, pregnancy and childbirth, dentistry, and methods for treating bone fractures.

Materia medica is a Latin term initiated by Pedanius Dioscorides (1 C.E.—[Christian/common era]) that means the material/substance of medicine. The term *materia medica* has since been replaced by the more modern term *pharmacology*. Dioscorides traveled with the Roman army to observe local healing customs and collect samples of **indigenous** plants used as drugs. He later wrote about his findings concerning over 600 plant species in a volume titled *De Materia Medica*.

During the Middle Ages (5–12 C.E.), monks who lived in secluded monasteries are credited with maintaining gardens filled with healing herbs. The monks were also responsible for translating, copying, and distributing manuscripts containing pharmacologic information. The first independently owned apothecary shop was believed to have been established in Baghdad (8 C.E.) and represents the beginning of the modern-day pharmacy and a separation of the professions of physicians and pharmacists.

Galen (129–199 C.E.), who was recognized primarily as a philosopher, was also well known as a physician and pharmacologist. Many of the preparations originated by Galen have modern counterparts that are still in use today.

A well-organized document written in Arabic in 869 C.E. by al-Agrabadhin tly Sabur bin Sahl gives detailed descriptions of various drug preparations including ointments, **electuaries** (sweetened pastes taken orally), powders, syrups, and tablets. The document also describes drug compounding and storage techniques including the need for weighing and measuring the components accurately as well as the importance of using pure ingredients. Many of the drugs mentioned in the document have origins in China; therefore it is believed that the establishment of trade routes through the Middle East influenced the apothecary practices locally and eventually westward to Europe. By the 13th century, the concept of distinct identities of physicians and pharmacists had spread across Europe, Africa, and Asia.

Over the next few centuries, new drugs from natural sources were identified and techniques for isolating and refining drug substances improved. As the body of knowledge concerning **anatomy**, **physiology**, and **pathophysiology** increased, theories about drug actions also emerged and were tested. The first official **pharmacopeia** was published in Italy in 1498 and contained a list of all of the approved drugs (called a **formulary**). The pharmacopeia also set the legal standard for drug formulas and manufacturing processes. The next major breakthrough in pharmacy practice occurred in 1828, when *Friedrich Wöhler* of Germany was able to **synthesize** urea (an organic substance) from inorganic materials in a laboratory; this branch of scientific research is called synthetic organic chemistry.

Experimental techniques involving chloroform, ether, and nitrous oxide inhalation **anesthesia** began to emerge in both dental and surgical settings in the mid-1800s. There is some controversy about who initiated the first successful anesthetic. Horace Wells, Crawford Williamson Long, and William Morton (among others) are all credited.

The first formal pharmacology education program is reported to have been established in 1847 at a university in Estonia (formerly part of Russia). The department chair, Rudolf Buchheim, built a laboratory and began gathering and reporting scientific pharmacologic data. Buchheim's student and successor Oswald Schmiedeberg is acknowledged as the founder of modern pharmacology because in his nearly 50 years as a pharmacology professor, he trained most of the pharmacology professors of the era and was responsible for writing a textbook titled the *Outline of Pharmacology*, which was published in 1878.

The dawn of the 20th century brought rapid advances in all areas of pharmacology. Vitamins (1912), insulin (1922), penicillin (1928—gained popularity after 1940), sodium pentothal (1936), sulfonamides (late 1930s), streptomycin (1944), gelatin foam (1945), anticancer drugs (late 1940s), polio vaccine (1954), measles vaccine (1963), microfibrillar collagen (1974), propofol (1986), and many other drugs, too numerous to list here, were all developed during this period.

Enhancements in surgical techniques could not evolve until the 20th century when physicians were able to implement pain control (anesthesia) methods, manage hemorrhage (via thermal, chemical/pharmacologic, and mechanical means), and prevent and treat infection (due to discoveries in microbiology, identification of the principles of asepsis, and recognition of the significance of antibiotics). Progress in all three areas is closely linked to innovations in pharmacology.

As technology progresses, discoveries in all fields of science will continue to lead to improvements in the delivery quality of patient care. Table 1-1 provides a brief time line of the history of pharmacology.

TABLE 1-1 History of Pharmacology Time Line

Date	Event
Ancient History	Rudimentary treatments—devised from animal, mineral, and plant sources. Information was passed by word of mouth from one generation to the next.
2600 B.C.E.	Mesopotamian clay tablets—contain medical texts describing the signs and symptoms of an illness, prescribed treatment, and a plea to the gods requesting healing.
Circa 2000 B.C.E.	*Pen Tsao*—contains information about the medicinal properties of 365 healing compounds made from plant (barks, herbs, roots), mineral, and animal sources.
Circa 1600 B.C.E.	*The Medical Book of Thoth* lists combinations of plant and animal mixtures as cures for many human complaints.
1552 B.C.E.	*Ebers Papyrus* contains roughly 700 formulas, remedies, and incantations designed to treat physical and mental illnesses.
1 C.E.	*De Materia Medica*—contains information concerning more than 600 medicinal plant species and local healing customs that were collected by Dioscorides as he traveled with the Roman army.
5–12 C.E.	Monks—lived in secluded monasteries and maintaining gardens filled with healing herbs; also translated, copied, and distributed manuscripts containing pharmacologic information.
8 C.E.	Establishment of the first independently owned apothecary shop (Baghdad).
129–199 C.E.	Galen—devised many pharmaceutical preparations still in use today.
869 C.E.	Al-Agrabadhin tly Sabur bin Sahl—provided detailed descriptions of various drug preparations, drug compounding, and storage techniques. Promoted use of pure ingredients and accurate measurement of ingredients. Chinese influence is seen as trade routes through the Middle East affect the apothecary practices locally and eventually westward to Europe.

900–1400	New drugs from natural sources were identified and techniques for isolating and refining drug substances improved.
1498	Italy—first official pharmacopeia.
1828	Wöhler (Father of organic chemistry—Germany)—synthesized an organic substance from inorganic materials in his laboratory.
Mid-1800s	Inhalation anesthesia—experimental techniques involving chloroform, ether, and nitrous oxide inhalation anesthesia were used in dental and surgical settings.
1847	Estonia (Russia)—first formal pharmacology education program established; department chair, Rudolf Buchheim.
1878	Oswald Schmiedeberg—acknowledged as the founder of modern pharmacology; wrote textbook titled the *Outline of Pharmacology*.
20th century	Rapid pharmacologic advances: • Vitamins (1912) • Insulin (1922) • Penicillin (1928—[gained popularity after 1940]) • Sodium pentothal (1936) • Sulfonamides (late 1930s) • Streptomycin (1944) • Gelatin foam (1945) • Anticancer drugs (late 1940s) • Polio vaccine (1954) • Measles vaccine (1963) • Microfibrillar collagen (1974) • Propofol (1986) And many other drugs, too numerous to list.
21st century	As technology progresses, discoveries in all fields of science will continue to lead to improvements in the delivery quality of patient care; the future!

LAWS, POLICIES, AND PROCEDURES

Several regulatory agencies, state and federal laws, and facility policies and procedures are in place to protect the patient from harm in the surgical environment. Typically, an individual facility's policies and procedures reflect agency regulations as well as the state and federal laws and in some instances the facility policies may be stricter. If there is a conflict between federal law, state law, or facility **policy**, the stricter rule must be applied. The surgical technologist must be aware of and follow all regulations that pertain, not only to medication safety, but to all aspects of surgical practice in their locale.

International Support

The World Health Organization (WHO) collaborates with agency representatives from several national governments to provide support to those agencies to allow each nation to create standards for drug safety, effectiveness, and quality thereby promoting patient safety; especially in developing nations. The goal is development and standardization of a set of international guidelines concerning drug manufacture, storage, distribution, and dispensation. The WHO is also involved in detecting and penalizing manufacturers and distributors of illegal drugs.

In 2009, the WHO published a document titled *Guidelines for Safe Surgery*. The guidelines address patient safety concerns such as ensuring correct patient/site surgery, safe administration of anesthesia, protecting the patient's airway, planning for potential blood loss, avoiding adverse drug reactions, preventing surgical site infection, avoiding retention of foreign bodies, accurate specimen care/identification, using communication, and reporting of errors to the appropriate agencies. Some of the guidelines that relate directly to medication use in the surgical environment are:

- Rapid recognition and response to adverse drug reactions

- Recommended practices to avoid drug delivery errors (such as labeling techniques)

- Administration of prophylactic antibiotics

The full *Guidelines for Safe Surgery* document contains a reproducible Surgical Safety Checklist (found on page 98 of the document) that may be adapted to meet the needs of each facility. The free checklist can be accessed and downloaded from the following **uniform resource locator (URL):** http://apps.who.int/iris/bitstream/10665/44185/1/9789241598552_eng.pdf

Federal Law

One of the first federal laws regulating the pharmaceutical industry was the Drug Importation Act of 1848, which allowed the United States Customs agency to prevent adulterated drugs from foreign markets from entering the United States. The Biologics Control Act of 1902 was implemented to ensure that proper contamination prevention procedures were followed during the manufacturing process for serums and vaccines. The entity currently known as the Center for Biologics Evaluation and Research that oversees safety and effectiveness of all biologic products including blood products and vaccines is a result of the Biologics Control Act.

The federal government became more active in regulation of medications in 1906 when the Pure Food and Drug Act (also known as the Wiley Act) was signed into law by President Theodore Roosevelt. The comprehensive new law became active in January of the following year and pertained to labeling of medications (particularly those containing morphine) and set quality and purity standards intended to prevent manufacturing, selling, or transporting of medications deemed unsafe because they were impure, untested, or otherwise harmful. Inspection of manufacturing plants and shipments of foreign and domestic drugs was assigned to the United States Bureau of Chemistry (which eventually became the United States Food and Drug Administration). Quality and purity standards and labeling requirements were dictated by the United States Pharmacopeia and/or the National Formulary. The Sherley Amendment was added to the Pure Food and Drug Act in 1912 to prevent manufacturers and drug merchants from making false claims about the therapeutic action(s) of a drug. The Harrison Narcotic Act of 1914 required a prescription for the purchase of narcotics such as codeine and opium (and any related compounds or derivatives) and also regulated the import, sale, and manufacture of narcotics. The Harrison Narcotic Act was replaced with the Comprehensive Drug Abuse Prevention and Control Act of 1970.

The Food, Drug, and Cosmetic Act of 1938 was signed into law by President Franklin Roosevelt and was intended to replace the 1906 law. Improved and expanded provisions of the new law included a requirement that all components of the drug must be safe and a condition that all drugs had to be approved by the newly established United States **Food and Drug Administration (FDA)** prior to marketing. The 1941 Amendment and the 1944 Penicillin Amendment required testing of each drug for potency and purity. The Penicillin Amendment was later expanded to include all antibiotics.

A 1952 provision (Durham-Humphrey Amendment) to the Food, Drug, and Cosmetic Act identified drugs that must be sold only by prescription of a medical professional and those that could remain available without a prescription over-the-counter (OTC). Labels of prescription only drugs were required to reflect the prescription only condition and state the intended use of the drug. The Kefauver-Harris Amendment was enacted in 1962 and added provisions for proof of drug effectiveness and required drug labels to include information concerning side effects. In 1966, the Fair Packaging and Labeling Act was put into effect to require all drug packaging to provide honest and informative information in a language that the patient or consumer could understand.

The Comprehensive Drug Abuse Prevention and Control Act of 1970, also known as the Controlled Substances Act of 1970, replaces the Harrison Narcotic Act of 1914. The Controlled Substances Act identifies drugs that are regulated as narcotics and established a classification system according to the intended use of the drug and the potential for dependence on the drug or for the drug to be abused. There are five categories or schedules for classification of controlled substances. The categories or schedules are identified using the Roman numerals I–V. Labels on controlled substance must reflect the category of the drug. This may be accomplished with an uppercase C followed by the appropriate Roman numeral or the Roman numeral may appear within the C (Figure 1-1). Refer to Chapter Three for additional information concerning the Controlled Substances Act. The United States **Drug Enforcement Administration (DEA)** was later founded to enforce the Controlled Substances Act. The Poison Prevention Packaging Act (also 1970) introduced legislation requiring the use of child-proof caps on medication containers.

In 1976 more amendments were made to the Food, Drug, and Cosmetic Act concerning potency of vitamin and mineral supplements. The Orphan Drug Act of 1983

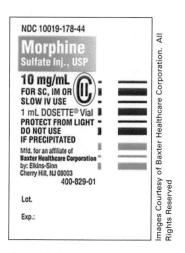

FIGURE 1-1 **Drug Label Identifying Controlled Substance Classification**

allows a streamlined process for approval of drugs used for treatment of rare diseases that would not be otherwise marketable. The Drug Price Competition and **Patent** Term Restoration Act (1984) allows manufacturers of brand name drugs to extend their patents for an additional five years and also provides a simplified application and approval process for generic drugs that have already been approved as brand name drugs without requiring performance of additional research.

In 1990, the Omnibus Budget Reconciliation Act (OBRA) changed the way that Medicaid and Medicare handle drug reimbursement and requires pharmacists to offer counsel to patients receiving new prescriptions and to provide written information concerning the prescribed drug. The Board of Pharmacy oversees OBRA compliance.

The Health Insurance Portability and Accountability Act (HIPAA) of 1996 ensures that a patient is able to continue health care coverage when changing employers and protects the patient's right to privacy in all areas related to health care.

Federal regulatory agencies will continue to monitor the processes involved with drug development, manufacturing, storage, distribution, and delivery and update the laws, as needed, to keep up with the advances. Table 1-2 provides an overview of federal drug regulations.

Regulatory Agencies

Two federal agencies are responsible for consumer protection by enforcing regulations related to the safety and **efficacy** of the pharmaceutical industry in the United States. The two agencies are the United States Drug Enforcement Administration and the United States Food and Drug Administration.

United States Drug Enforcement Administration   The United States Drug Enforcement Administration (DEA) was established in 1973 by President Nixon as a division of the Department of Justice. The DEA is responsible for enforcing the controlled substances (narcotics) laws by investigating those suspected of violating the laws and bringing criminal and civil charges against violators on the local, national, and international levels. Practitioners, such as physicians and pharmacists, must be registered with the DEA in order to be allowed to prescribe and/or dispense controlled substances or to perform research using controlled substances. Once the registration is approved, a certificate is issued and the practitioner is assigned a DEA number that must be printed on an official prescription form. The DEA number must be renewed every three years. There are nearly 230 DEA offices in 21 regions throughout the United States and more than 80 offices in 63 foreign countries. The DEA also offers drug abuse prevention programs.

United States Food and Drug Administration   The United States Food and Drug Administration (FDA) was formed in 1930 and is responsible for overseeing the effectiveness, safety, and security of all drugs (human and veterinary), biological agents (including blood and vaccines), medical devices, cosmetics, and radiation emitting devices. The jurisdiction of the FDA extends to safety and security of the nation's food supply as well.

All new drugs must meet strict guidelines set forth by the FDA prior to approval for use. It can take 12–15 years for a new drug to be developed and the related costs can be upward of 800 million dollars. Upon discovery, the new drug is tested extensively in a laboratory setting; which can include short- and long-term animal trials. During the laboratory testing period, the interaction of the drug molecules with the target cells (**pharmacodynamics**) is studied; as are the most effective route(s) for administering the drug, the dosage amount, and timing of additional doses (if needed). Any toxic effects, side effects, and adverse effects are noted. The way that the drug is processed through the body (**pharmacokinetics**) is also determined. When the drug is ready for clinical (human) testing, the FDA must approve and specific **protocols** must be followed. Due to the many legal and ethical issues surrounding drug trials, human subjects are informed of the potential risks and benefits of participating in the study and must give informed consent to be included in the trial. Human testing takes place in four phases.

- Phase 1—Takes approximately 1–2 years and involves a small number of subjects. The goals of phase 1 are to determine the ideal dosage and identify the best route(s) of administration. The subjects are observed to determine if the desired therapeutic effect on the body is produced and any unwanted effects are noted.

- Phase 2—Takes approximately 1–3 years and involves several hundred subjects. The goals of phase 2 are to determine if the drug is effective in providing the desired therapeutic effect and to identify any short-term risks.

- Phase 3—Takes several years and involves several hundred to several thousand subjects. The goals of phase 3 are to continue to determine the effectiveness of the drug's therapeutic effect and to identify any long-term risks.

- Phase 4—Length of time and number of participants varies. The goals of phase 4 are to further observe effectiveness of the drug and to determine long-term safety of the drug.

Once the human testing is complete and the drug is patented, an internal branch of the FDA, called the Center for Drug Evaluation and Research, reviews all known

TABLE 1-2 Overview of Federal Drug Regulations

Date	Act	Overview
1848	Drug Importation Act	• US Customs agents authorized to prevent adulterated drugs from foreign markets from entering the United States.
1902	Biologics Control Act	• Ensured proper contamination prevention procedures were followed when manufacturing serums and vaccines.
1906	Pure Food and Drug Act (Wiley Act)	• Pertained to labeling of medications (particularly those containing morphine). • Set quality and purity standards. • US Bureau of Chemistry was formed to inspect manufacturing plants and shipments of foreign and domestic drugs. • Quality and purity standards and labeling requirements were dictated by the United States Pharmacopeia and/or the National Formulary.
1912	Sherley Amendment	• Prevented manufacturers and drug merchants from making false claims about the therapeutic action(s) of a drug.
1914	Harrison Narcotic Act	• Required a prescription for the purchase of narcotics such as codeine and opium (and any related compounds or derivatives) and also regulated the imports, sales, and manufacturing of narcotics.
1938	Food, Drug, and Cosmetic Act	• Replaced the Pure Food and Drug Act. • All drug components must be safe. • All drugs must be approved by the FDA.
1941	Insulin Amendment	• Insulin must be tested for potency and purity.
1944	Penicillin Amendment	• Penicillin (and eventually all antibiotics) must be tested for potency and purity.
1952	Durham-Humphrey Amendment	• Identified drugs that must be sold only by prescription of a medical professional and those that could remain available without a prescription over-the-counter (OTC). • Labels of prescription only drugs were required to reflect the prescription only condition and state the intended use of the drug.
1962	Kefauver-Harris Amendment	• Required proof of drug effectiveness. • Required drug labels to include information concerning side effects.
1966	Fair Packaging and Labeling Act	• Required all drug packaging to provide honest and informative information in a language that the patient/consumer could understand.
1970	Comprehensive Drug Abuse Prevention and Control Act (Controlled Substances Act)	• Replaced Harrison Narcotic Act of 1914 • Identified drugs that are regulated as narcotics. • Established classification system according to the intended use of the drug and the potential for dependence on the drug or for the drug to be abused.
1970	Poison Prevention Packaging Act	• Required use of childproof caps on medication containers.
1976	Amendments to Food, Drug, and Cosmetic Act	• Regulated potency of vitamin and mineral supplements.
1983	Orphan Drug Act	• Streamlined approval process for treatment of rare diseases.
1984	Drug Price Competition and Patent Term Restoration Act	• Allowed manufacturers of brand name drugs to extend their patents for an additional five years. • Provided a simplified application and approval process for generic drugs that have already been approved as brand name drugs.
1990	Omnibus Budget Reconciliation Act (OBRA)	• Changed the way that Medicaid and Medicare handle drug reimbursement. • Required pharmacists to offer counsel patients receiving new prescriptions. • Written information concerning the prescribed drug must be provided. • Board of Pharmacy oversees compliance.
1996	Health Insurance Portability and Accountability Act (HIPAA)	• Ensured continuing health care coverage when changing employers. • Protected patient's right to privacy in all areas related to health care.
Ongoing	Under Development	• Processes involved with drug development, manufacturing, storage, distribution, and delivery will be monitored. • Laws will be updated, as needed.

TABLE 1-3 Roles/Responsibilities of the DEA and the FDA

Agency	Roles/Responsibilities
DEA (Established in 1973)	• Responsible for controlled substances only (legal/illegal) • Enforces controlled substance laws • Manages narcotic classifications
FDA (Established in 1930)	• Responsible for drugs (prescription/OTC), foods, and cosmetics • Enforces regulations • Inspects manufacturing facilities • Ensures proper labeling • Approves/removes drugs from market

information about the drug. The review process can take up to 2 years. Once the review is complete, the results are presented to the FDA through an advisory committee for final approval of the drug. Before the drug is marketable, the manufacturing site must be inspected, a brand (proprietary) name determined, a registered **trademark** obtained, and the wording of the drug label must be approved. Following release of the drug, studies concerning the effectiveness, dosing, and undesired effects continue; special attention is given to any populations (such as geriatric patients) that were not included in the human trials. If a problem is detected, the FDA may impose restrictions on the sale of the drug or the approval may be revoked and the drug removed from the market. Table 1-3 differentiates the roles and responsibilities of the DEA and the FDA.

State Law

Roles of various medical practitioners are spelled out in the individual state's practice acts. The purpose of a practice act is to protect the public by identifying the scope of practice, setting practice limits, and defining the responsibilities of the practitioner. Penalties for noncompliance with the practice act are also described. Information pertaining to tasks that can be delegated to the surgical technologist is usually found in the medical practice act and the nurse practice act, and although the title of surgical technologists may not be used, applicable terms include unlicensed assistive personnel and allied health professional. State law must conform to federal law; however, the state may impose stricter regulations. Laws contained within the practice acts vary from state to state, and it is the individual surgical technologist's personal duty to read, understand, and abide by the related practice acts. Most medical and nurse practice acts are accessible online.

Facility Policies and Procedures

Facility policies and procedures must comply with both federal and state law and may be even stricter. The stricter regulation always prevails. A policy is a written institutional rule or plan of action that addresses a specific need and requires compliance within that institution. The rationale for the policy and sanctions for noncompliance are frequently included in the document. A **procedure** outlines the steps necessary to implement the policy. The policies and procedures at each facility differ and are very specific to the institution. As part of the new employee orientation, all personnel should be given an opportunity to become familiar with the necessary policies and procedures. New policies and procedures should be introduced to all staff as soon as they become available. Policies and procedures should be readily available to all employees at all times. The surgical technologist should refer to the policy and procedure documents frequently to ensure compliance.

Verbal Orders as Accepted Practice

In the surgical environment, it may not always be practical for the physician to interrupt what he or she is doing to write a prescription. Therefore issuance of verbal orders is common and accepted practice. Additional information concerning verbal orders is available in Chapter Three.

MEDICATION PUBLICATIONS

Several publications are available that provide reference material concerning OTC and prescription medications. Each publication has a specific purpose and provides information related to that purpose. The surgical technologist should have easy access to detailed information about drugs frequently used in the surgical environment.

Physician's Desk Reference

The *Physician's Desk Reference* (PDR) is available online and in print and provides a **monograph** (complete and detailed description) of all labeling information for each drug that is approved by the FDA. The monograph includes the following information:

- Brand name/generic name/name of manufacturer

- Description (chemical composition/ingredients)

- Clinical pharmacology
  - Therapeutic classification
  - Mechanism of action (pharmacodynamics)
  - Movement of the drug through the body (pharmacokinetics)
  - Drug interactions
  - Carcinogenesis, mutagenesis, fertility impairment
  - Pregnancy category
  - Special populations
    - Labor and delivery
    - Nursing mothers
    - Pediatric/geriatric use

- Adverse reactions
- Indication(s)/usage
- Contraindications
- Warnings
- Precautions
- Abuse/dependence
- Overdosage
- Dosage (adult/pediatric) administration
  - Handling
- How supplied (drug forms)

United States Pharmacopeia and National Formulary

The first *United States Pharmacopeia* (USP) was published in 1820 and the first *National Formulary* (NF) was published in 1888. The two publications were originally intended to complement each other; however, duplications in the content resulted in an eventual merger (1975). The *United States Pharmacopeia* and *National Formulary* (USP–NF) is the combined document that is published annually and updated three times per year. A pharmacopeia is a reference book that is published by a recognized authority (such as the federal government) that sets the legal standards for drug quality, strength, and purity. Standards for drug strength and purity are enforced by the FDA and state agencies. A formulary is an official listing of approved drugs which may also provide the formulas for manufacturing the drug. The NF contains a list of all of the drugs approved by the FDA; however, a formulary may also be used by an insurance company to list all of the drugs covered by the plan or by a pharmacy listing all of the drugs that should be in stock.

The USP–NF contains a monograph for each drug, which contains the name(s) of the ingredient(s) in the preparation; all labeling, packaging, and storage information; and the specification. The specification indicates the testing that must be performed on the drug to demonstrate conformity to the stipulated USP Reference Standards (purity, quality, and strength) as well as the procedures that must be followed during testing and the criteria for acceptance. When a drug manufacturer demonstrates that all specifications have been met, the USP Verified Mark (Figure 1-2) may be added to the package label and the consumer is assured that the quality of the product is consistent and that the manufacturing processes are of high quality.

National Drug Code Directory

The *National Drug Code Directory* is a database that contains information about all drugs and insulin products. Each product is assigned a ten-digit, three-segment

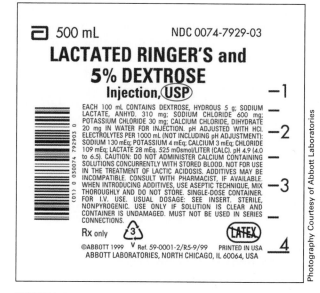

FIGURE 1-2 Drug Label Identifying USP Verified Mark

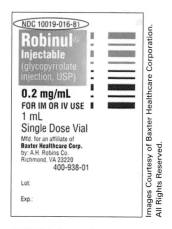

FIGURE 1-3 Drug Label Identifying National Drug Code (NDC)

national drug code (NDC) that appears in the following format (*****-***-**), which allows universal identification of all human drugs (Figure 1-3). The first segment identifies the manufacturer, the second segment identifies the product (name, strength, dosage form), and the third segment identifies the packaging (size, type). In addition to the information contained within the NDC, the directory also provides information concerning the route(s) of administration, active ingredients, unit of measurement, major drug classification, and the FDA application number.

American Hospital Formulary Service (AHFS) Index

The *American Hospital Formulary Service* (AHFS) *Index* is published by the American Society of Health-System Pharmacists. The American Society of Health-System

Pharmacists is a professional society, established in 1959, that is independent of the drug manufacturers. The AHFS publishes the advantages and disadvantages of various drug therapies and examines claims of drug efficacy. Information for the publication is gathered from existing evidence-based drug studies which is then assimilated and scientifically analyzed by the editorial staff and a report is generated. The report evaluates the drug's performance, often by employing comparative analysis techniques. **Off-label uses** for **antineoplastic** drugs are also evaluated and reported. The AHFS is also responsible for the therapeutic drug classification system that serves both as a widely recognized database and a numeric system that is used when billing for pharmaceuticals.

The Medical Letter on Drugs and Therapeutics

The Medical Letter on Drugs and Therapeutics is a newsletter that is published every two weeks in print and online formats. *The Medical Letter on Drugs and Therapeutics* provides independent, peer-reviewed evaluations of drugs newly approved drugs by the FDA and also offers reviews of any changes made to existing drugs. Evaluations include assessments of the efficacy, cost, and toxic effects, and may provide suggestions for possible alternative drugs.

The Joint Commission

The Joint Commission (TJC) is formerly known as the Joint Commission on Accreditation of Healthcare Organizations (JCAHO). In 1910, Dr. Ernest Codman proposed a system, called the End Result System for Hospital Standardization, for tracking patients released from hospitals to determine if the treatment received was effective. If the treatment was not effective, an analysis of the outcome was conducted and recommendations for improvement were made with the hope that subsequent patients with similar diagnoses would experience better outcomes based on the enhanced treatment. When the American College of Surgeons (ACS) was founded in 1913 improving the end result tracking system was one of their objectives. A one-page document titled *The Minimum Standard for Hospitals* was developed by the ACS in 1917 and in 1918, the ACS inspected 692 hospitals and only 89 facilities met the minimum standard. Through the years, more standards were developed and TJC evolved from the ACS. Today, TJC is a private, nonprofit organization whose goal is to evaluate health care organizations to ensure that the care provided is safe, effective, and of the highest quality. Nearly 20,000 organizations are accredited by TJC. Following initial accreditation, a health care organization must be inspected (surveyed) every three years or sooner in order to remain accredited.

National Patient Safety Goals

In addition to providing accreditation services, TJC has developed several policies that relate to patient safety including the *National Patient Safety Goals* that were instituted in 2002. One of the goals relates to the use of abbreviations that should not be used in the health care setting. Another recommendation is that health care facilities develop a list of look-alike/sound-alike drugs. Additional information concerning the "do not use" list and look-alike/sound-alike drugs is found in Chapter Three. Other TJC elements of performance that relate to the surgical environment include:

- Patient identification
- Blood transfusion
- Medication labeling (on the sterile field)
- Hand hygiene
- Infection control practices
- Prevention of surgical site infections
- Catheter associated urinary tract infections
- Pre-procedure verification (correct patient, correct site)/time-out

MEDICATION/SOLUTION VIOLATIONS

Any violation of federal law, state law, or facility policy and procedure is a very serious offense. Precautions must be taken to ensure that no violations occur. Failure to follow the law or facility policy may result in harm to the patient and severe consequences for all surgical team members involved, including the surgical technologist.

Narcotic Precautions

Techniques for handling narcotics in the operating room are described in detail in Chapter Nine.

Personal Negligence

A surgical technologist who does not comply with federal law, state law, and/or facility policies and procedures is at risk of receiving disciplinary action up to and including termination of employment, loss of national certification, and may face civil and criminal charges.

Consequences to Patient

As a result of noncompliance with federal, law, state law, and/or facility policies and procedures, the patient may suffer mild to severe consequences up to and including death.

Summary

I. Definition of the term *pharmacology*
   a. The study of drugs—Pertaining to composition, properties, and uses of the drug—especially those that make it medically effective, and the effects or characteristics of the drug.

II. Brief history (time line) of pharmacology
   a. Ancient History—Rudimentary treatments; formulas passed by word of mouth
   b. 2600 B.C.E.—Mesopotamian clay tablets
   c. Circa 2000 B.C.E.—*Pen Tsao*
   d. Circa 1600 B.C.E.—*The Medical Book of Thoth*
   e. 1552 B.C.E.—*Ebers Papyrus*
   f. 1 C.E.—*De Materia Medica*
   g. 5–12 C.E.—Middle Ages; monks in secluded monasteries maintained medicinal gardens
   h. 8 C.E.—First independently owned apothecary shop established in Baghdad
   i. 129–199 C.E.—Galen
   j. 869 C.E.—Al-Agrabadhin tly Sabur bin Sahl; detailed descriptions of various drug preparations, compounding, and storage techniques; promoted use of pure ingredients and accurate measurement; Chinese influence seen as trade routes through the Middle East affect the apothecary practices locally and eventually westward to Europe.
   k. 900–1400—New drugs from natural sources; improved techniques for isolating and refining drug substances
   l. 1498—First pharmacopeia (Italy)
   m. 1828—Wöhler synthesized an organic compound from inorganic materials
   n. Mid-1800s—Inhalation anesthesia
   o. 1847—First formal pharmacology education program (Estonia)
   p. 1878—*Outline of Pharmacology* by Schmiedeberg (founder of modern pharmacology)
   q. 20th century—Rapid pharmacologic advances
   r. 21st century—Future developments

III. Laws, policies, and procedures—If there is a conflict, the stricter rule must be applied
   a. International support
      i. World Health Organization
   b. Federal law
      i. Regulatory agencies
         1. DEA
            a. Responsible for controlled substances only
            b. Enforces controlled substance laws
            c. Manages narcotic classifications
         2. FDA
            a. Responsible for prescription and OTC drugs, foods, and cosmetics
            b. Enforces regulations
            c. Inspects manufacturing facilities
            d. Ensures proper labeling
            e. Approves/removes drugs from the market
   c. State law
      i. State practice acts
      ii. Vary from state to state
   d. Facility policies and procedures
      i. Vary between facilities
      ii. Policy—Written rule; plan of action
      iii. Procedure—Steps necessary to implement policy
      iv. Provide rationale; sanctions for noncompliance
   e. Verbal orders as accepted practice
      i. Common and accepted practice in the surgical environment
      ii. Not practical to write orders during a procedure

IV. Medication publications
   a. *Physician's Desk Reference* (PDR)—Contains monographs of all FDA-approved drugs
   b. *Pharmacopeia of the United States of America and National Formulary* (USP–NF)—National drug reference book; contains legal standards for drug quality, strength, and purity; enforced by the FDA; lists all drugs approved by the FDA
   c. *National Code Directory*—National data base that provided universal identification codes for all human drugs
   d. *American Hospital Formulary Service Index* (AHFS)—Provides information concerning various drug therapies and examines claims of efficacy
   e. *The Medical Letter*—Provides evaluations of newly approved drugs and reviews of changes to existing drugs

V. The Joint Commission—Private, nonprofit organization whose goal is to evaluate health care organizations to ensure that the care provided is safe, effective, and of the highest quality. TJC accredited nearly 20,000 organizations
   a. *National Patient Safety Goals*—Developed policies related to patient safety; several goals related to safe surgical practices

VI. Medication/solution violations—Violation of federal law, state law, or facility policy and procedure is a very serious offense. Take precautions to ensure that no violations occur. Failure to follow the law or facility policy may result in harm to the patient and severe consequences
   a. Narcotic precautions—Refer to Chapter Nine
   b. Personal negligence
      i. Disciplinary action (including termination of employment)
      ii. Loss of national certification
      iii. Civil and criminal charges
   c. Consequences to patient—May be mild to severe (including death)

Critical Thinking Review

1. Break down the term *pharmacology* and provide definitions for the word root and the suffix.
2. The drug propofol (Diprivan®) was discovered in 1986. Identify the drug classification and provide a brief description of how the drug is used.
3. What is the role of the WHO in international drug safety?
4. List three of the WHO *Guidelines for Safe Surgery* that relate directly to medication use in the surgical environment and explain the importance of each.
5. Which federal agency was created as a result of the Controlled Substances Act of 1970?
6. Briefly describe the role of the United States Food and Drug Administration (FDA).
7. Why is it important for a surgical technologist to be familiar with the content of the state practice acts in the state where he or she is employed?
8. Differentiate between a policy and a procedure.
9. If there is a conflict between federal law, state law, and facility policy and procedure; to which regulation must the surgical technologist adhere?
10. List three or more possible consequences of a medication or solution violation.

References

American Society of Health-System Pharmacists. (2011). *American hospital formulary service pharmacologic therapeutic classification system.* Retrieved from http://www.ahfsdruginformation.com/class/index.aspx

American Society of Health-System Pharmacists. (2011). *Drug information.* Retrieved from http://www.ahfsdruginformation.com/products_services/di_ahfs.aspx

Ballentine, C. (1981). *Sulfanilamide disaster.* Retrieved from http://www.fda.gov/AboutFDA/WhatWeDo/History/ProductRegulation/SulfanilamideDisaster/default.htm

Bixler, C. (n.d.). *The history of pharmacology.* Retrieved from http://www.ehow.com/about_5399506_history-pharmacology.html

Frey, K. et al. (2008). *Surgical technology for the surgical technologist: a positive care approach* (3rd ed.). Clifton Park, NY: Delmar Cengage Learning.

Glen, I. (n.d.). *Propofol, past, present and future…* Retrieved from http://analysis3.com/PROPOFOL,-PAST,-PRESENT-AND-FUTURE…-pdf-e23060.html

The Joint Commission. (2011). *National patient safety goals.* Retrieved from http://www.jointcommission.org/standards_information/npsgs.aspx

The Joint Commission. (2011). *History of the Joint Commission.* Retrieved from http://www.jointcommission.org/about_us/history.aspx

Junge, T. (2009). "From concept to creation: A look at the drug discovery, development, and approval process." *The Surgical Technologist*, January 2009, Volume 41, Number 1, pp. 13–20.

Meadows, M. (2006). *Promoting safe and effective drugs for 100 years.* Retrieved from http://www.fda.gov/AboutFDA/WhatWeDo/History/ProductRegulation/PromotingSafeandEffectiveDrugsfor100Years/default.htm

The Medical Letter Online. (2011). *The medical letter on drugs and therapeutics.* Retrieved from http://secure.medicalletter.org/medicalletter

The Medical Letter Online. (2011). *Treatment guidelines from the medical letter.* Retrieved from http://secure.medicalletter.org/treatmentguidelines

Moini, J. (2009). *Fundamental pharmacology.* Clifton Park, NY: Delmar Cengage Learning.

Mugler, M. (1996). *A brief history of the FDA.* Retrieved from http://keithlynch.net/les/doc8.html

North, M. (2004). *Pure food and drug act (1906).* Retrieved from http://www.ncbi.nlm.nih.gov/books/NBK22116

Pharmacology. (n.d.). *Webster's Revised Unabridged Dictionary.* Retrieved from http://dictionary.reference.com/cite.html?qh=pharmacology&ia=web1913

Regents of the University of Minnesota. (2010). *What is pharmacology?* Retrieved from http://www.pharmacology.med.umn.edu/whatispharm.html

Scheindlin, S. (2001). *A brief history of pharmacology.* Retrieved from http://pubs.acs.org/subscribe/journals/mdd/v04/i05/html/05timeline.html

United States Drug Enforcement Administration. (n.d.). *DEA Mission Statement.* Retrieved from http://www.justice.gov/dea/agency/mission.htm

United States Food and Drug Administration. (n.d.). *About FDA.* Retrieved from http://www.fda.gov/AboutFDA/CentersOffices/default.htm

United States Food and Drug Administration. (2011). *National drug code directory.* Retrieved from http://www.accessdata.fda.gov/scripts/cder/ndc/default.cfm

United States Pharmacopeial Convention. (2011). *About USP.* Retrieved from http://www.usp.org/aboutUSP

United States Pharmacopeial Convention. (2011). *USP–NF—An overview.* Retrieved from http://www.usp.org/USPNF

United States Pharmacopeial Convention. (2011). *USP Reference Standards—An overview.* Retrieved from http://www.usp.org/referenceStandards

United States Pharmacopeial Convention. (2011). *USP verified pharmaceutical ingredients.* Retrieved from http://www.usp.org/USPVerified/pharmaceuticalIngredients

Washington State University College of Pharmacy. (2011). *History of pharmacy.* Retrieved from http://www.pharmacy.wsu.edu/history/history01.html

Woodrow, R. (2007). *Essentials of pharmacology for health occupations* (5th ed.). Clifton Park, NY: Thomson Delmar Learning.

World Health Organization. (2009). *WHO guidelines for safe surgery 2009.* Retrieved from http://whqlibdoc.who.int/publications/2009/9789241598552_eng.pdf

World Health Organization. (2011). *Medicines regulatory support.* Retrieved from http://www.who.int/medicines/areas/quality_safety/regulation_legislation/en

Chapter
TWO

DIMENSIONAL ANALYSIS

Student Learning Outcomes

After studying this chapter, the reader should be able to:

- Define the term *dimensional analysis*.
- Perform basic mathematical calculations to allow conversion between the various measurement systems.
- Identify the seven symbols represented in the Roman numeral system and apply the rules that relate to the Roman numeral system to accurately identify numbers expressed using the Roman numeral system.
- Differentiate between military time and standard or civilian time and accurately state the time using either system.
- Describe the international unit measurement system and identify the types of drugs measured in international units.
- Describe the milliequivalent measurement system and identify the types of drugs measured in milliequivalents.
- Describe the apothecary measurement system and note the circumstances in which the apothecary system is employed.
- Describe the household measurement system and note the circumstances in which the household system is employed.
- Identify terminology related to the metric system and describe the value of each term.
- Accurately perform temperature conversions between the Celsius and Fahrenheit scales.
- Calculate correct drug dosages.

Key Terms

Additive	Dehydrated	Hyperthermia	Rankine temperature scale
Ante meridiem (AM)	Diluent	Hypothermia	Reconstitute
Antibiotics	Dilute	Incident report	Roman numeral system
Apothecary system	Dimensional analysis	Incompatibility	Shelf life
Arabic numerals	Dose	Instability	Solute
Biological	Dye	International unit	Solution
Biological potency	Enzyme	Kelvin temperature scale	Solvent
Blood pressure	Equivocal	Mass	Stain
Celsius	Fahrenheit	Metabolic rate	Standard time
Civilian time	Fat-soluble vitamin	Military time	Symbol
Compatibility	Heart rate	Milliequivalent	Turbidity
Complexation	Hemostasis	Posology	Vital signs
Concentrate	Hemostatic agent	Post meridiem (PM)	
Contrast media	Hormone	Potency	
Decimal system	Household system	Precipitate	

DIMENSIONAL ANALYSIS

The term *dimensional analysis* is used to describe the process of understanding and applying the relationships between the qualities of various items (such as drugs and systems for identifying and measuring drug dosages) based on the physical characteristics (dimensions) of each item. Dimensional analysis that often occurs in the surgical setting includes comparisons of weight, size (length, width, height, or volume), distance, temperature, and time between various systems (such as the **household** system versus the metric system, Roman versus Arabic numbering systems, military versus standard time).

BASIC MATH

As a vital surgical team member, the surgical technologist is responsible for all of the medications, solutions, tissue **dyes** and **stains, contrast media, hemostatic agents,** and any other type of chemical within the sterile field. This responsibility is shared with other surgical team members and includes procuring, preparing, handling, and managing all substances according to federal law, state law, and facility policy and procedure. Fundamental knowledge of the commonly used numbering systems and application of accurate basic mathematical skills applied to calculating drug dosages and concentrations in the surgical setting is critical. A calculation error could produce a devastating result for the patient.

Symbols and terminology important to understanding basic mathematical concepts include:

- − Symbol that represents the term *subtraction*
- − Symbol that indicates division; separates the numerator and denominator of a fraction
- % Symbol that represents the term *percent*
- . Symbol that represents a decimal point
- / Symbol that separates the numerator and denominator of a fraction; indicates division
- ⟯ Symbol that represents long division; long division bracket
- : Symbol that represents a ratio (colon)
- + Symbol that represents the term *addition*
- < Symbol that represents the term *less than*
- = Symbol that represents the term *equals*
- > Symbol that represents the term *greater than*
- × Symbol that represents the term *multiplication*
- ÷ Symbol that represents the term *division*
- √ Symbol that represents the term *square root*

- ° Symbol that represents the term *degrees*
- Addend—Number that is added to another (augend) to obtain one sum
- Addition—Unification of two or more numbers to obtain one sum
- Augend—Number to which another is added (addend) to obtain one sum
- Constant—Fixed; unchanging
- Denominator—Lower number of a fraction
- Difference—Result of subtraction
- Dividend—Number that is to be portioned or divided; numerator of a fraction; contained within the long division bracket
- Division—Splitting or dividing a number into equal groups
- Divisor—Number of desired portions of the dividend; denominator of a fraction; number to the left of the long division bracket; may be a factor of another number
- Equal—Two numbers or other items that are alike in degree, quantity, or volume
- Equation—Mathematical statement showing that two expressions are alike
- Equivalency—Expression of relationships between two mathematical statements that are alike
- Express—To represent using a character, figure, formula, or symbol
- Extremes—Two outer terms of a proportion that are cross multiplied when solving for an unknown
- Factor—An integer that can be divided into another integer without producing a remainder
- Fraction—Equal divisions of an item or a portion that is less than the whole item or number
- Integer—A positive or negative whole number including zero
- Long division bracket—Symbol (⟯) that separates the dividend from the divisor when performing long division
- Means—Two inner terms of a proportion that are cross multiplied when solving for an unknown
- Minuend—Number from which another number (subtrahend) is subtracted
- Multiplicand—Number that will be multiplied by another number (multiplier)

- Multiplication—Mathematical calculation performed with two numbers to obtain a product; consists of addition of a number (multiplicand) to itself the number of times specified

- Multiplier—Number by which another number (multiplicand) is multiplied

- Numerator—Upper number of a fraction

- PEMDAS—Acronym that represents the terms (*parenthesis*, *exponents*, *multiplication*, *division*, *addition*, and *subtraction*) which serves as a reminder to employ the order of operations when solving an algebraic problem. Perform the operations inside the parenthesis first, then the exponents, next multiplication and division (from left to right), and finally addition and subtraction (also from left to right)

- Percent—Parts per hundred

- Product—Result of multiplication

- Proportion—Comparison of two ratios that are equal

- Quotient—Result of division

- Ratio—Expression of a relationship between two numbers or components by comparing them to one another

- Reciprocal—Number that when multiplied by a given number or quantity results in a product of one; synonymous with the term *multiplicative inverse*

- Reduce to lowest terms—Cancellation of all common terms (factors) in the numerator and denominator of a fraction until no common terms remain; synonymous with the term *simplify*

- Remainder—Portion that is left after the mathematic process is complete

- Simplify—Cancellation of all common terms in the numerator and denominator of a fraction until no common terms remain; synonymous with the term *reduce to lowest terms*

- Square root—A divisor of a number that when squared results in the same number. For example, the square roots of 9 are 3 and 3 because $3 \times 3 = 9$

- Subtraction—Calculation of the difference between two numbers

- Subtrahend—Number to be subtracted from another (minuend)

- Sum—Result of addition

Fractions

The word *fraction* is derived from the Latin term *fractio* that was used to describe breaking an object into pieces. Fractions are equal divisions of an item or a portion that is less than the whole item or number. Fractions are used in pharmacology to indicate medication doses that are not whole numbers and in everyday activities such as food preparation, making purchases and receiving change, telling time, analyzing survey information, among other uses. A fraction can be written as a common fraction (e.g., ½), a decimal fraction (e.g., 0.5), or a percentage (e.g., 50%); all three numbers (½, 0.5, and 50%) represent the same value (one half).

Common Fractions

Common fractions are written as a numerator over a denominator (e.g., a/b in which *a* is the numerator and *b* is the denominator). A diagonal line (/) or a horizontal line (−) may be used to separate the numerator from the denominator. The denominator is the bottom number that represents the total number of equal divisions of the whole item or number. The numerator is the top number that represents the number of equal parts of the whole that are currently available. The line (diagonal or horizontal) separating the numerator and the denominator is a division sign meaning that the numerator is divided by the denominator. When the numerator and denominator are the same number (equal to each other), the fraction is equal to one (e.g., 1/1 = 1 and 50/50 = 1).

There are seven variations of the common fraction (examples are shown in parenthesis):

- Simple fraction—contains only one numerator and one denominator (½)

- Compound fraction—requires a mathematical calculation in either the numerator or the denominator (2 × 6/14 = 8/14)

- Complex fraction—contains a simple fraction in the numerator, denominator, or both (simple fraction in the numerator 2½/5; simple fraction in the denominator 5/2½; simple fraction in both the numerator and the denominator 5½ /1½)

- Proper fraction—numerator is smaller than the denominator (1/2)

- Improper fraction—numerator is larger than the denominator (4/3)
  - To express an improper fraction as a mixed number, divide the numerator by the denominator and note the whole number (4/3 = 4 ÷ 3 = 1 with a remainder of 1); and write the remainder (if any) to the right of the whole number as a fraction and reduce to lowest terms as needed (4/3 = 1 1/3)

- Mixed number—contains a whole number and a fraction (1½)

- Equivalent fraction—has the same value as another fraction (8/14 = 4/7)

- To identify an equivalent fraction, reduce the fraction to lowest terms by finding the largest whole number that will divide evenly both the numerator and denominator and performing the calculation (the number 2 was used to reduce [divide] 8/14 to 4/7). Equivalent fractions may also be identified by multiplying the fractions (refer to the upcoming segment concerning multiplying fractions)

When adding proper fractions, the denominators must be the same number and only the numerators are added (1/2 + 1/2 = 2/2 = 1; when reduced to lowest terms); the denominator remains constant. If the denominator is not the same, the fractions must first be changed to equivalent fractions with the same denominator before they can be added (to add 1/3 + 2/6, 1/3 must first be changed to the equivalent fraction of 2/6 so that the two fractions have the same denominator and the fractions are added: 2/6 + 2/6 = 4/6 = 2/3; when reduced to lowest terms). To add mixed number fractions, the denominators must be the same. Then the fractions are added first and any whole numbers are added to the results of addition of the fractions (5 1/4 + 4 2/4 = 9 ¾ if the denominators are the same and 5 1/4 + 4 1/2 = 5 1/4 + 4 2/4 = 9 3/4 if the denominators are different).

When subtracting proper fractions, the denominators must be the same before they can be subtracted and only the numerators are subtracted (2/4 − 1/4 = 1/4); the denominator remains constant. If the denominator is not the same, the fractions must first be changed to equivalent fractions with the same denominator before they can be subtracted (to subtract 1/2 − 1/4, 1/2 must first be changed to the equivalent fraction of 2/4 so that the two fractions have the same denominator before the fractions are subtracted 2/4 − 1/4 = 1/4). To subtract mixed number fractions, the denominators must be the same. Then the fractions are subtracted first and the whole numbers are subtracted next (5 2/3 − 2 1/3 = 3 1/3 if the denominators are the same and 5 4/6 − 2 1/3 = 5 2/3 − 2 1/3 = 3 1/3 if the denominators are different).

When multiplying proper fractions, the numerators are multiplied first, the denominators are multiplied next, and reduced to lowest terms as needed (2/4 × 2/4 = 2 × 2/4 × 4 = 4/16 = 1/4; when reduced to lowest terms). To multiply mixed number fractions, first change the mixed number fraction to an equivalent improper fraction, multiply next (numerators first and then the denominators), and reduce to lowest terms as needed (1½ × 1¼ = 3/2 × 5/4 = 3 × 5/2 × 4 = 15/8 = 1 7/8; when reduced to lowest terms).

When dividing proper fractions, the second fraction is inverted (the inverted fraction is called the reciprocal), multiply the fractions, and reduce to lowest terms (5/8 ÷ 3/16 = 5/8 × 16/3 = 5 × 16/8 × 3 = 80/24 = 10/3 = 3 1/3; when reduced to lowest terms). To divide mixed number fractions, first change the mixed number fraction to an equivalent improper fraction, invert the second fraction, multiply the numerators followed by the denominators, and reduce to lowest terms as needed (1½ ÷ ½ = 3/2 ÷ 1/2 = 3/2 × 2/1 = 3 × 2/2 × 1 = 6/2 = 3/1 = 3; when reduced to lowest terms).

Decimal System

The **decimal system** is part of the metric system and relies on a place value system that is based on multiples of 10 and uses a decimal point to separate the whole numbers (also called integers; includes all positive and negative numbers and zero) from the fractions. The decimal system is preferred over common fractions in medical, scientific, and international trade settings because it is accurate and easy to use.

The following rules are applied when using the decimal system. (Examples are shown in parenthesis.)

- Ten symbols (called **Arabic numerals**) are used to represent the entire decimal system and all other numbers are created by placing the symbols in an assigned place value column. The 10 symbols and the numbers they represent are:
  - 0—Zero
  - 1—One
  - 2—Two
  - 3—Three
  - 4—Four
  - 5—Five
  - 6—Six
  - 7—Seven
  - 8—Eight
  - 9—Nine

- The decimal point is represented by a period (.) and the term *point* is spoken to represent the decimal point (the decimal term 1.5 is spoken as one point five); the term *and* may also be used to represent the decimal point (the decimal term 1.5 could also be spoken as one and five tenths).

- Decimal numbers are read from left to right.

- Figure 2-1 demonstrates the place values assigned to each column of the decimal system and identifies the related terminology.
  - Place value to the left of the decimal point represents whole numbers that increase in value 10 times for each place value column that is added. From the decimal point moving to the left, the whole number in each column is spoken as:
    - One(s) or unit(s) (say the Arabic numeral)
    - Ten or teen (when combined with the ones or units column)
    - Hundred(s)
    - Thousand(s)
    - Ten thousand(s)
    - Hundred thousand(s)
    - Million(s)

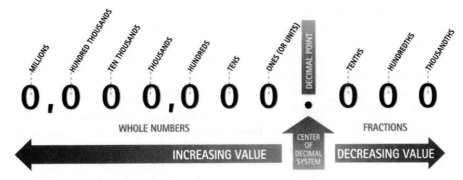

FIGURE 2-1 Decimal System Place Values and Terminology

- Place value to the right of the decimal point represents fractions that decrease in value 10 times for each place value column that is added. From the decimal point moving to the right, the fraction in each column is spoken as:
  - Tenth(s)
  - Hundredth(s)
  - Thousandth(s)
  - Ten thousandth(s)
  - Hundred thousandth(s)
  - Millionth(s)
- The Institute for Safe Medication Practices (ISMP) (refer to Chapter Three; Table 3-3) recommends use of a zero before the decimal point if the decimal number is a fraction only ("point 5 milligrams" should be written as "0.5 mg") and use of a trailing zero following a whole number is not recommended (5 milligrams should be written as 5 mg) to reduce the risk of error.
- The ISMP also recommends use of a comma to identify dosing units at or above 1,000 (one thousand) and a second comma when expressing dosing units at or above 1,000,000 (one million) to reduce the risk of error.
- In pharmacology, decimal fractions typically do not extend beyond the hundredth(s) column and facility policy may allow rounding of a decimal fraction to the nearest tenth. If the fraction is five or greater, round up to the next higher tenth (1.45 could be rounded up to 1.5) and if the fraction is four or less, round down to the nearest tenth (1.44 could be rounded down to 1.4).
- When converting a common fraction to a decimal fraction, divide the numerator by the denominator (1/2 = 1 ÷ 2 = 0.5).
- When converting a decimal fraction to a common fraction, read the decimal fraction by stating the value of the column to the right of the decimal point

(0.25 would be stated as twenty-five hundredths), then rewrite the decimal fraction as a common fraction using the decimal number as the numerator and the column value as the denominator (25/100), and reduce to lowest terms as needed (1/4).

- Zeros may be added to the right of the decimal point for convenience and do not change the value of the decimal fraction (0.5 may be changed to 0.50 or 0.500; however the value remains five tenths).

When adding decimals, arrange the numbers to be added in vertical columns and ensure that the decimal points of each number are in alignment, find the sum (perform addition) as if the decimal numbers were whole numbers (carry over numbers, if necessary), and insert the decimal point directly under the decimal points in the problem. For example:

$$\begin{array}{r} 0.50 \\ +\underline{0.25} \\ 0.75 \end{array}$$

When subtracting decimals, arrange the numbers to be subtracted in vertical columns and ensure that the decimal points of each number are in alignment, find the difference (perform subtraction) as if the decimal numbers were whole numbers (regroup or borrow, if necessary), and insert the decimal point directly under the decimal points in the problem. For example:

$$\begin{array}{r} 0.50 \\ -\underline{0.25} \\ 0.25 \end{array}$$

When multiplying decimals, arrange the numbers to be multiplied in vertical columns and ensure that the digits to the right are aligned, find the product (perform multiplication) as if the decimal numbers were whole numbers, count the total number of decimal places in the multiplicand (top number) and the multiplier (bottom number), and count the appropriate number of decimal places from right to left to identify the location in which to apply the decimal point in the product (answer). For example:

$$0.25 \quad \text{(two decimal places)}$$
$$\underline{\times\ 0.5} \quad \text{(plus one decimal place)}$$
$$125$$
$$\underline{0000}$$
$$0.125 \quad \text{(equals three decimal places)}$$

When dividing a decimal by a whole number, set up the division process by using the long division bracket ($\overline{)}$), place a decimal point in the quotient in alignment with the decimal point of the dividend (number inside the bracket), and find the quotient (perform division) as if the decimal number were a whole number.

$$1.5 \div 2$$

$$
\begin{array}{r}
0.75 \quad \text{(quotient)} \\
\text{(divisor)} \quad 2\overline{)1.50} \quad \text{(dividend)} \\
\underline{14} \\
10 \\
\underline{10} \\
0
\end{array}
$$

When dividing a whole number by a decimal, set up the division process by using the long division bracket ($\overline{)}$), make the decimal (divisor) a whole number by moving the decimal point to the right as many place values as needed to eliminate the decimal point. The same process must also be applied to the whole number (dividend) by placing a decimal point after the whole number and moving it to the right an equal number of place values that the decimal point of the divisor was moved. Moving the decimal point is the same as multiplying the divisor and dividend by multiples of 10 (if the decimal point is moved one place value, multiply each number by 10; if the decimal point is moved two place values, multiply each number by 100, etc.). Once the location of the decimal point is determined, place a decimal point in the quotient in alignment with the decimal point of the dividend (number inside the bracket), and find the quotient (perform division) of the whole numbers.

$$4 \div 1.25$$

$$400 \div 125$$

$$
\begin{array}{r}
3.2 \quad \text{(quotient)} \\
\text{(divisor)} \quad 125\overline{)400.00} \quad \text{(dividend)} \\
\underline{375} \\
250 \\
\underline{250} \\
0
\end{array}
$$

Percentages

The term *percent* is from the Latin per centum, which means "by the hundred." When stating a percentage,

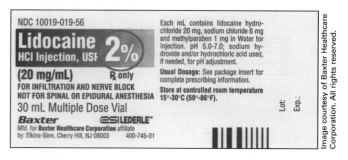

FIGURE 2-2 Lidocaine Label Demonstrating Dosage in Percent (2%)

the number is written as parts of one hundred with one hundred considered the whole. The number preceding the percent symbol (%) indicates quantity or how many parts per hundred are available (50% would be stated as fifty percent and means that fifty parts per hundred are available). A space is not used between the number and the percent symbol. Percentage is another way of expressing a fraction in which the numerator is the number preceding the percent symbol and the denominator is always 100 (1% = 1/100). A percentage can easily be expressed as a decimal simply by moving the decimal point (a decimal point always follows a whole number; although it is often not written) two place values to the left (1% = 0.01). In pharmacology, percent is often used to identify the strength of a medication. A larger percent represents a stronger medication. Strength of the drug lidocaine is identified with the use of percent (Figure 2-2); 2% lidocaine is twice as strong as 1% lidocaine.

Ratios

A ratio is a way of expressing a relationship between two numbers or components by comparing them to one another. When stating a ratio, the two numbers are separated by a colon (:). The relationship between 1 and 10 is written as 1:10 and stated as a 1-to-10 ratio. A ratio is always reduced to lowest (simplest) terms (2:20 would be reduced to 1:10). Ratios can also be expressed as a quotient, a fraction, or a decimal. To express a ratio as a quotient (the result of dividing); divide the number to the left of the colon by the number to the right of the colon (1:10 = 1 ÷ 10 = 0.1). To express a ratio as a fraction, write the number to the left of the colon as the numerator and the number to the right of the colon as the denominator (1:10 = 1/10). To express a ratio as a decimal, divide the numerator by the denominator and reduce to lowest terms as needed (1:10 = 1/10 = 0.1).

In pharmacology, ratios are often used to express the relationship of the components of a solution. The drug (**solute**) is usually added to a liquid (**solvent**) and the ratio compares the amount of the solute to the

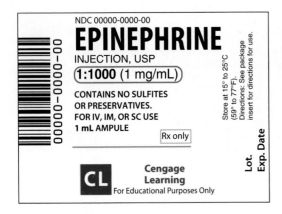

FIGURE 2-3 Epinephrine Label Demonstrating Dosage as a Ratio (1:1000)

amount of solvent. In Figure 2-3 the strength of the drug adrenaline (epinephrine) is identified through the use of the ratio 1:1000; meaning that there is one part adrenaline to one thousand parts of liquid. Another example of the use of ratios in the surgical environment is when the surgeon intends to expand a skin graft; expansion ratios range from 1.5:1 (graft size is expanded to 1.5 times the original size) to 9:1 (graft size is expanded to 9 times the original size).

Proportions

Proportion compares two ratios that are equal (2:20 = 1:10). In pharmacology, proportion is used to compare medication dosage equivalencies (to calculate the dosage of a medication as it relates to the patient's weight) or to calculate dosage when the dose ordered differs from the dose available. The following rules are applied when working with proportions:

- Terms of each ratio must be labeled

- Terms of both ratios must be stated in the same sequence

- Known terms are stated as a ratio on the left side of the equation and the unknown term (represented by X) is stated as a ratio on the right side of the equation

- To find the unknown term (X), set up the proportion as a fraction and cross multiply (2/20 = 1/10). When cross multiplying, multiply the extremes (two outer terms [in bold]); (**2**:20 = 1:**10**) and then the means (two inner terms ([in bold]); (2:**20** = **1**:10)

- Solve for X by dividing both sides of the proportion by the same number to leave X alone on one side of the equation

The following example shows the procedure used to calculate the dosage of a medication as it relates to the

patient's weight: A physician ordered one milligram of a medication per kilogram of body weight and the patient weighs 30 kilograms. How many milligrams of the medication will the patient receive?

- The terms of each ratio are labeled and in the same sequence

  dose ordered:per measure of weight = dose needed:patient's weight

  mg:kg = mg:kg

- The known terms are stated as a ratio on the left side of the equation and the unknown term is represented by X on the right side of the equation

  1mg:1kg = Xmg:30kg

- Convert to a fraction

  1mg/1kg = Xmg/30kg

- Cross multiply the extremes (in bold; **1**mg/1kg = Xmg/**30**kg) and then the means (in bold; 1mg/**1**kg = **X**mg/30kg)

  $1 \times 30 = 1 \times X$
  (product of the extremes) 30 = 1X
  (product of the means)

- Solve for X by dividing both sides of the proportion by the same number, which in this example is 1

  30/1 = X/1
  30 = X
  The patient will be given 30mg of the drug

The following example shows the procedure used to calculate the dosage when the dose ordered differs from the dose available: A surgeon ordered 100,000 units of bacitracin for irrigation of a surgical wound. Bacitracin is available only in vials that contain 50,000 units. How many vials of bacitracin will be needed?

- The terms of each ratio are labeled and in the same sequence

  dose available:known quantity = dose needed: unknown quantity

  units:vial = units:vials

- The known terms are stated as a ratio on the left side of the equation and the unknown term is represented by X on the right side of the equation

  50,000 units:1 vial = 100,000 units:X vials

- Convert to a fraction

  50,000 units/1 vial = 100,000 units/X vials

- Cross multiply the extremes (in bold; **50,000** units/1 vial = 100,000 units/**X** vials) and then the means (in bold; 50,000 units/**1** vial = **100,000** units/X vials)

$$50,000 \times X = 1 \times 100,000$$

(product of the extremes) $50,000X = 100,000$
(product of the means)

- Solve for X by dividing both sides of the proportion by the same number, which in this example is 50,000

$$50,000X/50,000 = 100,000/50,000$$

$$X = 2$$

Two vials of bacitracin will be needed

NUMBERING AND MEASUREMENT SYSTEMS

Several numbering and measurement systems are employed in the surgical environment. Numbering systems that are different from the Arabic numeral and standard/civilian time systems used daily include the Roman numeral system and military time system. Measurement systems used in pharmacology that have additional applications in the surgical environment include international units, milliequivalent measures, the metric system (especially length, weight, and volume), Celsius temperature, the apothecary system, and the household system. It is important that all surgical team members be familiar with each system and are capable of easily and accurately performing conversions between the systems.

Roman Numeral System

The **Roman numeral system** originated in ancient Rome and is still used today in pharmacology to designate narcotic classifications and on written prescriptions. Roman numerals are also used to number pages in the preface of a textbook, number items contained within an outline, to express the year of a copyright, on clock faces, for counting or numbering annual events (the Super Bowl, for example), and to indicate generational relationships when selecting names for a newborn. The Roman numeral system uses letters (may be upper or lower case) to represent numbers but does not include a symbol to represent zero and a separate system is used to denote fractions.

The following rules are applied when using the Roman numeral system (examples are shown in parenthesis):

- Only seven symbols are used to represent the entire Roman numeral system and all other numeric values are created by combining the seven symbols. The seven symbols and the numbers they represent are:
  - I—One
  - V—Five
  - X—Ten
  - L—Fifty
  - C—One hundred
  - D—Five hundred
  - M—One thousand
- Roman numerals are read from left to right
- Numerals placed to the right of a larger numeral add value (II means I plus I equals II or $1 + 1 = 2$ and VI means V plus I equals VI or $5 + 1 = 6$)
- Numerals of a lesser value placed to the left of a larger numeral are negative or subtract value (IV means negative I plus V equals IV or negative 1 plus 5 equals 4; can also be solved by using V minus I equals IV or $5 - 1$ equals 4)
- Most numerals can be repeated up to three times; however symbols V, L, and D can never be repeated or subtracted
- When deciphering the Roman numeral system, the order of operations is as follows. First, identify and perform all subtraction(s) (smaller numeral to the left of a larger numeral). Then, add all remaining values (any numeral to the right of a larger numeral) (the order of operations used to identify the number XLVIII is to identify and perform the subtraction(s) $(X-L) + VIII$; and add all remaining values $(40) + 5 + 1 + 1 + 1 = 40 + 8 = (48)$

The Roman numeral system is difficult to use when attempting to perform mathematical calculations. Expressing large numbers when using the Roman numeral system can be cumbersome and difficult to interpret; therefore, the use of Roman numerals as they relate do pharmacology is limited.

Table 2-1 provides limited examples that demonstrate the relationship between the Roman numeral system and the Arabic numbering system that is commonly used in the United States.

Military Time

Military time uses a 24-hour clock while **standard time** (sometimes referred to as **civilian time**) uses a 12-hour clock with the additional designations of A.M. (acronym for the Latin term *ante meridiem*—meaning "before midday/noon") and P.M. (acronym for the Latin term *post meridiem*—meaning "after midday/noon"). Military time may be substituted for standard time to eliminate any potential confusion between A.M. and P.M. and is popular not only in military settings, but in emergency services settings as well as hospitals and surgery centers. Three o'clock in the morning (3:00 A.M.) could easily be confused with three o'clock in the afternoon (3:00 P.M.) when using standard time, but a potential error may be eliminated with the use of

TABLE 2-1 Relationship Between Roman Numeral and Arabic Numbering Systems

Roman Numeral	Interpretation	Arabic Numeral	English Term
Ṡ	Semi, semisis	½	One half
I	1	1	One
II	1 + 1	2	Two
III	1 + 1 + 1	3	Three
IV	− 1 + 5 or 5 − 1	4	Four
V	5	5	Five
VI	5 + 1	6	Six
VII	5 + 1 + 1	7	Seven
VIII	5 + 1 + 1 + 1	8	Eight
IX	− 1 + 10 or 10 − 1	9	Nine
X	10	10	Ten
XX	10 + 10	20	Twenty
XXX	10 + 10 + 10	30	Thirty
XL	− 10 + 50 or 50 − 10	40	Forty
L	50	50	Fifty
LX	50 + 10	60	Sixty
LXX	50 + 10 + 10	70	Seventy
LXXX	50 + 10 + 10 + 10	80	Eighty
XC	− 10 + 100 or 100 − 10	90	Ninety
C	100	100	One hundred
D	500	500	Five hundred
M	1,000	1,000	One thousand

military time because 3:00 A.M. would be represented as 0300 and 3:00 P.M. as 1500. The guidelines for using military time are (examples are shown in parenthesis):

- Military time is written as a four digit number.
  - The first two numbers indicate the hour (1000 in military time is the same as 10:00 A.M. in standard time).
  - The third and fourth numbers indicate the minutes (1047 in military time is the same as 10:47A.M. in standard time).
- Use of a colon separating the hour and minute is eliminated.
  - However, a colon may be used to separate minutes from seconds (1047:06 would be used to specify ten hundred forty seven and six seconds or 10:47:06 A.M.).
- If the time indicated is the top of the hour, the term *hours* is spoken after the time; otherwise use of the term *hours* is eliminated (five o'clock in the afternoon would be written as 5:00 P.M. and spoken as five P.M. in standard time and written as 1700 and spoken as seventeen hundred hours in military

time, but five twenty nine in the afternoon would be written in standard time as 5:29 P.M. and spoken as five twenty nine P.M. and written in military time as 1729 and spoken as seventeen twenty nine).

When converting standard time to military time, there is a direct correlation between the hours from midnight to noon; 1:00 A.M. becomes 0100, 2:00 A.M. becomes 0200, and the pattern continues until 12:00 P.M. or 1200. After noon, the process becomes a little more complex. When using standard time, numbering of the hours starts over again repeating the times with the P.M. designation. When using military time, for each hour after noon, the number one is added to twelve; therefore, 1:00 P.M. in standard time becomes 1300 hours in military time, 2:00 P.M. in standard time becomes 1400 hours in military time, and the pattern continues until midnight which can be expressed in military time as 0000 hours or 2400 hours (either is acceptable and the preference will be identified in the facility policy). An easy method for converting standard time to military time after noon is to add 12 hours to the standard time. For example, 2:00 P.M. plus 12 would make the military time equivalent 1400 hours. And to convert military

TABLE 2-2 Comparison of Standard and Military Timekeeping Systems

Standard (Civilian) Time Written	Standard (Civilian) Time Spoken (use of the term *o'clock* is optional)	Military Time Written	Military Time Spoken
12:00 A.M. (midnight)	twelve (o'clock) A.M.	0000 or 2400	zero hundred hours or twenty four hundred hours
1:00 A.M.	one (o'clock) A.M.	0100	zero one hundred hours
2:00 A.M.	two (o'clock) A.M.	0200	zero two hundred hours
3:00 A.M.	three (o'clock) A.M.	0300	zero three hundred hours
4:00 A.M.	four (o'clock) A.M.	0400	zero four hundred hours
5:00 A.M.	five (o'clock) A.M.	0500	zero five hundred hours
6:00 A.M.	six (o'clock) A.M.	0600	zero six hundred hours
7:00 A.M.	seven (o'clock) A.M.	0700	zero seven hundred hours
8:00 A.M.	eight (o'clock) A.M.	0800	zero eight hundred hours
9:00 A.M.	nine (o'clock) A.M.	0900	zero nine hundred hours
10:00 A.M.	ten (o'clock) A.M.	1000	ten hundred hours
11:00 A.M.	eleven (o'clock) A.M.	1100	eleven hundred hours
12:00 P.M. (noon)	twelve (o'clock) P.M.	1200	twelve hundred hours
1:00 P.M.	one (o'clock) P.M.	1300	thirteen hundred hours
2:00 P.M.	two (o'clock) P.M.	1400	fourteen hundred hours
3:00 P.M.	three (o'clock) P.M.	1500	fifteen hundred hours
4:00 P.M.	four (o'clock) P.M.	1600	sixteen hundred hours
5:00 P.M.	five (o'clock) P.M.	1700	seventeen hundred hours
6:00 P.M.	six (o'clock) P.M.	1800	eighteen hundred hours
7:00 P.M.	seven (o'clock) P.M.	1900	nineteen hundred hours
8:00 P.M.	eight (o'clock) P.M.	2000	twenty hundred hours
9:00 P.M.	nine (o'clock) P.M.	2100	twenty one hundred hours
10:00 P.M.	ten (o'clock) P.M.	2200	twenty two hundred hours
11:00 P.M.	eleven (o'clock) P.M.	2300	twenty three hundred hours

time after noon to standard time 12 hours is subtracted from the military time. For example 1500 hours minus 12 would make the standard time equivalent 3:00 P.M.

Table 2-2 provides a comparison between standard time and military time as well as a pronunciation guide.

International Units

An **international unit** (IU or unit) is an arbitrary type of measure that represents the **biological potency** (activity, action, or effect) of a drug within the body regardless of the **mass** (weight or volume) of the substance that is accepted globally. Because a unit is standardized according to the action of the drug, standardization of the unit pertains only to that drug (a unit of topical thrombin is different than a unit of bacitracin and from a unit of heparin sodium). There is no standard conversion

of drugs that are measured in units to another type of measure such as milligrams or milliliters. **Biologicals, enzymes, fat-soluble vitamins,** heparin, **hormones,** and some **antibiotics** are measured in international units.

The following rules are applied when working with international units (examples are shown in parenthesis):

- The number of units is written first, followed by a space, and the word units spelled out in lowercase letters (10 units).

- A comma is used if the number of units is four digits or greater (10,000 units).

Standards for international units are set forth by the International Conference for Unification of Formulae in collaboration with the WHO. The United States Pharmacopeia (USP) verified mark on the label indicates that the drug preparation meets the consistency standards related to purity, quality, and strength and that the manufacturing process of the drug is of high quality. Refer to Chapter One for additional information concerning the USP.

Milliequivalent Measures

A **milliequivalent** (mEq) is a unit of measure that represents one thousandth of a measure. For example, if a drug is measured in by weight in grams, then a milliequivalent is one thousandth (0.001) of a gram. Milliequivalents are often used when referring to electrolytes such as calcium gluconate, potassium chloride (KCl) (Figure 2-4), and sodium bicarbonate. Additionally, some lab test results (such as bicarbonate, chloride, potassium, and sodium) are reported in milliequivalents per liter of blood (mEq/l).

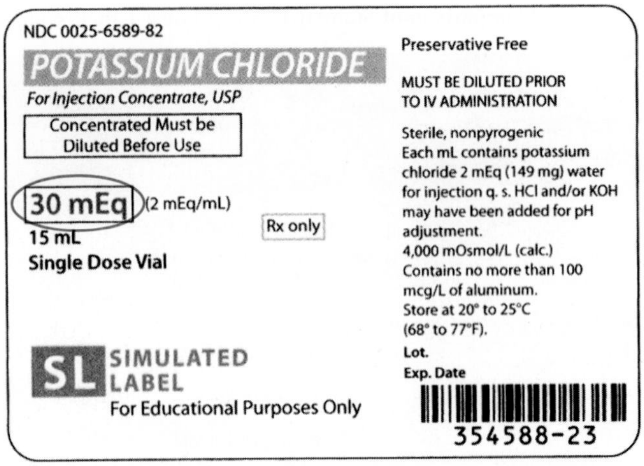

Apothecary System

The **apothecary system** is a system for measurement that originated in ancient Greece and was used by physicians to prescribe medicine and by pharmacists to formulate the prescribed compound. Because of inconsistencies in the apothecary system that could lead to potential patient harm, apothecary system was officially replaced (for pharmacologic applications) by the metric system in the United States in 1971; however, few medications (such as aspirin, codeine, digitalis, and phenobarbital) are still prescribed and labeled in both apothecary (grains) and metric (milligrams) terms (1 grain = 64.79 891 milligrams).

FIGURE 2-4 Potassium Chloride Label Demonstrating Dosage in Milliequivalents (20 mEq).

A complex set of symbols and Roman numerals are used to represent the measures of the apothecary system. Weight and volume in the apothecary system are based on the weight of a single grain of wheat. Note that the dram for measuring weight is not equal to a fluid dram for measuring volume and the apothecary measures should not be confused with other types of measures that use similar terminology. For example, an apothecary pound is 12 ounces and in the household system one pound equals 16 ounces. Table 2-3 identifies the measures and related terminology of the apothecary system.

TABLE 2-3 Apothecary System

Apothecary Measure	Abbreviation (symbol)	Equivalent
Weight		
grain	gr	Based on the weight of a single grain of wheat
scruple	(Ꝫ)	20 grains
dram/dracham	(ℨ)	3 scruples
ounce	(℥)	8 drams
pound	lb	12 ounces
Volume		
minim	(℔)	Quantity of water in a drop that weighs 1 grain
fluid scruple	(fℨ)	20 minims
fluid dram	(fℨ)	3 fluid scruples
fluid ounce	(f℥)	8 fluid drams
pint	pt	16 fluid ounces
quart	qt	2 pints
gallon	gal	4 quarts

Household System

The household measurement system is similar to the method that the colonists brought with them from England. The **household system** is primarily used in the United States to determine length (inches, feet, and yards), weight (ounces, pounds, tons), and volume (drops, teaspoons, tablespoons, ounces, cups pints, quarts, gallons). Household measurements are sometimes referred to as United States customary units. In most other countries, the metric system is used. Utensils for measurement using the household system can fluctuate in size making the household system less exact than the metric system.

Over-the-counter and prescription drugs that are intended for the patient to take at home may be ordered using the household system because the measuring devices are readily available and the risk of error is reduced because the patient or caregiver is familiar with household measurements. Cough syrup, for example, is often measured in teaspoons.

In the hospital setting, household measurements may be used when working with preparations that will be used externally as well as oral or rectal preparations that do not require exact measurements. Because household measurements are familiar, knowledge of the household system is useful when making comparisons with the metric system. When using the household system, measurements related to volume may be correlated with pharmacology; however, length and weight measurements that will be utilized in the surgical environment include length and weight of a neonate, size and weight of a specimen, size of a traumatic injury, length of an incision, among other uses. For example, parents may be told that a neonate is 19 inches long and weighs 6 pounds 4 ounces, but the information will likely be recorded in the patient's chart using the metric system as 48.26 centimeters of length and 100 kilograms of weight. Table 2-4 identifies the measures and related terminology of the household system.

Metric System/Systeme International d'Unites (SI)

The need for an international system of measurement was identified in the late 17th century and several ideas were proposed, but no action was taken to formalize or standardize any of the suggestions for over 100 years. In 1790, the National Assembly of France made a formal request to the French Academy of Sciences (Academy) for a system of weights and measures that could not be disputed. The Academy appointed a Commission to develop a system that was based on science and easy to use. The Commission determined that the decimal system would be the basis for all of the calculations and that the terms *meter*, *gram*, and *liter* would be used to identify length, weight, and volume respectively. At first, the metric system was not widely accepted, but in 1840, the French government mandated use of the system. Due to the standardization and accuracy of the weights and measures, the metric system was well suited for scientific, engineering, and industrial applications. Therefore, with the technological advances in industry and increased international trade due to enhanced global transportation options; use of the metric system became widespread. In 1875, at the Meter Convention, the Treaty of the Meter (Treaty) was signed by 17 countries and by 1900 that number had more than doubled. In 1960, at the General Conference on Weights and Measures (General Conference), the Treaty was revised and additional measures (such as the second related to time, the ampere related to electric current, the Kelvin related to thermodynamic temperature, mole related to the amount of substance, and candela related to luminous intensity) were added. Additionally the name of the system was changed to the Systeme International d'Unites (International System of Units), which is represented by the acronym SI. The General Conference meets periodically to review the standards and recommend improvements to the system.

Systeme International d'Unites is commonly known as the metric system and is the preferred system of weights and measures in pharmacology because of the accuracy and ease of use of the system. Most medications are prescribed and manufactured using weight or volume related to the metric system. Additionally, lab values as well as sizes of specimens, incisions, traumatic wounds, neoplasms, and neonates are reported using metric terminology. All units of measure in the metric system differ from one another in multiples of 10 and conversions are easily performed by simply moving the decimal point to the right to indicate the positive powers of 10 or to the left to indicate the negative powers of 10. Keep in mind that an error in decimal placement will cause a 10-fold increase or decrease in the strength of the dose; therefore accurate calculation skills are imperative.

The following rules are applied when working with the metric system (examples are shown in parenthesis):

- Three basic units of measure are commonly used in medical settings. (Table 2-5)

- Twenty prefixes (Table 2-6) are used to denote the size of each basic unit of measure; however, only the seven more central (closest to the decimal point) prefixes (from kilo- to micro-) are commonly used in the medical setting.

- Prefixes indicating whole numbers are to the left of the decimal point and prefixes indicating fractions are to the right of the decimal point.

- All prefixes may be affiliated with each of the three basic units of measure (millimeter, milligram, milliliter).

TABLE 2-4 Household System

Household Measure	Abbreviation (symbol)	Equivalent
Volume		
drop	gtt	None—drop size may vary according to: Amount of pressure applied to the bulb Angle at which the dropper is held Diameter of the opening of the dropper Temperature of the medication Viscosity of the medication
teaspoon	t or tsp	60 drops
tablespoon	T or tbsp	3 teaspoons
fluid ounce	fl oz or oz	2 tablespoons
cup	C	8 ounces
pint	pt	2 cups/32 ounces
quart	qt	2 pints/4 cups/32 ounces
gallon	gal	4 quarts/16 cups/128 ounces
Weight		
ounce	oz	Varies—related to: International avoirdupois ounce (most common—28.350 grams or 437.5 grains) International troy ounce (usually used to weigh precious metals—31.103 grams or 480 grains) Apothecary ounce (equivalent to a troy ounce)
pound	lb	16 ounces
Length		
inch	in (")	Unknown—inch size may be related to: Latin word *unica*, which means one-twelfth of a part (possibly the length of a human foot) Length of the distal portion of a human thumb Three grains of barley (taken from the center of the ear, dried, and laid end-to-end) One hundred points (.) lined up side-by-side
foot	ft (')	12 inches (possibly length of a human foot)
yard	yd	3 feet (possibly the girth of the waist of a Saxon King or the distance from the tip of Henry I's nose to the end of his outstretched thumb)
mile	mi	5,280 feet

TABLE 2-5 Metric Units of Measure

Unit of Measure	Symbol	Representation
meter	m	length
gram	g	weight
liter	l or L	volume

- Whole numbers are represented by Arabic symbols (0, 1, 2, 3, etc.).

- A decimal point is not used if only whole numbers are used (10).

- Metric measurements may include a whole number and a fraction (1.5).

- Quantities of less than one are represented by a decimal fraction and a zero is placed to the left of the decimal point if the fraction is not accompanied by a whole number (0.5).

- The unit of measure follows the number (2 milliliters).

- A space is used between the number and the unit of measure (1 gram).

- The entire prefix and unit of measure may be written out (5 milligrams) or abbreviations may be used for both the prefix and the unit of measure (5 mg).

TABLE 2-6 Metric System Prefixes (from Largest to Smallest)

Prefix/Symbol	Related Terminology	Numeric Representation
yotta-/Y	septillion	1,000,000,000,000,000,000,000,000
zetta-/Z	sextillion	1,000,000,000,000,000,000,000
exa-/E	quintillion	1,000,000,000,000,000,000
peta-/P	quadrillion	1,000,000,000,000,000
tera-/T	trillion	1,000,000,000,000
giga-/G	billion	1,000,000,000
mega-/M	million	1,000,000
kilo-/k	thousand	1,000
hecto-/h	hundred	100
deca-/da	ten	10
decimal point	point	.
deci-/d	tenth	0.1
centi-/c	hundredth	0.01
milli-/m	thousandth	0.001
micro-/μ or mc	millionth	0.0001
nano-/n	billionth	0.00001
pico-/p	trillionth	0.000001
femto-/f	quadrillionth	0.0000001
atto-/a	quintillionth	0.00000001
zepto-/z	sextillionth	0.000000001
yocto-/y	septillionth	0.0000000001

TABLE 2-7 Metric System Length Equivalencies

Length	Abbreviation	Equivalency
1 kilometer	1 km	1000 meters
1 hectometer	1 hm	100 meters
1 dekameter	1 dam	10 meters
1 meter	1 m	1 meter
1 decimeter	1 dm	0.1/one tenth of a meter
1 centimeter	1 cm	0.01/one hundredth of a meter
1 millimeter	1 mm	0.001/one thousandth of a meter

- A zero is not used at the end (to the right) of a decimal fraction.
- The space occupied by one milliliter is equal to one cubic centimeter therefore the terms are interchangeable; however, the ISMP recommends the use of milliliter when referring to volume.

Length

The Commission identified the term *meter*, based on the Greek word *metron* meaning "to measure," as the unit of length. The scientific basis for the meter is related to the size of the earth and represents one ten-millionth of the distance from the North Pole to the equator along the meridian nearest to Dunkirk, France. Table 2-7 identifies common metric system length equivalencies and Table 2-8 provides a comparison of metric length to those of the household system.

Weight

The Commission identified the term *gram* as the unit of weight. The scientific basis for the gram is related to the weight of a cubic centimeter (0.01 meter on each side of the cube) of water at its maximum density, which occurs

TABLE 2-8 Metric System Length Compared to Household System Length

Metric Length	Household Length (rounded to hundredths)
1 kilometer	0.62 mile/3,280.84 feet/39,370.08 inches
1 hectometer	0.06 mile/328.08 feet/3,937.01 inches
1 dekameter	0.01 mile/32.81 feet/393.7 inches
1 meter	3.28 feet/39.37 inches
1 decimeter	0.33 foot/3.94 inches
1 centimeter	0.03 foot/0.39 inch
1 millimeter	0.04 inch

TABLE 2-9 Metric System Weight Equivalencies

Weight	Abbreviation	Equivalency
1 kilogram	1 kg	1000 grams
1 hectogram	1 hg	100 grams
1 dekagram	1dag	10 grams
1 gram	1 g	1 gram
1 decigram	1 dg	0.1/one tenth of a gram
1 centigram	1 cg	0.01/one hundredth of a gram
1 milligram	1 mg	0.001/one thousandth of a gram
1 microgram	1 µg or 1mcg	0.000001/one millionth of a gram

TABLE 2-10 Metric System Weight Compared to Household and Apothecary System Weight

Metric Weight	Household Weight (rounded to hundredths)	Apothecary Weight (rounded to hundredths)
1 kilogram	2.2 pounds/35.27 ounces	2.68 pounds/32.15 ounces
1 hectogram	0.22 pounds/3.53 ounces	0.27 pound/3.22 ounces
1 dekagram	0.35 ounces	0.32 ounce/2.57 drams
1 gram	0.04 ounces	0.26 dram/0.77 scruple
1 decigram	n/a	0.08 scruple/1.54 grains
1 centigram	n/a	0.15 grain
1 milligram	n/a	0.02 grain
1 microgram	n/a	n/a

at 4°C. Table 2-9 identifies common metric system weight equivalencies and Table 2-10 provides a comparison of metric weight to those of the household and apothecary systems.

Volume

The Commission identified the term *liter* as the unit of volume. The scientific basis for the liter is related to the size of a cubic decimeter (0.1 meter on each side of the cube). Table 2-11 identifies common metric system volume equivalencies and Table 2-12 provides a comparison of metric volume to those of the household and apothecary systems.

Temperature Conversion

Over the years, several scales have been developed to measure temperature, but only four are currently in use. The **Kelvin and Rankine scales** are based on absolute zero (a theoretic temperature at which all molecular movement is thought to cease) and no number on either scale can be less than (below) zero. The Kelvin and Rankine scales are commonly used in scientific and industrial settings.

The **Celsius** (also known as centigrade) and **Fahrenheit** scales are based on the point at which water freezes and the point at which water boils. The Celsius scale is part of the metric system and is recognized

TABLE 2-11 Metric System Volume Equivalencies

Volume	Abbreviation	Equivalency
1 kiloliter	1 kl	1000 liters
1 hectoliter	1 hl	100 liters
1 dekaliter	1dal	10 liters
1 liter	1 l or 1 L	1 liter/1000 ml
1 deciliter	1 dl	0.1/one tenth of a liter/100 ml
1 centiliter	1 cl	0.01/one hundredth of a liter/10ml
1 milliliter	1 ml	0.001/one thousandth of a liter

TABLE 2-12 Metric System Volume Compared to Household and Apothecary System Volume

Metric Volume	Household Volume (rounded to hundredths)	Apothecary Volume (rounded to hundredths)
1 kiloliter	264.17 gallons	n/a
1 hectoliter	26.42 gallons	n/a
1 dekaliter	2.64 gallons/10.57 quarts	n/a
1 liter	1.06 quarts/2.11 pints	270.51 drams/32 ounces
1 deciliter	0.42 cup/3.38 ounces	27.05 drams/84.48 scruples
1 centiliter	0.34 ounces/0.68 tablespoon	2.70 drams/8.45 scruples
1 milliliter	0.20 teaspoon/20 drops	0.84 scruple/15 minims

TABLE 2-13 Comparison of Common Celsius and Fahrenheit Temperatures

	Celsius (C)	Fahrenheit (F)
Freezing point of water	0° C	32° F
Normal body temperature (measured orally)	37° C	98.6° F
Boiling point of water	100° C	212° F
Absolute zero	−273° C	−459° F

globally and the Fahrenheit scale is popular primarily in the United States. Both the Celsius and Fahrenheit scales are commonly used to measure air temperature, the temperature at which food is cooked and stored, temperatures employed when sterilizing surgical supplies, and to identify normal and abnormal body temperatures.

Identification of abnormal body temperature is important because an increase in body temperature (referred to as **hyperthermia**) could indicate the presence of an inflammatory or infectious process as well as an anesthetic complication called malignant hyperthermia. A decrease in body temperature is called **hypothermia**. Both hyperthermia and hypothermia can alter the patient's **metabolic rate, vital signs** such as **heart rate** and **blood pressure**, and circulatory status; thereby disrupting homeostasis. The surgical patient's vital signs, including temperature measurement, are monitored throughout all

three phases of surgical case management. The Celsius scale is preferred in medical settings. Table 2-13 provides a comparison of common temperatures between the Celsius and Fahrenheit scales.

Fahrenheit to Celsius

Two methods are available for use when converting Fahrenheit temperatures to the Celsius scale. Both methods involve use of an algebraic formula that involves use of a fraction. Remember to employ the order of operations when solving an algebraic problem. The acronym PEMDAS (PEMDAS represents the terms *parenthesis, exponents, multiplication, division, addition,* and *subtraction*) serves as a reminder to perform the operations inside the parenthesis first, then the exponents, next multiplication and division (from left to right), and finally addition and subtraction (also from left to right).

In the first example the fraction is expressed as a common fraction (°F − 32) × 5/9 = °C and in the second example a decimal fraction is used (°F − 32) / 1.8 = °C.

Celsius to Fahrenheit

Similar algebraic calculations are employed to convert Celsius temperatures to the Fahrenheit scale. A method using a common fraction (°C × 9/5) + 32 = °F and a method involving a decimal fraction °C × 1.8 + 32 = °F.

DOSAGE CALCULATION

The term *posology* is used to describe the study of dosages of drugs. The root word *posos* is from the Greek meaning "quantity" and the suffix—*logy* means "to study." The **dose** is the amount of medication that the patient receives. The physician will calculate the amount of the drug to be prescribed based on one of two primary factors; the patient's weight in kilograms or the patient's body surface area. Additional factors that must be considered in dosage calculation include the therapeutic action of the drug, the patient's ability to metabolize the drug effectively, known sensitivity to the drug, tolerance to the drug, age and sex of the patient, genetic factors, possible interactions with other drugs that the patient may be taking, maximum dose permitted, the patient's activity level, time of administration, route of administration, hepatic first pass effect, and any comorbid (metabolic, pathologic, and/or psychologic) conditions that may affect movement of the drug through the body and/or interaction of the drug with the target cells. In some instances, the manufacturer has determined the usual adult dosage for a specified drug which is based on the size of a normal adult. The USP defines a normal adult as a male or female who is 24 years of age and weighs 150 pounds/68.18 kilograms. Prior to calculating the drug dosage, it may first be necessary to convert the patient's weight in pounds to kilograms (refer to Table 2-10).

It is the surgical technologist's responsibility to keep track of the amount of medication used from the sterile field during the surgical procedure. The dosage delivered to the patient must be accurately recorded in the patient's operative record which becomes part of the permanent medical record/chart. If a medication dosing error occurs, the event must be reported immediately to the physician and an **incident report** completed. Additionally, it may be necessary to file medication error reports with appropriate state and federal agencies.

MIXING MEDICATIONS

Sometimes a drug or solution must be mixed with another drug or solution for medical use. One or more drugs or solutions may be combined to produce an enhanced effect. **Dehydrated** and **concentrated** drugs must be reconstituted prior to use.

Combining Medications

An **additive** is a substance that is combined with the primary drug or solution to produce synergistic or agonistic effects (refer to Chapter Eight for additional information). Synergists (sometimes called adjunctive agents) are drugs that work with one or more other drugs to enhance the effects of one or more of the drugs. Agonists are drugs that simulate or prolong the action of another drug or naturally occurring substance but do not have an independent action. Additives may also be used to **dilute**, **reconstitute**, activate, act as a preservative, give flavor to, or alter the pH of the initial drug.

When combining medications, the individual(s) preparing the drugs for use must ensure that the drugs or solutions are compatible. **Compatibility** can be determined by reading information packaged with the drug, referring to a printed or online drug reference (an **incompatibility** chart may be posted in the satellite pharmacy, medication room, or on the medication cart), or by asking another health care professional (physician, pharmacist, etc.). If two medications are inadvertently mixed that are incompatible, a negative reaction may occur outside of or inside the body. A medication mixture should never be used if there is any sign of incompatibility. Signs of incompatibility include:

- Visual changes—Incompatibilities may be seen as an unexpected color change, presence of **precipitates** (appearance of particles in the solution), formation of gas (appearance of bubbles), or **turbidity** (loss of clarity; cloudiness). **Equivocal** incompatibility occurs when a visual manifestation is uncertain, inconsistent, or lasts for only a short time.

- Chemical changes—Incompatibilities may not be visible. Quality or **potency** of the drug may be degraded and/or the solution may be toxic. The term *complexation* is used to describe a situation in which two or more compounds in the mixture form a chemical that inactivates one or more of the drugs.

- **Instability** of the mixture—Stability of the mixture may be influenced by the length of time elapsed from when the drug was mixed, exposure to light, and temperature variations.

- Therapeutic incompatibility—Occurs when a pharmacological reaction (undesirable) occurs within the patient because two or more incompatible medications were given concurrently. It is imperative that the patient disclose all medications (prescription, over-the-counter, and illegal) and dietary supplements (including herbs and vitamins) currently in use as well as any alcohol use/abuse in order to reduce the risk of therapeutic incompatibilities.

The following safe medication practices are applied in the surgical environment to prevent incompatibilities when mixing medications:

- Anytime that medications are mixed, consider the possibility that an incompatibility may occur.

- Read and carefully follow the manufacturer's instructions.

- Follow the most strict set of rules (includes federal or state law, agency requirements, or facility policies and procedures).

- If a drug or solution is to be given as a bolus through the intravenous line, be sure to consider the type of fluid (and any existing additives) in the solution bag or bottle for possible incompatibilities.

- Sterile technique must be applied.

- Be vigilant as visual incompatibility may be equivocal.

- All medications must be accurately labeled (each location of the drug).

- Once the drugs are mixed, it may be necessary to calculate the correct dose.

Reconstituting Medications

Some drugs are manufactured in a dehydrated or highly concentrated form to increase **shelf life**, ease storage concerns, and alleviate shipping problems. Prior to use, some dehydrated or concentrated drugs must be reconstituted (returned to the liquid form or diluted prior to use). Some drugs (such as topical thrombin and acetylcholine chloride intraocular solution) requiring reconstitution are prepared in a kit from the manufacturer. The kit may contain the medication, the **diluent**, and any necessary supplies.

The following safe medication practices are applied in the surgical environment when reconstituting medications:

- The manufacturer's instructions must be followed exactly to return the substance to the proper concentration (use the correct type and amount of diluent).

- All applicable federal laws, state laws, agency requirements, and facility policies and procedures must be implemented; follow the stricter rule.

- Sterile technique must be applied.

- Following reconstitution, the shelf life of the drug may be limited.

- The reconstituted form of the drug may need to be stored differently (refrigerated, protected from light, etc.) than the dehydrated or concentrated form.

- Accurately label all locations of each medication.

- Following reconstitution, it may be necessary to calculate the correct dose.

In addition to drugs that will be reconstituted, it will also be necessary to reconstitute various types of tissue grafts.

Concentrating and Diluting Medications

The term *concentration* refers to the strength of the medication. A medication may be manufactured in one or more concentrations or the concentration can be altered by increasing or decreasing the components. In the surgical environment, most medications are administered in the liquid form and the liquid is referred to as a solution. A **solution** is a mixture of two components; the solute (which in pharmacology is the medication) and the solvent which is the liquid portion. To increase the concentration (make stronger) of a medication, either more solute is added or less solution is used. To dilute, or decrease the concentration (make weaker) of a medication, either less solute is used or more solution is added.

Summary

I. Dimensional analysis—Process of understanding and applying the relationships between the qualities of various drugs and systems for identifying and measuring drug dosages based on the physical characteristics of each item

II. Basic math—Calculation skills necessary to ensure patient safety when managing drugs; includes dosage calculations and concentrations

   a. Fractions—Equal divisions of an item or a portion that is less than the whole item or number

     i. Common fractions—Written as numerator (top number that represents the number of parts available) over denominator (bottom number that represents the total number of equal divisions) using a diagonal or horizontal line to separate the two numbers

     ii. Decimal system—Place value numbering system that relies on multiples of 10 and uses a decimal point to separate the whole numbers from the fractions

     iii. Percentages—Parts per hundred; represented by the % symbol

   b. Ratios—Expression of a relationship between two numbers or components

   c. Proportions—Comparison of two ratios that are equal

III. Numbering and measurement systems—Specifically used in the surgical environment
   a. Roman numeral system—System of numbering that uses letters (upper or lower case) to represent numbers but does not include a symbol to represent zero
   b. Military time—Timekeeping system that uses a 24-hour clock to eliminate any potential confusion between A.M. and P.M. that may occur within the civilian timekeeping system
   c. International units—Arbitrary type of measure that represents the biological potency of a drug within the body regardless of the mass of the substance that is accepted globally; standardized according to the action of the drug, standardization of the unit pertains only to that drug
   d. Milliequivalent measures—Unit of measure that represents one thousandth of a measure
   e. Apothecary system—Measurement system that originated in ancient Greece and was used by physicians to prescribe medicine and by pharmacists to formulate the prescribed compound; few medications (such as aspirin, codeine, digitalis, and phenobarbital) are still prescribed and labeled in apothecary terms
   f. Household system—Measurement system primarily used in the United States to determine length, weight, and volume; also referred to as United States customary units
   g. Metric system/Systeme International d'Unites (SI)—Scientific system for measuring length, weight, and volume that uses Arabic numerals and is decimal based
      i. Length—Measured in meters; refer to equivalency and comparison tables
      ii. Weight—Measured in grams; refer to equivalency and comparison tables
      iii. Volume—Measured in liters; refer to equivalency and comparison tables
   h. Temperature conversion—Must be able to convert between Fahrenheit and Celsius scales
      i. Fahrenheit to Celsius—Use one of the following formulas: (°F − 32) × 5/9 = °C or (°F − 32) / 1.8 = °C
      Celsius to Fahrenheit—Use one of the following formulas: (°C × 9/5) + 32 = °F or °C × 1.8 + 32 = °F
IV. Dosage calculation—Study of dosage calculations is called posology
V. Mixing medications—One or more drugs or solutions may be combined to produce an enhances effect; dehydrated and concentrated drugs must be reconstituted prior to use
   a. Combining medications—An additive is combined with the primary drug or solution to produce a synergistic or agonist effect
   b. Reconstituting medications—Drugs manufactured in dehydrated or concentrated forms must be returned to the liquid state or diluted prior to use
   c. Concentrating and diluting medications—To concentrate a drug use less solution or more solute; to dilute a drug use more solution or less solute

Critical Thinking Review

1. Define the term *dimensional analysis* and describe the situations that dimensional analysis is applied in the surgical setting.
2. Differentiate between a proper and an improper fraction.
3. The Institute for Safe Medication Practices (ISMP) recommends use of a zero before a decimal point if the decimal number is a fraction only. Why? Use information found elsewhere in this textbook to answer this question.
4. What number does the Roman numeral II represent? Provide two examples of the use of Roman numerals in pharmacology.
5. Why is the military time–keeping system preferred in the health care setting? Write the equivalent of 0300 using civilian time.
6. Explain how to convert international units to milligrams.
7. What does the term *milliequivalent* mean? Provide two examples of the use of milliequivalent measures in the medical setting.
8. Explain why one milliliter is equal to one cubic centimeter. When referring to volume, use of which term (*ml* or *cc*) is recommended by the ISMP?
9. State the normal body temperature (measured orally) using both the Celsius and Fahrenheit scales.
10. List and describe the visual changes that can take place when mixing medications that would indicate incompatibility of the drugs. Should a drug mixture be used if an incompatibility occurs?

References

Association of Surgical Technologists. (2005). *Guideline statement for safe medication practices in the perioperative area*. Retrieved from http://www.ast.org/pdf/Standards_of_Practice/Guideline_Safe_Medication_Practices.pdf

Austin Community College. (2008). *Reconstituting medications*. Retrieved from http://www.austincc.edu/rxsucces/pdf/reconstructionpdf.pdf

Aylor, R. (2011a). *Apothecary system*. Retrieved from http://www.gpht.org/apothecary-system.html

Aylor, R. (2011b). *Household measurements*. Retrieved from http://www.gpht.org/household-measurements.html

Bedgood, A. (2008). *Pediatric dosage rules*. Retrieved from http://www.austincc.edu/rxsucces/ped1.html

Broyles, B., Reiss, B., & Evans, M. (2007). *Pharmacological aspects of nursing care* (7th ed.). Clifton Park, NY: Thomson Delmar Learning.

Cobb, S. (2007). *Integers and order of operations*. Retrieved from http://learn.midsouthcc.edu/learningObjects/algebraPrep/section_1/index.html

Curren, A. M. (2010). *Dimensional analysis for meds* (4th ed.). Clifton Park, NY: Delmar Cengage Learning.

Daniels, J. M. & Smith, L. M. (1999). *Clinical calculations: A unified approach* (4th ed.). Clifton Park, NY: Cengage Learning.

Decimal point. (n.d.). *The American heritage® science dictionary*. Retrieved from http://dictionary.reference.com/browse/decimal+point

Denominator. (n.d.). *The American heritage® science dictionary*. Retrieved from http://dictionary.reference.com/browse/denominator

Des Moines Area Community College. (2012). *The household system*. Retrieved from http://www.dmacc.edu/medmath1/HOUSEHOLD/hhold_intro.html

Dvorscak, B. (n.d.). *Proportion*. Retrieved from http://mypages.iit.edu/~smart/dvorber/lesson3.htm

Espinosa, R. (2008). *Dosage problems*. Retrieved from http://www.austincc.edu/rxsucces/dosage1.html

Felder, K. (1996). *One of these things is not like the other: A discussion of units*. Retrieved from http://www4.ncsu.edu/unity/lockers/users/f/felder/public/kenny/papers/units.html

Fraction. (n.d.). *The American heritage® Stedman's medical dictionary*. Retrieved from http://dictionary.reference.com/browse/fraction

Frey, K., et al. (2008). *Surgical technology for the surgical technologist: A positive care approach* (3rd ed.). Clifton Park, NY: Delmar Cengage Learning.

Gremanna Community College (n.d.). *How to solve drug dosage problems*. Retrieved from http://www.germanna.edu/tutor/Handouts/Nursing/Drug%20Dosage%20Calculation%20Packet.pdf

Gtt. (n.d.). *The American heritage® Stedman's medical dictionary*. Retrieved from http://dictionary.reference.com/browse/gtt

Heiserman, D. (2004). *Factors which influence drug dosage effects*. Retrieved from http://www.waybuilder.net/sweethaven/MedTech/Pharmacol/coursemain.asp?whichMod=module010305

Helmenstine, A. (2012). *What is absolute zero?* Retrieved from http://chemistry.about.com/od/chemistryfaqs/f/absolutezero.htm

Institute for Safe Medication Practices. (n.d.). *ISMP's list of error-prone abbreviations, symbols, and dose designations*. Retrieved from http://www.ismp.org/tools/errorproneabbreviations.pdf

Integer. (n.d.). *The American heritage® science dictionary*. Retrieved from http://dictionary.reference.com/browse/integer

Lack, J. & Stuart-Taylor, M. (1997). *Calculation of drug dosage and body surface area of children*. Retrieved from http://bja.oxfordjournals.org/content/78/5/601.full.pdf

Los Angeles Harbor College. (2012). *Reconstitution of solutions*. Retrieved from http://www.lahc.edu/classes/nursing/nurs302/Chapter_12.pdf

Mercer County Community College. (n.d.). *Decimals: Fast facts*. Retrieved from http://www.mccc.edu/~kelld/decff.htm

Michon, J. P. (2012). *Roman numerals*. Retrieved from http://www.numericana.com/answer/roman.htm

Military Connection. (2012). *Military time overview*. Retrieved from http://www.militaryconnection.com/military-time.asp

Milliequivalent. (n.d.). *The American heritage® Stedman's medical dictionary*. Retrieved from http://dictionary.reference.com/browse/milliequivalent

Moini, J. (2009). *Fundamental pharmacology for pharmacy technicians*. Clifton Park, NY: Delmar Cengage Learning.

Montgomery, J. (2008). *Conversion problems*. Retrieved from http://www.austincc.edu/rxsucces/conversion1.html

National Aeronautics and Space Administration. (2004). *Temperature scales and absolute zero*. Retrieved from http://cryo.gsfc.nasa.gov/introduction/temp_scales.html

National Institute of Standards and Technology. (2012). *International system of units*. Retrieved from http://physics.nist.gov/cuu/Units/introduction.html

National Institute of Standards and Technology. (n.d.). *A brief history of measurement systems*. Retrieved from https://standards.nasa.gov/history_metric.pdf

Nave, R. (n.d.). *Water density*. Retrieved from http://hyperphysics.phy-astr.gsu.edu/hbase/chemical/waterdens.html

Navy CyberSpace. (2009). *Military time conversion charts*. Retrieved from http://www.navycs.com/militarytime.html

Nelson, K. (2012). *Roman numerals*. Retrieved from http://www.pharmacy-tech-study.com/romannumerals.html

Numerator. (n.d.). *The American heritage® science dictionary*. Retrieved from http://dictionary.reference.com/browse/numerator

Okeke, C. (n.d.). *Pharmaceutical calculations in prescription compounding*. Retrieved from http://www.pharmacopeia.cn/v29240/usp29nf24s0_c1160.html

Percent. (n.d.). *The American heritage® science dictionary*. Retrieved from http://dictionary.reference.com/browse/percent

Peterson, D. (2012). *Military time, spoken*. Retrieved from http://mathforum.org/library/drmath/view/61445.html

Posology. (n.d.). *The American heritage® Stedman's medical dictionary*. Retrieved from http://dictionary.reference.com/browse/posology?s=t

Rice, J. (2006). *Principles of pharmacology for medical assisting* (4th ed.). Clifton Park, NY: Thomson Delmar Leaning.

Rosenthal, K. (2007). *Preventing IV drug incompatibilities*. Retrieved from http://www.resourcenurse.com/feature_incompatibilities.html

Rowlett, R. (2000). *The metric system in the United States*. Retrieved from http://www.unc.edu/~rowlett/units/usmetric.html

Simmons, B. (2011). *Mathwords: Terms and formulas from beginning algebra to calculus*. Retrieved from http://www.mathwords.com

Syracuse University. (n.d). *Operations in fractions*. Retrieved from http://cstl.syr.edu/fipse/fracunit/opfrac/opfrac.htm

Tennessee Wesleyan College. (n.d.). *Math review and basic pharmacology math*. Retrieved from www.twcnet.edu/lib/file/manager/Gail_Lambert/Math_Review.ppt

United States Metric Association. (2012). *Metric system temperature (Kelvin and degree Celsius)*. Retrieved from http://lamar.colostate.edu/~hillger/temps.htm

University of Minnesota. (2006). *Normal lab values (for reference only)*. Retrieved from http://www.student.med.umn.edu/wardmanual/normallabs.php

Walker, R. (2007). *Metric system prefixes*. Retrieved from http://simetric.co.uk/siprefix.htm

Woodrow, R. (2007). *Essentials of pharmacology for health occupations* (5th ed.). Clifton Park, NY: Thomson Delmar Learning.

World Health Organization. (2012). *WHO international biological reference preparations*. Retrieved from http://www.who.int/biologicals/reference_preparations/en

Chapter THREE

DRUG IDENTIFICATION AND CLASSIFICATION

Student Learning Outcomes

After studying this chapter, the reader should be able to:

- Differentiate between the three types of drug nomenclature.
- Describe various drug classifications and provide examples of one or more drugs from each classification.

Key Terms

Chemical name	Generic name	Pharmaceutical	Proprietary name
Controlled substance	Narcotics	Pharmacist	Prototype
Drug Enforcement	Nomenclature	Preference card	Standing orders
Administration	Official "Do Not Use" List	Prescription	Stat

DRUG NOMENCLATURE

The word *nomenclature* refers to a system for naming or the rules for naming. Therefore, when the term *drug nomenclature* is used, it pertains to the system or rules for naming pharmaceuticals. The term *pharmaceutical* pertains to a drug that is prepared commercially or in a pharmacy and/or dispensed by a retail or hospital pharmacist. A **pharmacist** is an individual who has passed the North American Pharmacist Licensure Examination (NAPLEX®) or the Multistate Pharmacy Jurisprudence Examination (MPJE®), which is administered by the National Association of Boards of Pharmacy (NAPB®) and is licensed by the appropriate State Board of Pharmacy to prepare and dispense drugs in that state. Most drugs have three names: the chemical name, the generic name, and the proprietary name.

Chemical Name

The **chemical name** provides the exact formula and molecular structure of the drug. Chemical names are lengthy, complicated, and difficult to pronounce and use. Typically the chemical name is not printed on the label of a drug, but is found in the package insert that accompanies the drug. Chemical names can also be located in the *Physician's Desk Reference*. An example of a chemical name is acetylsalicylic acid and it represents what is commonly known by its generic name, aspirin. Chemical names are most often utilized in the research setting.

Generic Name

The **generic name** is the nonproprietary name of the drug and often the generic name is the official name of the drug as it appears in the *United States Pharmacopeia–National Formulary* (USP–NF). The generic name is frequently a shortened version of the chemical name or may be a reference to the intended use of the drug that is selected by the original developer. The generic name is the preferred name for use in the health care setting because several manufacturers may market the same drug under different proprietary names. Health care facilities often change vendors to secure the best contracted price for pharmaceuticals. For example, the generic drug bupivacaine is marketed under the brand names of Sensorcaine® and Marcaine® (among others), so the hospital pharmacy may alternate between the brands according to which company is currently offering the best price for the item. The generic name is prominently displayed on the drug label and is not capitalized. Continuing with the acetylsalicylic acid example, aspirin is the generic name for the chemical preparation acetylsalicylic acid.

Proprietary (Brand or Trade) Name

The **proprietary name** is also known as the trade name and the brand name. This is the name that the manufacturer assigns to the drug for marketing purposes. The proprietary name of the drug is displayed on the drug label and is capitalized. The proprietary name may be followed by the superscripted symbol representing a registered trademark (®). Following through with the acetylsalicylic acid example, some brand names for aspirin are Bayer® and Anacin®. Manufacturing differences may occur, making the preparation of each brand slightly different. For example, a manufacturer of a brand name drug may include a preservative, buffer, flavoring, or other type of additive to the formula; however, the main component of the drug remains the same and the principal action is not altered.

Table 3-1 provides four examples of the three types of drug nomenclature.

DRUG CLASSIFICATIONS

In addition to the three types of nomenclature described earlier, drugs are classified in various other ways as well. For example, drugs are classified by the way that they are prescribed and purchased (OTC, prescription, and controlled substances).

Drugs may also be classified according to their principal action, body system affected, physiological action, and therapeutic action. Keep in mind that each main drug classification may also have several subclassifications. One drug (e.g., phenobarbital) may fall into several categories. Drugs in each classification are represented by a specific prototype. A **prototype** is a generalization about the characteristics of the drugs in that classification. For example, all drugs that are classified

TABLE 3-1 Examples of Types of Drug Nomenclature

Brand Name	Generic Name	Chemical Name
Bayer®, Anacin®, etc.	Aspirin	Acetylsalicylic acid
Demerol®	Meperidine hydrochloride	Ethyl 1-methyl-4-phenylisonipecotate hydrochloride
Marcaine®, Sensorcaine®	Bupivacaine	1-butyl-*N*-(2,6-dimethylphenyl)piperidine-2-carboxamide
Sublimaze®	Fentanyl citrate	*N*-Phenyl-*N*-(1-(2-phenylethyl)-4-piperidinyl) propanamide

as antiemetics (a subclassification of therapeutic action) fit the prototype of drugs that reduce the risk of vomiting. Detailed descriptions of drugs in several classifications are found in Chapter Ten.

Over-The-Counter

Over-the-counter (OTC) drugs are those that can be purchased directly by the consumer without a prescription from a physician. A drug must meet the following criteria in order to be classified as an OTC drug:

- The drug presents minimal risk and maximum benefit.

- It must have a low potential for abuse or misuse.

- The consumer should be able to use the drug for common conditions that do not require a physician to diagnose (e.g., low-grade fever or headache).

- The label contains adequate information in a user-friendly format.

- Monitoring of the condition or use of the drug by a physician is not necessary.

Aspirin is an OTC drug that meets the requirements above. An individual may be suffering from a headache or a fever and based on the knowledge that he or she has about the drug the individual may make a determination that taking aspirin as directed on the label may be an effective treatment for the self-diagnosed condition.

Occasionally, certain OTC drugs must be requested from the pharmacist because they must be kept in an environmentally controlled storage location such as a refrigerator or a dark location. Other OTC drugs may have restrictions on the quantity that can be purchased and must also be requested from the pharmacist. Some OTC drugs such as cough medicines, must be purchased by an individual who meets a certain age requirement.

Prescription

A **prescription** is an order outlining the care of a patient that is given by a physician or other licensed health care professional such as a physician's assistant or a nurse practitioner. Prescriptions may pertain to various types of therapy or treatments. In this textbook, the term *prescription* will pertain to the order that is required prior to preparing and dispensing certain medications. The notation "R_x," which is from the Latin—meaning "take thou," is often used to represent a prescription or a pharmacy (Figure 3-1).

Written Prescription

Typically, a written prescription is given to a patient during a visit to his or her physician for treatment of a specific problem. The patient then takes the written

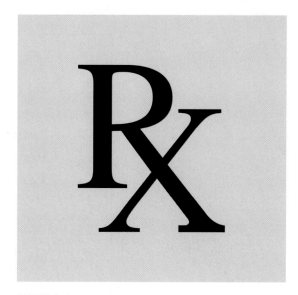

FIGURE 3-1 Symbol Representing a Prescription

prescription to the pharmacy of his or her choice (usually determined by the health insurance plan, if available) so that the pharmacist may fill the order and dispense the medication to the patient.

Preprinted forms containing the following information are the most common method for prescribing medications in the physician's office setting Figure 3-2.

- Name, address, and telephone number of the prescriber
  - May include the prescriber's license number and/or Drug Enforcement Agency number, especially if the prescription is for a controlled substance (refer to the controlled substance segment of this chapter)

- Name, address, and age or date of birth of the patient

- Current date

- Name, strength, and amount of the drug

- Instructions for the patient concerning the route of administration, frequency of administration, and any precautions or restrictions

- Number of refills allowed, if any

- Signature of the prescriber

- Brand or generic substitutions, if allowed

Medication Orders within a Hospital

In the hospital setting, medication orders are handled differently than they are in an office setting. When a patient is admitted to the hospital, the physician provides a set of orders to be carried out for the specific patient. The orders may be handwritten or computer generated.

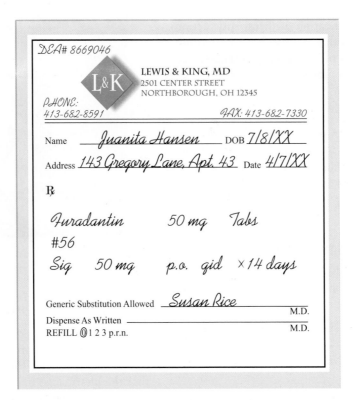

FIGURE 3-2 Prescription Example

Computer-generated orders are the preferred method because the number of transcription errors may be reduced and an interface with the billing department may be provided. The orders will pertain to all aspects of the care of the patient including (but not limited to) diet, diagnostic studies to be performed, frequency of measuring the patient's vital signs, and of course the list of medications prescribed for the patient. The order will contain the same type of information about each drug that would be included on a written prescription such as the date ordered, the name strength, and amount of the drug prescribed, instructions for administration of the drug, and the signature of the prescriber. In the hospital setting, the order is filled by the pharmacist and administered to the patient by qualified personnel.

In the surgical environment, it is typically the anesthesia provider, circulator, or surgeon who is responsible for medication administration. However, in certain situations the responsibility for administration of medication may fall to other team members as long as federal law, state law, and facility policies and procedures are followed. According to the Association of Surgical Technologists' Guideline Statement of Safe Medication Practices in the Perioperative Area, "A Certified Surgical Technologist (CST) and a Certified Surgical First Assistant (CSFA) are qualified to handle and administer medications in the O.R. under the direct supervision and order of the surgeon." The guideline in its entirety may be viewed online at http://www.ast.org/uploadedFiles/Main_Site/Content/About_Us/Guideline_Safe_Medication.pdf.

Standing Orders Some physicians, especially those who practice in specialty areas, who treat several patients with similar conditions, will frequently preestablish a set of orders for patients with that condition called **standing orders**. Standing orders are standard procedure and are always in force unless the prescriber indicates otherwise. For example, a general surgeon may have a set of standing orders that are applied to every adult patient who is referred to him or her with a diagnosis of possible appendicitis. A different set of standing orders might be available for every pediatric patient who is referred with the diagnosis of appendicitis. Upon the patient's admission to the hospital, the staff can begin administering the various treatments and medications immediately using the standing orders without contacting the physician to obtain new orders for each patient.

Surgeon Preference Cards In the operating room, the surgeon **preference card** is the tool utilized to prepare for the surgical procedure. The preference card is a form of standing orders. The preference card contains all of the pertinent information concerning a specific surgeon's requests for a specific surgical procedure including medication orders. An example of a surgeon preference card with a standing medication order is shown in Figure 3-3. Please note that the standing medication order contained within the preference card is highlighted. If any changes to the standing orders are required during the surgical procedure, they are most often issued verbally.

Preference Card

Surgeon:	**Dr. XYZ**
Procedure:	**Appendectomy – Adult (Traditional Approach)**
Position:	**Supine with arms extended on arm boards**
Glove Size/Style:	**8 white with 7½ ortho over** Dominant Hand: **Right**
Equipment:	**Electrosurgical unit with dispersive electrode** **Standard setting: 40/40 Blend 1** **Suction Apparatus** **Headlamp (available)**
Supplies:	**Laparotomy pack (customized, includes vertical lap sheet)** **Double basin set** **Towel packs x 2** **Gloves for all sterile team members** **Aerobic and anaerobic culture tubes (available)**
Instrumentation:	**Minor instrumentation set**
Suture and Usage:	**Ties:** **2-0 Vicryl Reel** **Pursestring:** **3-0 Vicryl SH** **Peritoneum:** **2-0 Vicryl CT-1** **Fascia:** **2-0 Vicryl CT-1** **Sub-Q:** **None or 3-0 Vicryl CT-1 (obese patient)** **Skin:** **Staples or 3-0 Nylon FSLX (if ruptured)**
Dressings:	**Triple antibiotic ointment** **Telfa** **4 x 4 Gauze** **2" Paper tape**
Skin Prep:	**Shave, if necessary** **Povidone Iodine – 5 minute**
Pharmaceuticals:	**Bupivacaine 0.5% (available for postoperative pain control)** **Control syringe (if needed)** **25 Gauge 1½" needle (if needed)**

FIGURE 3-3 Preference Card (with standing medication order highlighted)

Verbal Orders Verbal orders are those that are issued by the physician when it is not convenient to write them down. During a surgical procedure, the surgeon or anesthesia provider is not able to stop what he or she is doing and write a prescription to initiate or update an order. Therefore, the order is stated out loud and the surgical team members carry out the request. If a verbal order is not understood, the surgical team members involved must ask for clarification. The updated order is recorded in the operative record that becomes part of the patient's chart. Orders given over the telephone are another example of verbal orders.

Terminology Related to Medication Orders

Much of the terminology used to convey medication orders, whether in the written or verbal form, relate back to Latin. Initially, Latin was selected because it was considered a "dead" language that would not change over time and because the Latin words have exact meanings that cannot be misinterpreted. Latin terms that indicate the timing and frequency of drug administration as well as the route of administration are still in use today. Often, abbreviations, acronyms, and symbols are substituted instead of stating the full term. Table 3-2 contains many of the commonly used abbreviations, acronyms, and symbols along with the full Latin term and the English interpretation.

TABLE 3-2 Commonly Used Abbreviations, Acronyms, and Symbols

Abbreviation, Acronym, or Symbol	Latin Origin	English Meaning
ac	ante cibum	before meals
ad/as/au	auris dexter/auris sinister/auris utraque	right ear/left ear/each ear (both)
ad lib	ad libitum	at liberty/as much as desired
bid	bis in die	twice a day
cap(s)	n/a	capsule(s)
cc	cum cibo	with food/also cubic centimeter
da/daw	n/a	dispense/dispense as written
dc	n/a	discontinue/discharge
g/gm/GM	n/a	gram
gt/gtt/gtts	gutta/guttae	drop/drops/drops
h	hora	hour
hs	hora somni	hour of sleep (at bedtime)
IM	n/a	intramuscularly
IV	n/a	intravenously
kg	n/a	kilogram
l/L	n/a	liter
mcg	n/a	microgram
mEq	n/a	milliequivalent
mg	n/a	milligram
ml/mL	n/a	milliliter
npo	nil per os	nothing by mouth
od/os/ou	oculus dexter/oculus sinister/oculus utraque	right eye/left eye/each eye (both)
oz	n/a	ounce
pc	post cibum	after meals
per	per	by/through
po	per os	by mouth
prn	pro re nata	according to the circumstances/as needed
q	quaque	every
q3h (any number may be substituted, as prescribed)	quaque 3 hora	once every 3 hours
qd	quaque die	once every day
qid	quarter in die	four times per day
R_x	take thou	represents a prescription or a pharmacy
sc/sq	n/a	subcutaneous
sig	signa	write (usually an indication to the pharmacist that the directions that follow should be translated and written on the label for the patient)
soln	n/a	solution
stat	statum	immediately
susp	n/a	suspension
tab	n/a	tablet
tid	ter in die	three times per day

tr/tinc/tinct	n/a	tincture
U	n/a	unit
ung	unguentum	ointment
ut dict	ut dictum	as directed
w	n/a	with
w/o	n/a	without
@	n/a	at
>	n/a	greater than
<	n/a	less than
µ	n/a	micro
µg	n/a	microgram

Because many of the terms listed in Table 3-2 can look alike especially if handwritten or sound alike, the Institute for Safe Medication Practices (ISMP) has issued a List of Error-Prone Abbreviations, Symbols, and Dose Designations. The National Patient Safety Goals established by The Joint Commission (TJC) provides an **Official "Do Not Use" List** that identifies specific abbreviations that must appear on each accredited institution's do-not-use list. Of course, an individual institution's list may be more comprehensive than TJC requirement. Go to the ISMP web site at ISMP.org to review the "Do Not Use" list.

Commonly Confused Drug Names

Several OTC and prescription drugs have names that look or sound similar and can be easily confused. The ISMP has compiled a List of Confused Drug Names that also includes a list of look-alike and sound-alike names set forth by TJC. When health care providers are aware of a potential hazard, caution can be exercised to reduce the risk of committing an error.

Controlled Substances

The term *controlled substance* refers to a drug that is a narcotic. The United States **Drug Enforcement Administration** (DEA) is responsible for enforcement of the laws pertaining to controlled substances. The Controlled Substances Act identifies certain drugs that should be classified as narcotics and regulated. The Controlled Substances Act provides a classification system for narcotics according to their intended medical uses, the potential for an individual to abuse the drug, and its safety or the dangers that it poses. There are five categories or schedules for classification of controlled substances. The categories or schedules are numbered from I to V using Roman numerals. Refer to Chapter

Nine to learn more about handling of **narcotics** in the operating room.

Schedule I Controlled Substances

Schedule I drugs have no currently accepted medical use and have a high potential for abuse. Drugs in this category are highly addictive and are not considered safe for use even with medical supervision. The risk of physical or psychological dependence is serious.

Schedule II Controlled Substances

Schedule II drugs have a currently accepted medical use and have a high potential for abuse. Drugs in this category are severely restricted and are considered safe for use with medical supervision. The risk of physical or psychological dependence is serious.

Schedule III Controlled Substances

Schedule III drugs have a currently accepted medical use and have less potential for abuse than the drugs in Schedules I and II. The risk of physical or psychological dependence is moderate to low.

Schedule IV Controlled Substances

Schedule IV drugs have a currently accepted medical use and have less potential for abuse than the drugs in Schedule III. The risk of physical or psychological dependence is limited.

Schedule V Controlled Substances

Schedule V drugs have a currently accepted medical use and have less potential for abuse than the drugs in Schedule IV. The risk of physical or psychological dependence is low. Table 3-3 provides an overview of the Schedules as well as examples of drugs that fall into each category.

TABLE 3-3 Controlled Substances

Schedule	Overview	Examples
Schedule I	No current medical use Serious risk of physical or psychological dependence	heroin lysergic acid diethylamide (LSD) marijuana (in some areas) Note: In areas where marijuana is approved for medical use, it would be classified as a Schedule II controlled substance
Schedule II	Current medical use Serious risk of physical or psychological dependence	cocaine methamphetamine morphine
Schedule III	Current medical use Moderate to low risk of physical or psychological dependence	anabolic steroids aspirin or acetaminophen that contain codeine or hydrocodone certain barbiturates
Schedule IV	Current medical use Limited risk of physical or psychological dependence	alprazolam diazepam meprobamate pentazocine propoxyphene hydrochloride
Schedule V	Current medical use Low risk of physical or psychological dependence	cough medicines that contain codeine

Several factors are considered when the DEA makes a determination to place a drug on the controlled substances list. The factors are:

- The potential for abuse of the drug (actual or virtual)
- Knowledge of the potential properties and effects of the drug, especially its ability to cause hallucinations
- Knowledge of the pharmacologic effects of the drug
- History of the drug and any current patterns of abuse, if noted
- Identified or potential risk to public health
- Potential to cause physical or psychological dependence, if available
- Knowledge of related drugs that are controlled

Strict federal, state, and facility based policies and procedures are in place concerning obtaining, storing, dispensing, and discarding controlled substances. In some states, the law requires the prescriber to utilize a special tamper-resistant prescription form when ordering controlled substances.

Principal Action

The principal or main action of a drug is most often determined by the type of chemical used in preparing the drug. Principal action is sometimes referred to as chemical action. For example, all drugs made from the chemical barbituric acid are called barbiturates. The principal actions of all drugs in this classification (barbiturates) are similar because the base chemical is the same. Barbiturates depress the central nervous system. Phenobarbital fits the prototype of a barbiturate.

Body System Affected

Many drugs are classified according to the body system that is affected by the action of the drug. For example, all drugs that have an effect on the central nervous system would fall into this classification. Phenobarbital fits the prototype of a drug that affects the central nervous system.

Physiological Action

Drugs that change the function of the body (physiologic action) are placed in this category. For example, drugs that slow down the function of the central nervous system would be classified as central nervous system depressants. Phenobarbital fits the prototype of a central nervous system depressant.

Therapeutic Action

Drugs are also classified according to their therapeutic action (the benefits they provide). For example, drugs that reduce seizure activity are called anticonvulsants. Phenobarbital fits the prototype of an anticonvulsant.

Alternative and Complimentary Medications

Alternative medications are identified as those not considered part of conventional medical care. Alternative medications are used instead of standard Western medical practices. Herbal medicine and the use of nutritional (dietary) supplements are examples of alternative medications. Unfortunately, there has been very little regulation of the manufacturing processes for alternative medications, which has led to problems with dosage standardization and inconsistent use of additives (such as preservatives and flavorings). The consumer should carefully research the risks and benefits of alternative medications prior to initiating their use. Some patients benefit significantly from the use of alternative medications; however, their use can also be dangerous especially when mixed with conventional drugs or if the patient is pediatric, geriatric, pregnant, breast feeding, has chronic health problems, or is allergic. For example, ginger root is thought to reduce nausea and vomiting related to chemotherapy, general anesthesia agents, motion sickness, and pregnancy. Unfortunately, ginger also interferes with blood clotting. As a matter of routine, the health care provider should question the patient about the use of any alternative medications, along with questions about current conventional medications and any known allergies.

When conventional practices are paired with alternative options, the patient is said to be receiving complimentary or integrated care. In addition to herbal medicine and nutritional supplements, other forms of alternative and complementary medicine include acupuncture, hypnosis, and meditation. Scientific studies to determine the effectiveness of alternative and complementary therapies are underway.

Herbal Medicine

Herbs used in medicine are derived from plants that have healing properties. Herbal remedies have been in use for thousands of years, especially in Eastern cultures. Many herbs commonly used to add flavor when preparing meals also have medicinal uses. A few examples include allspice (antiemetic), basil (antidiarrheal), caraway (diuretic), cinnamon (antiseptic), garlic (antihypertensive), and turmeric (antiarthritic).

Nutritional Supplements

Nutritional supplements, also called dietary supplements, are designed to augment the patient's food intake especially if the individual is not meeting certain nutrient recommendations set forth by the Food and Nutrition Board of the Institute of Medicine in the Dietary Reference Intake (DRI). For easy reference, DRI reports and tables are available on the National Institutes of Health web site at http://ods.od.nih.gov/health_information/ Dietary_Reference_Intakes.aspx. Vitamins, minerals, fatty acids, fiber, amino acids, and certain hormones are all examples of nutritional supplements. Nutritional supplements are typically ingested in the form of a liquid, capsule, or tablet.

Summary

I. Drug nomenclature—System for naming pharmaceuticals
  a. Chemical name—Exact formula and molecular structure of the drug
  b. Generic name—Nonproprietary name of the drug (preferred name in the health care setting)
  c. Proprietary (brand or trade)—Name that the manufacturer assigns to the drug for marketing purposes
II. Drug classifications—Additional methods for identifying drugs
  a. Over-the-counter (OTC)—Drugs that can be purchased directly by the consumer without a prescription from a physician
  b. Prescription—Order outlining the care of a patient
    i. Written prescriptions—Order written by physician (or other licensed health care provider) that is required prior to preparing and dispensing certain medications
    ii. Medication orders within a hospital—List of medications prescribed for the patient
      1. Standing orders—Preestablished set of orders for patients with similar conditions
        a. Surgeon preference cards—Form of standing orders used specifically in the operating room
      2. Verbal orders—Spoken orders issued by the physician when it is not convenient to write them down
    iii. Terminology related to medication orders— Latin abbreviations and acronyms that indicate the timing and frequency of drug administration as well as the route of administration (to avoid errors, certain abbreviations, acronyms, and symbols should not be used)
    iv. Commonly confused drug names—Use caution not to confuse look-alike and sound-alike drugs
  c. Controlled substances —Narcotics
    i. Schedule I—No currently accepted medical use and a high potential for abuse
    ii. Schedule II—Currently accepted medical use and a high potential for abuse
    iii. Schedule III—Currently accepted medical use and less potential for abuse than the drugs in Schedules I and II
    iv. Schedule IV—Currently accepted medical use and less potential for abuse than the drugs in Schedule III
    v. Schedule V—Currently accepted medical use and less potential for abuse than the drugs in Schedule IV

d. Principal action—Main action of a drug determined by the type of chemical used in preparing the drug

e. Body system affected—Drug classification according to the body system that is affected by the action of the drug

f. Physiological action—Drugs that change the function of the body

g. Therapeutic action—Drugs are provide a therapeutic or beneficial action

h. Alternative and complementary medications—used instead of or in addition to conventional drugs

   i. Herbal medicine—Medicinal herbs derived from plants that have healing properties

   ii. Nutritional supplements—Augment the patient's food intake especially if the individual is not meeting the Recommended Daily Intake (RDI) of certain nutrients set forth by the FDA

Critical Thinking Review

1. List the three types of drug nomenclature and provide a brief description of each.
2. Which type of drug nomenclature is preferred in the health care setting? Why?
3. List the generic and the chemical names for the brand name drug Demerol®.
4. Is a prescription necessary to purchase an OTC drug? Why or why not?
5. List the information that must be present on a written prescription.
6. The surgeon preference card is a form of standing orders. If there is a change in the order because of the patient's special circumstances, how will the change most likely be communicated to the surgical team members?
7. On his preference card (Figure 3-3), Dr. XYZ is requesting bupivacaine 0.5% to be available for postoperative pain control. What are the brand and chemical names for this product?
8. What is the classification of the drug bupivacaine 0.5%? Use information found elsewhere in this textbook to answer this question.
9. The drug morphine is a controlled substance. According to the Controlled Substances Act, what is the schedule? Why?
10. Think about drugs that are classified according to the body system affected. Limited information is presented in this chapter. Use information contained elsewhere in this textbook or from outside resources to identify at least three more drugs that affect three additional body systems.

References

Association of Surgical Technologists. (2005). *Guideline statement for safe medication practices in the perioperative area.* Retrieved from http://www.ast.org/pdf/Standards_of_Practice/Guideline_Safe_Medication_Practices.pdf

Eustice, C. (2006). *What do the prescription abbreviations mean?* Retrieved from http://arthritis.about.com/od/arthritismedications/f/rxabbreviations.htm

Frey, K., et al. (2008). *Surgical technology for the surgical technologist: a positive care approach* (3rd ed.). Clifton Park, NY: Delmar Cengage Learning.

Harrison, K. (2007). *Chemistry, structures, and 3D molecules.* Retrieved from http://www.3dchem.com

Institute for Safe Medication Practices. (n.d.). *ISMP's list of confused drug names.* Retrieved from http://www.ismp.org/tools/confuseddrugnames.pdf

Institute for Safe Medication Practices. (n.d.). *ISMP's list of error-prone abbreviations, symbols, and dose designations.* Retrieved from http://www.ismp.org/tools/errorproneabbreviations.pdf

The Joint Commission. (2011). *Facts about the official "do not use" list.* Retrieved from http://www.jointcommission.org/assets/1/18/Official_Do_Not_Use_List_6_111.PDF

Junge, T. (September 2007). "Antiemetic properties of ginger." *The Surgical Technologist* vol. 39 no. 9. Association of Surgical Technologists.

Leonard, M. (2010). *Herbal supplements: helpful or harmful?* Retrieved from http://my.clevelandclinic.org/heart/prevention/alternative/herbals_theheart.aspx

MedlinePlus. (2007). Barbiturate intoxication and overdose. Retrieved from http://www.nlm.nih.gov/medlineplus/ency/article/000951.htm

National Association of Boards of Pharmacy. (n.d.). Retrieved from http://www.nabp.net

National Institutes of Health National Center for Complementary and Alternative Medicine. (n.d.). *What is complementary and alternative medicine?* Retrieved from http://nccam.nih.gov/health/whatiscam/#safety

Nomenclature. (n.d.). *The American heritage® dictionary of the English language* (4th ed.). Retrieved from http://dictionary.reference.com/browse/nomenclature

Pharmaceutical. (n.d.). *WordNet® 3.0.* Retrieved from http://dictionary.reference.com/browse/pharmaceutical

United States Drug Enforcement Administration. (n.d.). Retrieved from http://www.usdoj.gov/dea/index.htm

United States Food and Drug Administration. (n.d.). Center for drug evaluation and research office of nonprescription drugs. Retrieved from http://www.fda.gov/cder/Offices/otc/default.htm

Woodrow, R. (2007). *Essentials of pharmacology for health occupations* (5th ed.). Clifton Park, NY: Thomson Delmar Learning.

Chapter
FOUR

DRUG SOURCES

Student Learning Outcome

After studying this chapter, the reader should be able to:

- Identify the five main drug sources and provide examples of drugs from each source.

Key Terms

Amino acid	Chromosome	Microorganism	Porcine
Antibody	Deoxyribonucleic acid	Mineral	Protein
Antigen	(DNA)	Mitosis	Recombinant
Avian	Enzyme	Nucleotides	Synthesis
Biological	Equine	Nucleic acids	Synthetic
Biotechnology	Genetic engineering	Opioid	Vaccine
Botanic	Hormone	Ovine	Vitamin
Bovine	Ichthyoid	Pathogen	Zoologic
Caprine	Immune serum (antiserum)	Plasma	

DRUG SOURCES

There are five main sources from which drugs are derived. The five sources are animal (**zoologic**), **biotechnology** (recombinant DNA technology), laboratory **synthesis**, **mineral**, and plant (**botanic**). Drugs that are derived from living cells (botanic or zoologic—[including molds and **microorganisms**]) are said to come from **biological** sources. More than half of all pharmaceuticals currently in use are from biological sources. A brief description of each source and examples of drugs from each source are provided in this chapter.

Animal (Zoologic) Sources

Typically the term *zoologic* typically distinguishes lower animals from humans but keep in mind that a few drugs classified as having an animal origin are derived from human sources. An example of a drug derived from a human source is human antihemophilic factor (Hemofil M®), which is obtained from pooled human **plasma**, and is used in the treatment of certain blood clotting disorders.

Substances that naturally occur in the human body are often found in animals and can be obtained from the fluids, tissues, glands, and/or organs of various animals. For the most part, drugs commonly derived from animal sources include certain **enzymes** and some **hormones** but can include antibiotics, **vitamins**, **vaccines**, and **immune serum** (**antiserum**). The desired substance is extracted from the source, purified by chemical or physical means, formulated for human intake, packaged, shipped, and stored for future use. Table 4-1 provides examples of drugs derived from animal sources.

Additional terminology that relates to animal sources includes:

- **Avian**—bird
- **Bovine**—cattle
- **Caprine**—goat
- **Equine**—horse
- **Ichthyoid**—fish
- **Ovine**—sheep
- **Porcine**—swine (pig)

For some individuals, drugs derived from animal sources are cause for concern. Here are some of the reasons:

- Some individuals feel that using animals for the manufacture and testing of drugs is wrong.

- Drugs from animal sources could contain a substance, such as a **pathogen**, that may be harmful to the recipient. Even though drugs from animal sources are refined and may come from controlled environments, there is no guarantee of 100% purity. Researchers are attempting to replace many drugs from animal sources with **synthetic** alternatives.

- In some belief systems, religions, and cultures consumption or implantation of animal elements or animal derivatives is forbidden.

- Introduction of foreign **proteins** (**antigens**) may induce production of antibodies (including mild to severe allergic reactions that may include anaphylaxis and death).

Biotechnology (Recombinant DNA Technology)

The terms *biotechnology* and *recombinant DNA* (rDNA) technology are used interchangeably. The technology was developed as a subspecialty of molecular biology beginning in the early 1970s and is used to create pharmaceuticals that are typically derived from zoologic sources. The technology also has other medical and agricultural applications. The term *genetic engineering* is also used to describe rDNA technology.

Deoxyribonucleic acid (**DNA**) is contained within the **chromosomes** of a cell and houses genetic information that is transferred to the new cell during cell division (**mitosis**) (Figure 4-1). Refer to an anatomy and physiology book for more information concerning DNA, chromosomes, and mitosis. The term *recombinant* is used to describe genetic material (DNA) that is taken from one source (donor) and combined with DNA from a second source (host) to create DNA with only the desired trait or traits.

TABLE 4-1 Drugs Derived from Animal Sources

Drug Name	Classification	Source
Adrenalin (epinephrine)	Vasoconstrictor	Large animal adrenal gland
Heparin	Anticoagulant	Bovine lung
Insulin (regular; NPH)	Hormone (antidiabetic)	Bovine or porcine pancreas
Thrombin, topical	Procoagulant	(Thrombostat®) Bovine (Evithrom®) Human

The process of creating a pharmaceutical product with rDNA technology is complex and requires several steps to accomplish. The explanation provided here is a simplified overview of the rDNA process. When using recombinant DNA technology, a specific restricted portion of DNA that contains the desired trait is removed from the donor cell and is combined with the DNA of a live host (which may also be known as a vector) cell such as yeast or a nonpathogenic bacteria. The host cell containing the recombinant DNA is allowed to reproduce by fermentation or in a culture environment. When a sufficient quantity of the new cells has accumulated, the desired portion of the DNA is disrupted and extracted from the host, purified by chemical or physical means, formulated for human intake, packaged, shipped, and stored for future use. Table 4-2 provides examples of drugs derived from biotechnology.

Some of the benefits of rDNA technology include minimizing or eliminating the risk of transmission of pathogens and reducing the risk of allergic reaction because the rDNA product contains minimal (or is free of) human and animal antigens.

Laboratory Synthesis

In chemistry, the term *synthesis* is used to describe the process of combining simple chemical elements and/or compounds to create a more complex chemical. Synthesized drugs are typically manufactured in a laboratory setting using chemicals from organic (botanic and zoologic) sources. Synthesized drugs are designed to resemble substances that occur naturally but are less costly, easier to produce, and/or can be produced in greater quantity than the natural substance. The synthesized drug is purified by chemical or physical means, formulated for human intake, packaged, shipped, and stored for future use. An example of a drug synthesized in a laboratory is the drug meperidine sulfate (Demerol®), which is a narcotic analgesic (used to treat moderate or severe pain). Meperidine is also classified as an **opioid**, meaning that it resembles an opiate drug such as

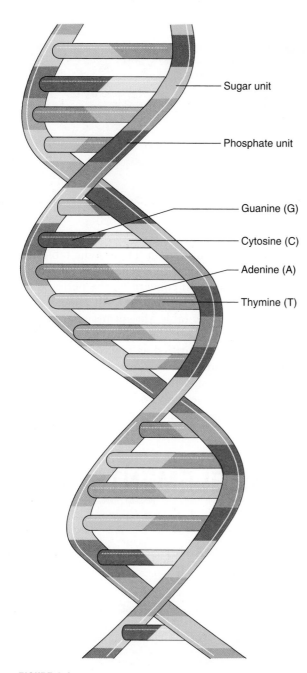

- Sugar unit
- Phosphate unit
- Guanine (G)
- Cytosine (C)
- Adenine (A)
- Thymine (T)

FIGURE 4-1 Recombinant DNA Technique

TABLE 4-2 Drugs Derived from Biotechnology

Drug Name	Classification	Source
Insulin, Human (Humulin®)	Hormone (antidiabetic)	rDNA (human/bacteria)
Hepatitis B Vaccine (Recombivax HB®)	Vaccine	rDNA (human/yeast)
Thrombin, topical (Recothrom®)	Procoagulant	rDNA (human/hamster)
Tissue Plasminogen Activator (tPA)	Thrombolytic	rDNA (human/bacteria)

TABLE 4-3 Drugs Derived from Laboratory Synthesis

Drug Name	Classification	Resembles
Cephalexin (Keflex®)	Antibiotic (semi-synthetic cephalosporin)	Penicillin
Methylprednisolone (Depo-Medrol®)	Steroidal anti-inflammatory	Corticosteroids manufactured in the adrenal cortex
Ketamine hydrochloride (Ketalar®)	Dissociative anesthetic agent	n/a
Ketorolac tromethamine (Toradol®)	Nonsteroidal anti-inflammatory	n/a

morphine. The concept of laboratory synthesis is not only used to manufacture pharmaceuticals, but has applications that are used commercially, in industry, and in agriculture as well. Table 4-3 provides examples of drugs derived from laboratory synthesis.

Mineral Sources

Minerals are inorganic elements that are naturally found in the earth and in water as well as in plants and animals that acquire the minerals from soil and water. All minerals are identified on the periodic table of elements (Figure 4-2). Refer to a general science book for additional information concerning the periodic table, the elements, and their properties. All minerals found listed on the periodic table are not necessary to maintain homeostasis within the body. The minerals that are necessary are identified as macrominerals, which are needed in significant amounts, and trace minerals, which are needed only in very small amounts. Minerals are needed by the body to regulate the heart rate, produce hormones, and maintain bone strength, among

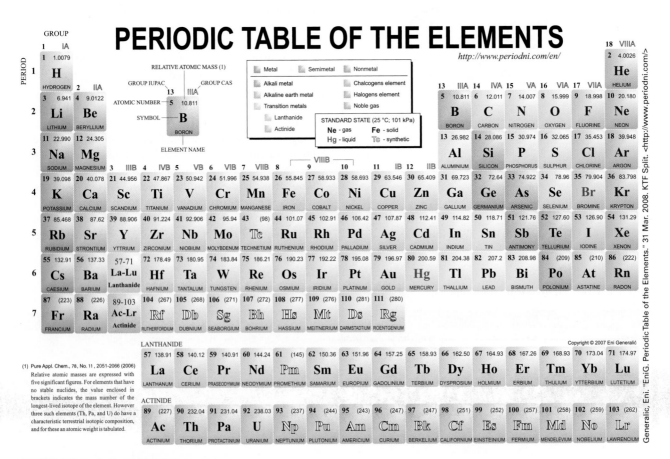

FIGURE 4-2 Periodic Table of Elements

other functions. Minerals are typically obtained by including plants and animals that have acquired the minerals from their original sources in our diet. When the Daily Reference Intake (DRI), established by the United States Department of Agriculture (USDA) Food and Nutrition Information Center (FNIC), is not being met through dietary intake of minerals, it may be necessary for an individual to take mineral supplements. The DRI for each mineral is established and varies according to life stage group (age) and sex. DRI tables can be found on the USDA and FNIC web sites: http://fnic.nal.usda .gov. Excessive consumption of certain minerals may have adverse effects. Minerals contained within the supplements are excavated (mined) from the earth or extracted from water, purified, formulated for human intake, packaged, shipped, and stored for future use.

Table 4-4 provides a brief overview of the minerals (macro and trace) necessary for human intake, their functions, and the related dietary sources.

Plant (Botanic) Sources

Hundreds of drugs are derived from plant (botanic) sources. In fact, several drugs that produce very different effects may be extracted from a single plant species. All parts of the plant (flowers, fruits, berries, leaves, bark, sap, roots, resin, etc.) may be a source for a drug. Once extracted, the plant substance is purified by chemical or physical means, formulated for human intake, packaged, shipped, and stored for future use. Table 4-5 provides examples of drugs derived from plant sources.

TABLE 4-4 Mineral Functions and Sources

Mineral Name	Function(s)	Dietary Source(s) (Macro)
Calcium (Ca) Atomic #20	• Blood clotting • Immunity • Muscle contraction • Production of energy • Tooth and bone formation and strength • Transmission of nerve impulses	• Dairy products • Green vegetables
Chlorine (Cl) Atomic #17 (Exists as chloride when combined with sodium to form salt)	• Digestion • Maintenance of fluid and electrolyte balance	• Salt
Magnesium (Mg) Atomic #12	• Energy production • Function of certain enzymes • Glucose use	• Fish • Grains • Green leafy vegetables • Legumes • Meat • Milk • Nuts
Phosphorus (P) Atomic #15	• Energy storage and transfer • pH maintenance • Synthesis of **nucleotides**	• Dairy products • Fish • Meat • Poultry • Vegetables
Potassium (K) Atomic #19	• Energy production • Muscle contraction • Synthesis of proteins and **nucleic acids** • Transmission of nerve impulses	• Fruits • Vegetables
Sodium (Na) Atomic #11	• Fluid and electrolyte balance	• Salt
Sulfur (S) Atomic #16	• Function of **amino acids**	• Dairy products • Garlic • Meat • Onions

(Continues)

TABLE 4-4 *(Continued)*

Mineral Name	Function(s)	Dietary Source(s) (Macro)
Cobalt (Co) Atomic #27	• Necessary component of vitamin B complex function	• Legumes (especially pulses) • Vegetables
Copper (Cu) Atomic #29	• Iron metabolism	• Cocoa • Organ meats (e.g., calf liver) • Seafood • Whole grains (especially bran)
Fluorine (F) Atomic #9 (exists as Fluoride (F), when reduced)	• Bone formation • Prevention of dental carries (cavities)	• Fluoridated water • Seafood
Iodine (I) Atomic #53	• Thyroid function	• Seafood
Iron (Fe) Atomic #26	• Component of hemoglobin	• Fortified grain products • Fruits • Meat and poultry • Vegetables
Manganese (Mn) Atomic #25	• Bone formation • Metabolism of amino acids, carbohydrates, and cholesterol	• Legumes • Nuts • Whole grains
Selenium (Se) Atomic #34	• Stress management • Thyroid hormone regulation	• Organ meats • Plants (according to soil content of selenium) • Seafood
Zinc (Zn) Atomic #30	• Component of certain enzymes and proteins • Gene expression	• Fortified cereals • Meat • Seafood

TABLE 4-5 Drugs from Plant Sources

Drug Name	Classification	Plant Species (common name)
Cocaine hydrochloride	Narcotic analgesic (Class II), local anesthetic, and vasoconstrictor	Erythroxylon coca (coca)
Morphine sulfate	Narcotic analgesic (Class II)	Papaver somniferum (poppy)
Papaverine hydrochloride	Smooth muscle relaxant	Papaver somniferum (poppy, but not a derivative of morphine)
Theophylline ethylenediamine (Aminophylline®)	Bronchodilator	Theobroma cacao (cocoa)

Summary

I. Animal sources
  a. Also known as zoologic sources
    i. Includes human sources
  b. Drugs that may be derived from animal sources
    i. Antibiotics
    ii. Enzymes
    iii. Hormones
    iv. Immune serum (antiserum)
    v. Vaccines
    vi. Vitamins
  c. Terminology related to animal sources
    i. Avian—bird
    ii. Bovine—cattle
    iii. Caprine—goat
    iv. Equine—horse
    v. Ichthyoid—fish
    vi. Ovine—sheep
    vii. Porcine—swine (pig)

II. Biotechnology
   a. Also known as recombinant DNA (rDNA) technology and genetic engineering
      i. The term *recombinant* refers to donor DNA that is combined with host DNA to produce DNA with specific desired components.
   b. Simplified overview of rDNA process
      i. Specific restricted portion of DNA containing desired trait is removed from the donor cell
      ii. Donor DNA is combined with DNA of a live host
      iii. Host cell containing the recombinant DNA is allowed to reproduce
      iv. Desired portion of the DNA is disrupted and extracted from the host, purified, and formulated for human intake
III. Laboratory synthesis
   a. Process of combining simple chemical elements and/or compounds to create a more complex chemical (drug)
   b. Typically organic substances are used to create synthesized drugs
IV. Mineral sources
   a. Inorganic elements naturally found in earth and water
      i. Plants and animals acquire minerals from soil and water
   b. Minerals necessary to maintain homeostasis (refer to Table 4-4)
      i. Macrominerals
         1. Calcium
         2. Chlorine
         3. Magnesium
         4. Phosphorus
         5. Potassium
         6. Sodium
         7. Sulfur
      iii. Trace minerals
         1. Cobalt
         2. Copper
         3. Fluorine
         4. Iodine
         5. Iron
         6. Manganese
         7. Selenium
         8. Zinc
V. Plant sources
   a. Also known as botanic sources
   b. Several drugs with different effects may be extracted from a single plant species.
   c. All parts of the plant may be a source for a drug
      i. Bark
      ii. Berry
      iii. Flower
      iv. Fruit
      v. Leaf
      vi. Resin
      vii. Root
      viii. Sap

Critical Thinking Review

1. The term *zoologic* is used in this chapter to identify drugs from animal sources. Does this description include drugs from human sources?
2. Differentiate between vitamins and minerals. Use information from an outside source to answer this question.
3. What are some of the benefits of rDNA technology?
4. Briefly describe the antigen/**antibody** response. Use information from an outside source to answer this question.
5. What is anaphylaxis? Use information from an outside source to answer this question.
6. Which organization is responsible for development of the Daily Reference Intake (DRI)?
7. List four body functions that are regulated by minerals.
8. What is the importance of an adequate intake of potassium in the diet?
9. What are the dietary sources of calcium?
10. List four parts of a plant that may be used as sources for drugs.

References

American Academy of Family Physicians (2009). *Vitamins and minerals: How to get what you need.* Retrieved from http://familydoctor.org/online/famdocen/home/healthy/food/general-nutrition/914.printerview.html

Aschenbrenner, D. & Venable, S. (2009) *Drug therapy in nursing.* Philadelphia, PA: Lippincott, Williams, & Wilkins.

Broyles, B., Reiss, B., & Evans, M. (2007). *Pharmacological aspects of nursing care* (7th ed.). Clifton Park, NY: Thomson Delmar Learning.

Chivian E. & Bernstein A. (2008). *Sustaining life: How human health depends on biodiversity.* New York: Oxford University Press.

Frey, K. et al. (2008). *Surgical technology for the surgical technologist: A positive care approach* (3rd ed.). Clifton Park, NY: Delmar Cengage Learning.

Kuure-Kinsey, M. & McCooey, B. (2000). *The basics of recombinant DNA.* Retrieved from http://www.rpi.edu/dept/chem-eng/Biotech-Environ/Projects00/rdna/rdna.html

Los Alamos National Laboratory (1999). *What is the periodic table of the elements?* Retrieved from http://periodic.lanl.gov/about.shtml

Merchant, B. (2009). *First drug made from genetically engineered animals approved by FDA.* Retrieved from http://www.treehugger.com/files/2009/02/first-drug-genetically-engineered-animals-approved-fda.php

Moini, J. (2009). *Fundamental pharmacology for pharmacy technicians.* Clifton Park, NY: Delmar Cengage Learning.

National Human Genome Research Institute (2009). *Deoxyribonucleic Acid (DNA).* Retrieved from http://www.genome.gov/25520880

National Institutes of Health (2009). *Minerals.* Retrieved from http://www.nlm.nih.gov/medlineplus/minerals.html#cat1

Rice, J. (2006). *Principles of pharmacology for medical assisting* (4th ed.). Clifton Park, NY: Thomson Delmar Leaning.

RxList (n.d). *Hepatitis B vaccine (recombinant).* Retrieved from http://www.rxlist.com/recombivax-drug.htm

RxList (n.d.). *FDA approves human thrombin for use in surgery.* Retrieved from http://www.rxlist.com/script/main/art.asp?articlekey=83642

Saul, S. (2006). *Seeking alternatives to animal-derived drugs.* Retrieved from http://www.nytimes.com/2008/04/01/business/01pigdrugs.html

Saxton, D., Ercolano-O'Neill, N., & Glavinspiehs, C. (2004). *Math and meds for nurses* (2nd ed.). Clifton Park, NY: Cengage Learning.

Synthesis (n.d.). *The American heritage® Stedman's medical dictionary.* Retrieved from http://dictionary.reference.com/browse/synthesis

Texas Heart Institute (2009). *Minerals: What they do and where to get them.* Retrieved from http://texasheart.org/HIC/Topics/HSmart/mineral1.cfm?&RenderForPrint=1

Texas Heart Institute (2009). *Trace elements: What they do and where to get them.* Retrieved from http://texasheart.org/HIC/Topics/HSmart/trace1.cfm

United States Department of Agriculture Food and Nutrition Information Center (2009). *Dietary guidance: DRI tables.* Retrieved from https://fnic.nal.usda.gov/dietary-guidance/dietary-reference-intakes/dri-tables-and-application-reports

United States National Library of Medicine (2009). *What is DNA?* Retrieved from http://ghr.nlm.nih.gov/handbook/basics/dna

University of Delaware (n.d.). *rDNA.* Retrieved from http://webapps.css.udel.edu/biotech/rDNA.html

Vajo, Z., Fawcett, J., & Duckworth, W. (2001). *Recombinant DNA technology in the treatment of diabetes: Insulin analogs.* Retrieved from http://edrv.endojournals.org/cgi/citemap?id=edrv;22/5/706

WebMD. (2005). *Wonder drugs using pharmazooticals.* Retrieved from http://www.medicinenet.com/script/main/art.asp?articlekey=52324

Woodrow, R. (2007). *Essentials of pharmacology for health occupations* (5th ed.). Clifton Park: Thomson Delmar Learning.

Chapter FIVE

DRUG FORMS

Student Learning Outcomes

After studying this chapter, the reader should be able to:

- Differentiate among the three main types of drug forms.
- Identify one or more drugs that are available in each form.

Key Terms

Aqueous solution	Homogenous	Semisolid	Syrup
Diffusion	Liquid	Solid	Tincture
Elixir	Mass	Solute	Viscosity
Emulsion	Matter	Solution	Volatile liquid
Gas	Mixture	Solvent	
Heterogenous	Reconstitute	Suspension	

DRUG FORMS

In science, **matter** is defined as any substance that has **mass** (takes up space). Drugs are found in the three basic forms of matter: **gas**, **liquid**, and **solid**. The drug form determines the way that the drug is given to the patient (route of administration), the movement of the drug throughout the body (pharmacokinetics), and the interaction of the drug with the target receptor, membrane, cell, tissue, organ, or whole body (pharmacodynamics).

Many drugs are a physical combination of two or more substances, called a **mixture**. In a mixture, each substance retains its own characteristics (properties). Mixtures can be classified as **heterogenous** (meaning that the substances are not equally distributed) or **homogenous** (meaning that the substances are equally distributed). An example of a mixture (homogenous) is 1% lidocaine (Xylocaine®) with epinephrine: 1:100,000. Table 5-1 identifies drug forms found in the medical setting and provides examples in each category.

Additional forms of matter (such as plasma) exist, however, there are currently no pharmacological applications for them; therefore, they will not be discussed in this textbook.

Chapter Ten contains a comprehensive listing of drug substances (in all forms) used in the medical setting.

Gas

Gases are actually liquids in their vapor form. To be in its vapor form, the liquid must evaporate or the temperature must be above the boiling point. For example, the boiling point for oxygen is −183.0°C (−297.4°F). Therefore, in the atmosphere of the earth, oxygen always exists in the vapor form. Gases have no shape or definite volume unless they are contained. If not contained, gases are able to extend indefinitely by a process called **diffusion**. To make storage and transportation easier, oxygen and other medical gases can be contained and cooled to their liquid state. Typically, gases are stored in pressurized cylinders (also called tanks). Chapter Nine contains information concerning storage and dispensing of gases.

Oxygen is not technically considered a pharmaceutical, but because it is a gas that is necessary for life, and is frequently administered in patient care settings, it is listed in this category (Figure 5-1). Nitrous oxide is an example of a medical gas.

Liquid

A liquid is described as the fluid form of matter. Fluids have the ability to flow and do not have a fixed shape, but their volume does not change. Liquids will take on the shape of the vessel in which they are contained (Figure 5-2). A pure liquid has no additives. Water is an example of a pure liquid.

Volatile Liquid

Volatile liquids are those that vaporize or evaporate easily. Several inhalation anesthesia agents are volatile liquids. A vaporizer, which is a component of the anesthesia delivery system, is needed to convert the volatile liquid to its vapor form and add the vaporized anesthetic agent

TABLE 5-1 Drug Forms

Category	Subcategory	Definition	Example(s)
Gas		Liquid in its vapor form	Nitrous oxide Oxygen
Liquid (Pure)		Fluid	Water
	Volatile Liquid	Liquid that is easily vaporized	Isoflurane (Forane®)
	Emulsion	Two liquids that cannot mix	Propofol (Diprivan®)
	Suspension	Mixture of a liquid and one or more solids that do not dissolve	Hydrocortisone, neomycin, and polymyxin B otic (Cortisporin Otic®)
	Solution	Mixture of two or more substances that combine easily	Normal saline (0.9% sodium chloride)
	Aqueous	Solution made with water	Dextrose 5% in water (D5W)
	Elixir	Solution made with ethyl alcohol that has been sweetened	Diphenhydramine elixir (Benadryl Elixir®)
	Syrup	Aqueous solution that has been sweetened	Guaifenesin and Codeine (Robitussin Ac®)
	Tincture	Alcohol-based solution	Benzoin tincture
Solid		Particulate form of matter	Bacitracin injection (Baci-IM®)
	Semisolid	Consistency between a solid and a liquid	Povidone iodine (Betadine®) ointment

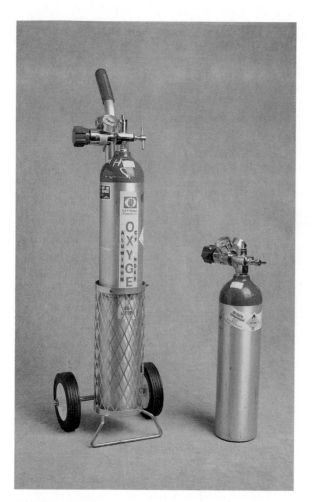

FIGURE 5-1 Oxygen—Stored in a Cylinder

to the mixture of oxygen and other agents that flow to the patient's lungs. Isoflurane (Forane®) is an example of a volatile liquid.

Emulsion

An **emulsion** consists of two liquids that cannot combine, for example, oil in water. This type of liquid is referred to as heterogenous. Droplets of one liquid are dispersed throughout the other liquid. Because settling of one of the liquids may occur, redistribution of the liquids may be necessary prior to use. Redistribution may be accomplished by gently shaking or rolling the drug container. Propofol (Diprivan®) is an example of an emulsion.

Suspension

A **suspension** consists of a liquid and one or more solids that do not dissolve. This type of liquid is also referred to as heterogenous. Solid particles are dispersed throughout the liquid. Because settling of the undissolved particles may occur, redistribution of the particles may be necessary prior to use. The redistribution procedure for a suspension is the same as that described for an emulsion. The drugs hydrocortisone, neomycin, and polymyxin B otic are combined with a liquid to form the drug Cortisporin Otic® which is an example of a suspension.

Solution

A **solution** is a mixture of two or more substances that combine easily. This type of liquid is referred to as homogenous. The substance in the larger amount is called a **solvent**. The solvent is typically the liquid portion of the mixture. The substance in the smaller amount is called a **solute**. The solute may be another liquid or a solid that is dissolved by the solvent. Normal saline (0.9% sodium chloride) is an example of a solution.

Aqueous   An **aqueous solution** is one in which the solvent is water. Water is known as the universal solvent because it is capable of dissolving many substances. Dextrose 5% in water is an example of an aqueous solution.

Elixir   An **elixir** is a sweetened solution in which the solvent is ethyl alcohol. When diphenhydramine is added to a sweetened alcohol-based liquid the drug Benadryl Elixir®, which is an example of an elixir, is formed.

Syrup   A **syrup** is an aqueous solution that has been sweetened with sugar to enhance the taste. The drugs guaifenesin and codeine are combined with a sweetened aqueous solution to form the drug Robitussin Ac® which is an example of a syrup.

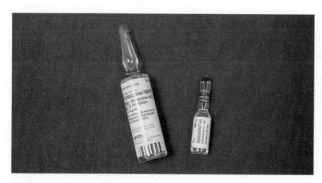

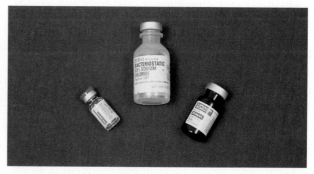

FIGURE 5-2 **Examples of Liquid Medications**

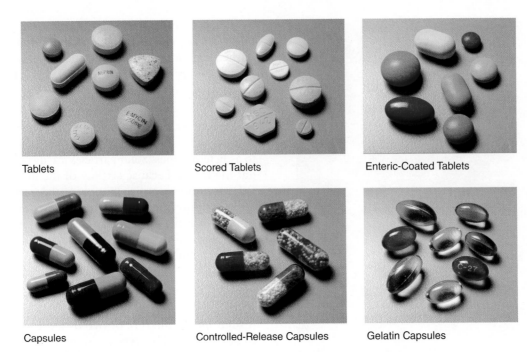

FIGURE 5-3 Examples of Solid and Semisolid Medications

Tincture   A **tincture** is an alcohol-based solution. Benzoin added to an alcohol-based solution is an example of a tincture called benzoin tincture (or tincture of benzoin).

Solid

A solid is described as the particulate form of matter. The chemicals of the solid may be separate particles or the particles may be bound together to form a larger unit. A solid has a fixed shape and the volume does not change. Many solid medications are manufactured in powder form. Powders may be contained within a capsule, compressed into a tablet, be in the form of a troche or a lozenge (a small medicated disc that dissolves when placed in the mouth), and some powders may require reconstitution (reconstitution involves addition of a liquid to a dried substance to return the substance to its former condition and strength) prior to use (Figure 5-3). Bacitracin for injection (Baci-IM®) is an example of a drug that is manufactured in the solid form and must be **reconstituted** prior to use.

Semisolid

Semisolids are of a consistency that is between a solid and a liquid. Creams, foams, gels, lotions, suppositories, and unguents (ointments) are examples of medications in the semisolid form. The term *viscosity* refers to the thickness of a liquid or a semisolid. A substance that is highly viscous is very thick. Many semisolids are emulsions. Povidone iodine (Betadine®) ointment is an example of a semisolid.

Summary

I. Gas—Liquid in its vapor form
II. Liquid—Fluid
    a. Volatile liquid—Liquid that is easily vaporized
    b. Emulsion—Two liquids that cannot mix
    c. Suspension—Mixture of a liquid and one or more solids that do not dissolve
    d. Solution—Mixture of two or more substances that combine easily
        i. Aqueous—Solution made with water
        ii. Elixir—Solution made with ethyl alcohol that has been sweetened
        iii. Syrup—Aqueous solution that has been sweetened
        iv. Tincture—Alcohol-based solution
III. Solid—Particulate form of matter
    a. Semisolid—Of a consistency that is between a solid and a liquid

Critical Thinking Review

1. List the three main drug forms and provide a brief description of each.
2. Briefly explain the process of diffusion. You may need to utilize an outside source, such as your anatomy and physiology book, to fully understand and convey this concept.
3. If oxygen is not technically considered a pharmaceutical, why is it discussed in this textbook?

4. Provide three examples of a volatile liquid. Give the generic and brand names of each. Use information found elsewhere in this textbook to answer this question.

5. Prior to using an emulsion or a suspension, why may it be necessary to redistribute the droplets or particles? How will redistribution be accomplished?

6. Describe the differences and similarities between heterogenous and homogenous mixtures.

7. Explain the meaning of the term *viscosity*. Describe the appearance of a semisolid that is slightly viscous.

8. Provide an example of a drug that is reconstituted prior to use. What does the term *reconstitution* mean?

9. What is the fourth state of matter and how is it used in the medical setting? Use information from an outside source, such as your surgical technology textbook, to answer this question completely.

10. Will all of the drug forms described in this chapter be utilized in the surgical setting? Why or why not? Use information found elsewhere in this textbook to answer this question.

References

Bennington, L. (2002). *Gale encyclopedia of nursing and allied health*. Detroit: The Gale Group. Retrieved from http://www.healthline.com/galecontent/medical-gases

Cohen, B. (2005). *Memmler's the human body in health and disease* (10th ed.). United States: Lippincott Williams & Wilkins.

DeTurck, D., Gladney, L., and Pietrovito, A. (1994). *Classification of matter*. Retrieved from http://www.physics.upenn.edu/courses/gladney/mathphys/subsubsection1_1_3_1.html

Frey, K., et al. (2008). *Surgical technology for the surgical technologist: a positive care approach* (3rd ed.). Clifton Park, NY: Delmar Cengage Learning.

Matter. (n.d.). *The American Heritage® Science Dictionary*. Retrieved from http://dictionary.reference.com/browse/matter

MedlinePlus. (2007). *Dictionary*. Retrieved from http://www.nlm.nih.gov/medlineplus/mplusdictionary.html

MedlinePlus. (2008). *Drugs, Supplements, and Herbal Information*. Drugs and supplements. Retrieved from http://www.nlm.nih.gov/medlineplus/druginformation.html

National Aeronautics and Space Administration. (2008). *States of matter*. Retrieved from http://www.grc.nasa.gov

O'Leary, D. (2000). *Oxygen*. Retrieved from http://www.ucc.ie/academic/chem/dolchem/html/elem/elem008.html

Ophardt, C. (2003). *Virtual chembook*. Retrieved from http://www.elmhurst.edu/~chm/vchembook/106Amixture.html

Chapter SIX

ROUTES OF ADMINISTRATION

Student Learning Outcome

After studying this chapter, the reader should be able to:

- Name and describe drug administration routes.

Key Terms

Auricular (otic)	Instillation	Intrathecal	Subcutaneous
Buccal	Intra-arterial	Intratracheal	Sublingual
Dermal	Intra-articular	Intravenous	Topical
Enteral	Intracardiac	Intravesicular	Transcutaneous
Epicutaneous	Intradermal	Intravitreal	Transdermal
Epidural	Intralaryngeal	Nasogastric (NG) tube	Transmucosal
Feeding tube	Intramuscular	Ocular	Urethral
Gastrostomy tube (G-tube)	Intranasal	Oral	Vaginal
Implantation	Intraocular	Parenteral	
Ingestion	Intraosseous	Rectal	
Inhalation	Intraperitoneal	Route of administration	

ROUTES OF ADMINISTRATION

The method that is used to convey a drug into the body is referred to as the **route of administration**. Several routes of administration are described in this chapter. One drug may be formulated in several different ways to allow for administration by various routes. For example, the drug furosemide (Lasix®), which is a loop diuretic, is manufactured in the tablet form to be administered by the oral (enteral) route and also in the liquid form for administration by the **parenteral** (by injection) route. Not all routes of administration are appropriate for use in the surgical environment because of NPO (nil per os or nothing by mouth) restrictions; however, there are a few exceptions to the NPO rule. The routes of administration are summarized in Table 6-1. Chapter Ten contains a comprehensive listing of drug substances commonly used in the surgical environment, a description of the drug action, as well as the route(s) of administration for each.

Once a drug is administered, an action is expected. The action of a drug upon the target receptor, membrane, cell, tissue, organ, or whole body is called pharmacodynamics. The concept of pharmacodynamics is explained in Chapter Eight. In some situations a drug is intended to act at the site of administration and in other situations, the drug must be absorbed by the capillaries and distributed (transported) to the target cells via the circulatory system. Movement of the drug throughout the body is a four-step process called pharmacokinetics. Absorption and distribution are the first two steps in the pharmacokinetics process. In this chapter, information concerning absorption will be presented. All four steps of the process of pharmacokinetics are presented in detail in Chapter Seven.

Enteral

The term *enteral* pertains to the intestine. The intestinal tract begins at the mouth and ends at the anus. Any route of administration involving the intestinal tract is considered enteral. The two main enteral routes of administration are oral and rectal.

TABLE 6-1 Summary of the Routes of Administration

Route	Description
Enteral	Involving the intestinal tract
Oral	Pertaining to the mouth
Buccal	Between the cheek and the gum
Sublingual	Under the tongue
Ingestion	To take in by swallowing
Feeding Tube	Tube inserted directly into the stomach
Nasogastric (NG) Tube	Tube inserted into the stomach via the nasal portal
Gastrostomy (G) Tube	Tube inserted into the stomach percutaneously (through the skin)
Rectal	Pertaining to the rectum
Inhalation	Forced or drawn into the lungs
Instillation	Dripped into the body
Ocular	Pertaining to the eye
Auricular (otic)	Pertaining to the ear
Parenteral	Other than enteral (usually by injection)
Intradermal	Into the skin
Subcutaneous	Pertaining to the adipose tissue
Intramuscular	Within a muscle
Intravenous	Within a vein
Intra-arterial	Within an artery
Intraosseous	Within a bone
Epidural	Above or outside of the dura mater
Intrathecal (spinal)	Within the dura mater
Intra-articular	Within a joint
Intracardiac	Within the heart

Topical	Applied to a surface
Epicutaneous/Dermal	Pertaining to the surface of the skin
Intranasal	Within the nose
Transcutaneous/Transdermal	Through the skin
Transmucosal	Through a mucous membrane
Intraperitoneal	Within the abdominal (peritoneal) cavity
Other	
Intralaryngeal/Intratracheal	With the larynx/within the trachea
Implantation	Inserted beneath the skin or into a body structure
Intraocular	Within the eye
Intravitreal	Within the vitreous humor
Urethral	Pertaining to the urethra
Intravesicular	Within the bladder
Vaginal	Pertaining to the vagina

Oral

The term *oral* pertains to the mouth. Medications that enter the body through the mouth are said to be administered orally. However, there are several subtypes of oral routes of administration including buccal, sublingual, and ingestion.

Sublingual The term *sublingual* means under the tongue. Medication usually in the tablet form is administered sublingually. The tablet is placed under the tongue (Figure 6-1A). The tablet is then dissolved by the saliva and the medication is absorbed topically by the capillaries of the mucous membrane under the tongue and on the floor of the mouth. Nitroglycerin (Nitrostat®), which is used to prevent or relieve angina pectoris by dilating the coronary arteries, is an example of a medication that may be administered via the sublingual route.

Buccal The term *buccal* means pertaining to the cheek or in the direction of the cheek. Medication in the tablet form is administered buccally. The tablet is placed between the cheek and the upper or lower gum (Figure 6-1B). The tablet is then dissolved by the saliva and the medication is absorbed topically by the capillaries of the mucous membrane on the inside of the cheek. Glucose tablets, which are used to raise a patient's blood sugar level in the case of hypoglycemia, are an example of a medication that may be administered via the buccal route. Note that glucose is also available in other forms for administration via other routes.

Ingestion The term *ingestion* means to take in or to swallow. Medication that is administered by ingestion may be in the liquid or solid forms. The medication is taken in through the mouth and swallowed. When the medication reaches the stomach it acts on the stomach contents, acts upon the mucous membrane lining of the stomach, is absorbed by the capillaries of the mucous membrane in its current form, or is broken down by the gastric juices and the byproducts are absorbed by the capillaries of the mucous membrane of the stomach or the first portion of the small intestine called the duodenum. Sodium citrate (Bicitra®), which is used preoperatively to neutralize gastric acid, is an example of a liquid medication that may be administered by ingestion. Typically the term *PO* (per os—by mouth) means that a medication is to be ingested.

Feeding Tube If a patient is temporarily or permanently unable to swallow, medication may be administered directly into the stomach through a **feeding tube**; however, the primary purpose of a feeding tube is to provide nutrition. The feeding tube is placed into the stomach or duodenum (first segment of the small intestine) either by inserting it through the nose and passing it through the pharynx and esophagus into the stomach (called a **nasogastric [NG] tube**) (Figure 6-2 A) or percutaneously

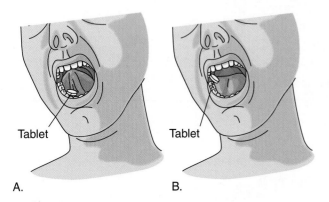

Tablet

A.

Tablet

B.

FIGURE 6-1 A. Sublingual Administration B. Buccal Administration

through the abdominal wall into the stomach (called a **gastrostomy tube or G-tube**) (Figure 6-2 B).

Rectal

Medications that are administered rectally are inserted through the anus into the rectum where they act on the contents of the rectum, act upon the mucous membrane lining of the rectum, or are absorbed by the capillaries of the mucous membrane of the rectum. **Rectal** medications may be in the liquid form such as an enema that is administered with the use of an applicator with an elongated tip. Enemas are used to perform a diagnostic study (e.g., barium enema) or to cause evacuation of the contents of the bowel. Alternatively, rectal medications may be inserted in the form of a suppository. A suppository is a medication that is in a solid form and has been shaped cylindrically for insertion into the rectum. (Note: suppositories can also be administered via the urethral or vaginal routes; however, in that situation, the route of administration would not be considered enteral.) Prochlorperazine (Compazine®), which may be used postoperatively to reduce nausea and vomiting, is an example of a medication that may be administered rectally.

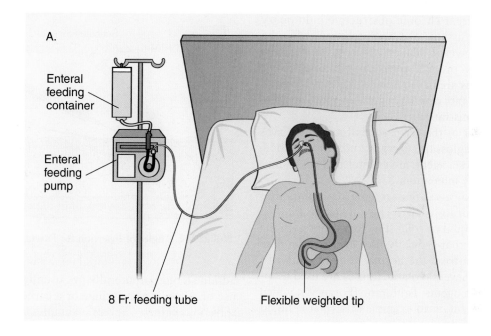

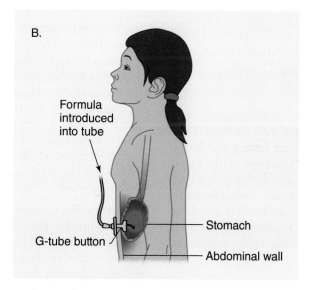

FIGURE 6-2 Feeding Tube
A. Nasogastric (NG) Tube
B. Gastrostomy Tube (G-tube)

Inhalation

Medications that are inhaled are pulled or forced into the lungs during the inspiration phase of respiration. Inspiration may occur naturally or in the case of a patient who is not breathing on his or her own (such as a patient under general anesthesia) the medication may be forced into the lungs mechanically with the use of a ventilator. Once the medication is in the lungs, it may act upon the mucous membrane lining of the respiratory tract, be absorbed by the capillaries of the mucous membrane, or enter the capillaries surrounding the alveoli.

In some situations, an inhaler is used as a storage and delivery mechanism for the medication. Inhalers are typically used to treat chronic obstructive pulmonary disease (COPD) or asthma and are rarely utilized in the operating room; however, inhalers are frequently used to enhance respiration preoperatively and postoperatively. Inhaled medications are in the form of a gas, a vapor, or an aerosol. Propellants may be added to vapors or aerosols to aid in administration.

The definition of the term *gas* is found in Chapter Five and in the glossary. Oxygen and nitrous oxide, which is an anesthesia agent, are examples of gasses that are administered by **inhalation**.

In pharmacology, vapors are volatile liquids that vaporize or evaporate easily. The substance may be changed from its liquid or solid state to a vapor with the use of a vaporizer that typically uses heat to stimulate the transformation from the normal state of matter to the gaseous form. Several volatile liquids are used as inhalation anesthesia agents. Isoflurane (Forane®), which is an anesthesia agent, is an example of a volatile liquid that is administered by inhalation.

An aerosol contains small liquid or solid particles that are suspended in a gas. The particles are dispensed from a pressurized container or with the use of an atomizer. Benzocaine, butamben, and tetracaine HCl (Cetacaine®), which is a **topical** anesthesia agent, is an example of an aerosol.

Instillation

Liquids that are instilled are dripped into the body. Once instilled, the medication acts upon the surface to which it was applied or is absorbed by the capillaries in the tissue. **Ocular** (eye) drops (Figure 6-3) and **auricular or otic** (ear) drops are examples of medications that are instilled. Hydrocortisone, neomycin, and polymyxin B otic (Cortisporin Otic®), which is an anti-inflammatory/antibiotic ear drop, is an example of a drug that is administered by **instillation**.

Parenteral

The term *parenteral* means other than enteral. Any route of administration that does not involve the intestinal tract is referred to as parenteral. Medications that are

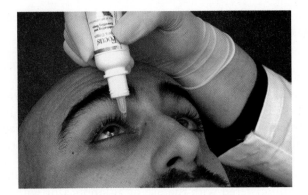

FIGURE 6-3 Instillation of Eye Drops

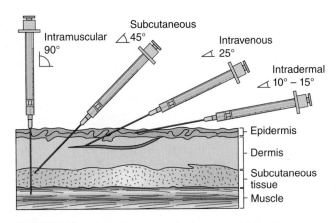

FIGURE 6-4 Angles of Insertion for Parenteral Injections

administered parenterally are usually injected with the use of a needle and syringe or a catheter, such as an intravenous catheter. Several examples of parenteral medication will be presented.

Intradermal

The term *intradermal* means within the skin. Medications administered intradermally are injected into the dermis, which is the deeper of the two main layers of the skin, with the help of a needle and syringe (Figure 6-4). The medication acts upon the dermis or is absorbed by the capillaries of the dermis. The Mantoux tuberculin skin test (also known as purified protein derivative or PPD) is an example of a medication that is administered via the intradermal route.

Subcutaneous

The term *subcutaneous* means under the cutaneous membrane (skin). The tissue located beneath the skin is the fat or adipose. A needle attached to a syringe is utilized to pierce both of the two main layers of the skin and then the medication is injected into the subcutaneous layer (Figure 6-4). The medication acts upon the subcutaneous tissue or is absorbed by the capillaries within the subcutaneous tissue. Two acceptable abbreviations for the term *subcutaneous* are sub-Q and SC. Insulin (used to lower the blood sugar) and heparin sodium (an anticoagulant) are examples of medications that may be administered subcutaneously. Note: both insulin and heparin may also be given by other routes of administration.

Intramuscular

The term *intramuscular* means within the muscle. A needle attached to a syringe is utilized to pierce the two main layers of the skin: the subcutaneous layer and then the medication is injected into the muscle layer (Figure 6-4). The medication acts upon the muscle or is absorbed by the capillaries of the muscle. IM is an acceptable abbreviation for intramuscular. Ketorolac tromethamine (Toradol®), which is a nonsteroidal anti-inflammatory agent, is an example of a medication that may be administered intramuscularly.

Intravenous

The term *intravenous* means within a vein. A needle attached to a syringe is utilized to pierce the two main layers of the skin—the subcutaneous layer and the superficial (closest to the surface of the body) wall of the vein allowing the medication to be injected into the vein and act upon the inner surface of the vein, the blood, or be transported to the target location by the blood. If fluids are to be administered, multiple doses of a medication will be necessary, or the need for administration of several different medications exists; a temporary catheter may be placed within the vein and the fluid or medication is infused (Figure 6-4). The term *infusion* means that the medication is inserted into the vein to produce the desired therapeutic effect. Sometimes intravenous fluids are said to be instilled because they do enter the body drop by drop, but intravenous administration is a better example of infusion. IV is an acceptable abbreviation for intravenous. Blood and normal (0.9%) saline are examples of fluids that are administered intravenously and mannitol (Osmitrol®) (an osmotic diuretic) is an example of a medication that is administered intravenously. Because intravenous medications are administered directly into the circulatory system, absorption related to the process of pharmacokinetics does not occur.

Intra-Arterial

The term *intra-arterial* means within an artery. Accidental administration of some drugs into an artery may be harmful, but there are times intra-arterial administration may be necessary when venous access may not be possible. Some of the latest treatments for certain types of advanced cancers require surgical implantation of an intra-arterial device or catheter for delivery of chemotherapeutic (antineoplastic) drugs directly to the site of the tumor. For example, the drug 5—Fluorouracil (5 FU) may be injected into the hepatic artery to treat metastatic colon cancer that has spread to the liver.

Intraosseous

The term *intraosseous* means within a bone. When intravenous access is not immediately available, especially in pediatric emergency situations, a specialized needle called a Cook-type screw tip (Sur-Fast®) or Jamshidi intraosseous needle may be inserted into the bone marrow to allow administration of fluids (colloid, crystalloid, and blood products) as well as medications. The proximal tibia is the preferred access point; however, other locations such as the distal femur and distal tibia may be used. The intraosseous route is effective because the vessels of the medullary canal drain into general venous circulation via medullary venous sinuses. Intraosseous access is considered a short-term solution to vascular collapse because of the risk of infection and the potential for the needle to become dislodged. Once necessary fluid resuscitation has been achieved, it is recommended that an attempt be made to access a peripheral or central vein to meet the patient's ongoing fluid and medication needs. A pictorial presentation showing the necessary supplies and the steps involved with insertion of an intraosseous access device is available on the WebMD web site at http://reference.medscape.com/article/80431-overview.

Epidural

The term *epidural* means outside of or above the dura mater, which is the outer layer of the covering of the central nervous system (meninges). A needle or catheter attached to a syringe is used to inject a steroidal anti-inflammatory agent, a narcotic, or an anesthetic agent into the epidural space (Figure 6-5). A combination of agents may also be used. Epidural injections typically occur in the region of the lumbar spine. The injected medication comes in contact with the spinal nerve roots, the facet joints, passes through the dura into the cerebrospinal fluid by osmosis and is expected to produce pain relief (analgesia) or loss of sensation (anesthesia). Methylprednisolone, which is a corticosteroid, is an example of a medication that may be administered epidurally.

Intrathecal (Spinal)

The term *intrathecal* means within a sheath. In this case, the sheath that is referred to is the dura mater, which is the outer layer of the covering of the central nervous system (meninges). A needle attached to a syringe is used to inject contrast media, a steroidal anti-inflammatory agent, a narcotic, or an anesthetic agent into the cerebrospinal fluid (Figure 6-6). A combination of agents may also be used. Intrathecal injections also known as spinal injections typically occur in the region of the lumbar spine. The injected medication mixes with the cerebrospinal fluid and comes in contact with the nerve roots and spinal cord to produce analgesia or anesthesia. Lidocaine (Xylocaine®), which is a local anesthetic agent, is an example of a medication that may be administered intrathecally.

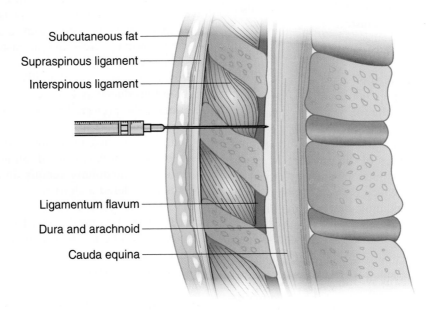

Subcutaneous fat
Supraspinous ligament
Interspinous ligament

Ligamentum flavum
Dura and arachnoid
Cauda equina

FIGURE 6-5 Epidural Administration

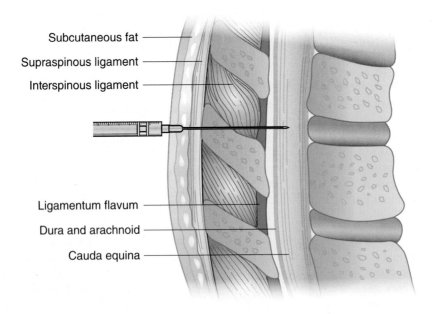

Subcutaneous fat
Supraspinous ligament
Interspinous ligament

Ligamentum flavum
Dura and arachnoid
Cauda equina

FIGURE 6-6 Intrathecal (Spinal) Administration

Intra-Articular

The term *intra-articular* means within a joint. A needle attached to a syringe is used to inject contrast media, a steroidal anti-inflammatory agent, or an anesthetic agent into the synovial fluid (Figure 6-7). The injected medication comes in contact with the joint surfaces or soft tissues surrounding the joint to enhance an imaging study, provide analgesia, or produce anesthesia. Bupivacaine (Marcaine®/Sensorcaine®), which is a local anesthetic agent, is an example of a medication that may be administered via the intra-articular route.

Intracardiac

The term *intracardiac* means within the heart. A needle attached to a syringe is used to inject the drug into the heart muscle (myocardium) or the left lower chamber of the heart (ventricle) (Figure 6-8). Adrenalin (epinephrine) is an example of a drug that may be injected via

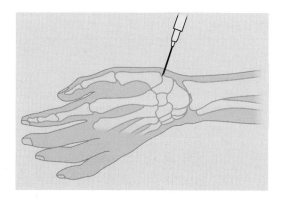

FIGURE 6-7 **Intraarticular Administration**

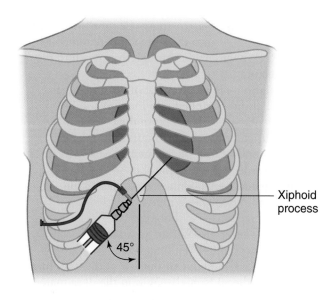

Xiphoid process

45°

FIGURE 6-8 **Intracardiac Administration**

the intracardiac route. In the case of a cardiac emergency, adrenalin acts as a cardiac stimulant to increase the strength of the heartbeat, increase the heart rate, and raise the blood pressure. Adrenalin also has other uses.

Topical

Drugs administered topically are placed on a surface, such as the skin (called **epicutaneous** or **dermal** administration) or on a mucous membrane, such as the nasal mucosa (**intranasal** administration). The drug may be expected to act locally on the surface to which it is applied or it may be expected to be absorbed through the skin (**transcutaneous** or transdermal) or the mucous membrane (transmucosal) to produce a systemic effect. During surgery, the topically administered drug is placed on an exposed body surface such as a blood vessel. Topical thrombin (Thrombostat®), which is a hemostatic agent (procoagulant) that is applied to a bleeding surface, is an example of a medication that is administered topically. Another example of medication administered topically in the operating room setting is an antibiotic irrigation solution. For example, bacitracin (Baci-IM®), which is an antibiotic, is often administered via the **intraperitoneal** (within the peritoneal cavity) route.

Several of the routes of administration that have already been presented in this chapter involve topical administration; examples include buccal, inhalation, instillation, sublingual, and rectal.

Other

In the operating room, the surgical technologist observes medication administration via a number of other routes that are less commonly seen in other clinical settings.

Intralaryngeal/Intratracheal

The term *intralaryngeal* means within the larynx and the term *intratracheal* means within the trachea. Prior to insertion of an oral or nasal endotracheal tube, the anesthesia provider may apply topical lidocaine hydrochloride (Xylocaine®) topical solution 4% (brand name examples include the Laryngeal Tracheal Anesthesia [LTA®] Kit and the Laryng-O-Jet®), which is an anesthetic agent, to numb the mucous membrane of the larynx (intralaryngeal) and trachea (intratracheal). The medication is sprayed onto the tissue via the use of a syringe and a specialized cannula and is expected to act topically upon the surface of the mucous membrane.

Implantation

The term *implantation* is used to describe medications (usually solids) that are inserted under the skin or into a body structure. The drug may be absorbed into the capillaries to achieve a systemic effect or it may act directly upon the tissue that it contacts. Some contraceptives, such as etonogestrel implant (Implanon®), which is about the size of a matchstick, are implanted. Antibiotic-impregnated polymethyl methacrylate beads that are impregnated with various antibiotics such as tobramycin (Nebcin®) or vancomycin (Vancocin®), which may be used to treat osteomyelitis, are also implanted. Brachytherapy for cancer treatment involves implantation of small pieces of radioactive metal called "seeds" that are about the size of a grain of rice. Additionally, pumps that deliver various medications, such as insulin for treatment of diabetes may be implanted.

Intraocular

The term *intraocular* means within the eye. Intraocular medications include balanced salt solution (BSS) that is used to provide moisture to the cornea and maintain the shape of the anterior cavity of the eye, and acetylcholine chloride intraocular solution (Miochol-E®), which is a miotic, is applied directly to the iris to constrict the pupil. Intraocular medications are expected to expand the eye or act topically on the internal structures of the eye. Another form of intraocular medication administration is intravitreal.

Intravitreal The term *intravitreal* means within the vitreous humor that is located in the posterior cavity of the eye. Intravitreal medications are expected to expand the contents of the posterior cavity or act topically. Viscoelastics, such as sodium hyaluronate (Healon®) are used intravitreally to separate tissues and as a replacement for the vitreous humor. During repair of a retinal detachment, an oil or gas (that is absorbed by the body after a period of time) may be injected into the vitreous humor to put pressure on the area of the retina that has been repaired with a laser or cryotherapy until healing occurs.

Urethral

The term *urethral* means pertaining to the urethra. Medications administered urethrally are inserted into the male or female urethra usually from a tube that has been fitted with a urethral applicator tip and are expected to act topically upon the mucous membrane of the urethra. Two percent lidocaine (Xylocaine®) jelly is a topical anesthetic agent that may be used during catheterization. A lubricant effect is also noted.

Intravesicular The term *intravesicular* means within the bladder. In this situation, the term pertains to the urinary bladder. A cystoscope or a catheter is inserted through the urethra into the bladder to allow administration of fluid or medications. The pharmaceutical is expected to expand the bladder or act topically on the bladder tissue. Examples of intravesicular medications include irrigation fluids such as sterile water and glycine, antibiotics

such as bafilomycins, and chemotherapy agents such as thiotepa (Thioplex®) and mitomycin C (Mutamycin®).

Vaginal

The term *vaginal* means pertaining to the vagina. The medication is expected to act topically on the vaginal tissue. Examples of medications that are administered vaginally include medications to modify the vaginal pH such as boric acid or acetic acid (Aci-gel®), medications for treatment of yeast infections such as miconazole (Monistat®), or antibiotics for the treatment of vaginal bacterial infections such as clindamycin (Cleocin®). During cervical biopsy or colposcopy a Schiller's test may be performed. During a Schiller's test a solution of iodine (5 grams) and potassium iodide (10 grams) in 100 ml of water called Lugol's® solution is applied to the cervix to help differentiate abnormal from normal tissue. Lugol's solution also has bacteriocidal and fungicidal properties.

Summary

I. Enteral—Involving the intestinal tract
  a. Oral—By mouth
    i. Buccal—Between the teeth and the gum
    ii. Sublingual—Under the tongue
    iii. Ingestion—To take in by swallowing
      1. Feeding tube—Tube placed into the stomach that is primarily used to provide nutrition to a patient who is unable to swallow but may also be used as a medication administration route
        a. Nasogastric (NG) tube—Tube inserted into the stomach via the nasal portal
        b. Gastrostomy (G) tube—Tube inserted into the stomach percutaneously
  b. Rectal—Insertion through the anus into the rectum
II. Inhalation—Forced or drawn into the lungs
III. Instillation—Dripped into the body
  a. Ocular—Instillation into the eye
  b. Auricular (otic)—Instillation into the ear
IV. Parenteral—Other than enteral (usually by injection)
  a. Intradermal—Into the skin
  b. Subcutaneous—Into the adipose tissue
  c. Intramuscular—Within a muscle
  d. Intravenous—Within a vein
  e. Intra-arterial—Within an artery
  f. Intraosseous—Within a bone
  g. Epidural—Above or outside of the dura mater
  h. Intrathecal (spinal)—Within the dura mater
  i. Intra-articular—Within a joint
  j. Intracardiac—Within the heart

V. Topical—Applied to a surface
   a. Epicutaneous/Dermal—Pertaining to the surface of the skin
   b. Intranasal—Within the nose
   c. Transcutaneous/Transdermal—Through the skin
   d. Transmucosal—Through a mucous membrane
   e. Intraperitoneal—Within the abdominal (peritoneal) cavity
VI. Other
   a. Intralaryngeal/Intratracheal—Within the larynx/within the trachea
   b. Implantation—Inserted beneath the skin or into a body structure
   c. Intraocular—Within the eye
      i. Intravitreal—Within the vitreous humor
   d. Urethral—Pertaining to the urethra
   e. Intravesicular—Within the bladder
   f. Vaginal—Pertaining to the vagina

Critical Thinking Review

1. Which term is used to describe the action of a drug upon the target cells?
2. Which term is used to describe the four-step process of movement of a drug throughout the body?
3. What piece of equipment may be needed to transform a volatile liquid into vapor? Which process is used to allow the transformation from the liquid to the vapor state?
4. List the two main routes of enteral administration.
5. Explain the difference between instillation and infusion.
6. Do the terms *spinal* and *epidural* mean the same thing? Why or why not?
7. What is the definition of the term *gas*? Use information contained elsewhere in this textbook to answer this question.
8. When a drug is administered intravenously, does absorption related to pharmacodynamics occur? Why or why not?
9. Provide three examples of parenteral routes of administration and provide a description of each.
10. What is a loop diuretic? Use information contained elsewhere in this textbook to answer this question.

References

Aerosol. (n.d.). *The American heritage® Stedman's medicaldictionary*. Retrieved from http://dictionary.reference.com/browse/aerosol

Buccal. (n.d.). *The American heritage® Stedman's medical dictionary*. Retrieved from http://dictionary.reference.com/browse/buccal

Cleveland Clinic. (n.d.). *Nitroglycerin tablets, capsules, and sprays*. Retrieved from http://my.clevelandclinic.org/drugs/nitroglycerin/hic_Nitroglycerin_Tablets_Capsules_and_Spray.aspx

Enteral. (n.d.). *The American heritage® Stedman's medical dictionary*. Retrieved from http://dictionary.reference.com/browse/enteral

Epidural. (n.d.). *The American heritage® Stedman's medical dictionary*. Retrieved from http://dictionary.reference.com/browse/epidural

Eslami, P. (2008). *Intraosseous access*. eMedicine from WebMD. Retrieved from http://emedicine.medscape.com/article/940993-overview

Frey, K., et al. (2008). *Surgical technology for the surgical technologist: A positive care approach* (3rd ed.). Clifton Park, NY: Delmar Cengage Learning.

Infusion. (n.d.). *The American heritage® Stedman's medical dictionary*. Retrieved from http://dictionary.reference.com/browse/infusion

Ingestion. (n.d.). *The American heritage® Stedman's medical dictionary*. Retrieved from http://dictionary.reference.com/browse/ingestion

Inhale. (n.d.). *The American heritage® Stedman's medical dictionary*. Retrieved from http://dictionary.reference.com/browse/inhalation

Instill. (n.d.). *The American heritage® Stedman's medical dictionary*. Retrieved from http://dictionary.reference.com/browse/instill

Intrathecal. (n.d.). *Merriam-Webster's medical dictionary*. Retrieved from http://dictionary.reference.com/browse/intrathecal

Joshi, G. & Tobias, J. (2007). *Intentional use of intra-arterial medications when venous access is not available*. Pediatric Anesthesia. Retrieved from http://www.scribd.com/doc/2061875/Intentional-Use-of-IntraArterial-Medications-When-Venous-Acess-in-Not-Available

Lugol's solution. (2009). *Encyclopedia Britannica*. Retrieved from http://www.britannica.com/EBchecked/topic/350973/Lugols-solution

Medline Plus. (2007). *Furosemide*. Retrieved from http://www.nlm.nih.gov/medlineplus/druginfo/meds/a682858.html

Medline Plus. (2007). *Nitroglycerin tablets, capsules, and sprays*. Retrieved from http://www.nlm.nih.gov/medlineplus/druginfo/meds/a601086.html

National Library of Medicine (n.d.). *Lidocaine hydrochloride spray*. Retrieved from http://dailymed.nlm.nih.gov/dailymed/fdaDrugXsl.cfm?id=1164&type=display

Parenteral. (n.d.). *The American heritage® Stedman's medical dictionary*. Retrieved from http://dictionary.reference.com/browse/parenteral

Ridley, M., Kingsley, G., Gibson, T., & Grahame, R. (2008). *Outpatient lumbar epidural corticosteroid injection in the management of sciatica.* Retrieved from http://rheumatology.oxfordjournals.org/cgi/content/abstract/27/4/295

Roh, M. (n.d.). *Chemotherapy.* The Liver Cancer Network. Retrieved from http://www.livercancer.com/treatments/chemotherapy.html

RxList (n.d). *Miochol.* Retrieved from http://www.rxlist.com/script/main/art.asp?articlekey=4393

Stöppler, M. (n.d.). *Tuberculosis skin test (PPD skin test).* Retrieved from http://www.medicinenet.com/tuberculosis_skin_test_ppd_skin_test/article.htm

Ting, P. (2001). *How does anesthesia work?* Retrieved from http://www.anesthesiologyinfo.com/articles/01062002.php

Vapor. (n.d.). *The American heritage® Stedman's medical dictionary.* Retrieved from http://dictionary.reference.com/browse/vapor

Chapter SEVEN

PHARMACOKINETICS

Student Learning Outcomes

After studying this chapter, the reader should be able to:

- Define the term *pharmacokinetics*.
- Outline the process of pharmacokinetics.

Key Terms

Absolute bioavailability
Absorption
Active transport
Anabolism
Anatomy
Baricity
Bioavailability
Catabolism
Circadian rhythm
Clearance
Comorbid condition
Diffusion

Distribution
Excretion
Facilitated passive diffusion (transport)
Fat soluble
Fat soluble vitamins
Half-life
Hepatic first pass effect
Hepatic portal system
Hemodynamic changes
Hydrophilicity
Immediate-release system

Ionization state
Liberation
Lipophilicity
Metabolism (biotransformation, biodegradation)
Metabolite
Modified-release system
Molecular weight
Osmosis
Passive transport
Pharmacodynamics
Pharmacokinetics

Physiology
Pinocytosis
Plasma protein binding
Protein channel
Relative bioavailability
Semipermeable membrane
Tissue binding (depot storage)
Transporters
Vesicle
Water soluble

PHARMACOKINETICS

Pharmacokinetics is the term used to describe the way the body processes a drug. The term *kinetic* refers to movement. Movement of the drug within the body is traced from introduction of the drug into the circulatory system through elimination of the drug from the body. The time needed for processing of the drug within the body is an important factor in determining necessary dosage and timing of future doses of the drug. Many factors or conditions can enhance or impede movement of the drug through the body, which in turn speed or slow pharmacokinetics of a particular drug.

The four main processes involved in pharmacokinetics are absorption, distribution, **metabolism (biotransformation)**, and excretion (Figure 7-1). The acronym ADME; "A" for absorption, "D" for distribution, "M" for metabolism, and "E" for excretion is often used to serve as memory tool as a reminder of the four processes involved in pharmacokinetics.

Pharmacokinetic processes occur in the order listed; however, more than one process may take place simultaneously. For example, as initial absorption of the drug into the circulatory system occurs, the portion of the drug absorbed is being transported (distributed) to the target cells; while the remainder of the drug is still being absorbed. Therefore, it is possible that a portion of the drug could be distributed, metabolized, and excreted before the entire process of absorption of the drug has occurred; especially when a **modified-release system** is in use.

Liberation

Drugs that must be freed from their administration form are said to be "liberated" prior to absorption. Most drugs requiring **liberation** are administered via the enteral route (usually by ingestion). Drugs are formulated **to be liberated immediately or on a** modified-release schedule. The term *immediate-release system* is used to describe drug forms that are easily broken down allowing the active ingredients to be available for absorption without delay (e.g., a capsule that dissolves rapidly and releases the medication quickly). Modified-release systems are designed to delay or extend liberation of the drug. Modified-release systems are designed to maintain the peak effect of the drug or reduce the number of times the drug must be administered. Examples of modified-release systems include delayed-release, extended-release, and sustained-release systems. A delayed-release system allows the drug to be liberated at a time other than immediately following administration. An extended-release system allows liberation of the drug over a prolonged period. Extended release systems may be sustained or controlled. Sustained-release systems allow steady liberation of the drug for a prolonged period and controlled-release systems, which are a form of sustained-release, are designed to maintain a steady concentration of the drug within the body. When liberation occurs, an "L" may be added to the beginning of the ADME acronym to form the new acronym LADME (Table 7-1).

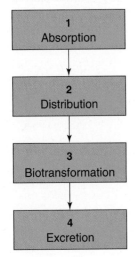

Four Processes Involved in Pharmacokinetics

1 Absorption

2 Distribution

3 Biotransformation

4 Excretion

FIGURE 7-1 Pharmacokinetic Processes

TABLE 7-1 Four Main Processes of Pharmacokinetics

Acronym	Name of Process	Description of Process
L (used only when needed)	Liberation	Freeing of the drug from its administration form
A	Absorption	Drug molecules are taken into the circulatory system by the capillaries
D	Distribution	Delivery of the drug to the target cells by the circulatory system
M	Metabolism	Chemical changes that a drug substance undergoes as it is being broken down (catabolism) within the body in preparation for excretion
E	Excretion	Elimination of the drug from the body

Absorption

Absorption is the first step in the process of pharmacokinetics. Absorption occurs when the drug is taken into the circulatory system by the capillaries. The site of absorption can be the site of administration, but that is not always true. For example, a drug given intramuscularly will be absorbed by the capillaries in the muscle, but a drug that is ingested may not be absorbed in the mouth but rather in the stomach or the small intestine once it has been liberated. A drug that is given intravenously is already in the circulatory system and absorption is not necessary. It may be desirable for drugs that act upon the tissue to which they are administered topically or locally to remain at the site of administration for a prolonged period of time (an agonist [refer to Chapter Eight] may be used). However, eventually the drug must still be absorbed and transported to allow for metabolism (biotransformation) and excretion.

Passive Transport

Most drugs enter the circulatory system at the site of absorption by a process called **passive transport**. In passive transport, the drug molecules (in solution) move from an area of high concentration across a **semipermeable membrane** (one that allows some molecules to pass through, but not all) to an area of low concentration by **osmosis** (a form of **diffusion**) until the concentration on both sides of the membrane is equal (Figure 7-2). No energy is expended during passive transport.

Facilitated Passive Diffusion (Transport) **Facilitated passive diffusion (transport)** also moves the drug molecules from an area of high concentration to an area of low concentration and uses no energy. However, proteins are used to develop a pathway (called a **protein channel**) to help transport the drug molecule across the semipermeable membrane (Figure 7-3).

Active Transport

A few drugs and certain electrolytes enter the circulatory system at the site of absorption by a process called **active transport**. In active transport, the drug molecules (in solution) move from an area of low concentration across a semipermeable membrane to an area of high concentration. Energy, usually in the form of adenosine triphosphate (ATP), is expended during active transport (Figure 7-4).

Pinocytosis The process of pinocytosis involves taking a small amount of fluid containing the drug molecule(s) into a cell by formation of a small sac called a **vesicle** from a portion of the cell wall. (Figure 7-5). Pinocytosis is a form of active transport that is used in very specific circumstances, such as absorption of **fat-soluble vitamins**.

Bioavailability

The term *bioavailability* is used to describe the amount of the drug that enters the circulatory system and is available to the target tissue cells. A drug given intravenously is said to have 100% bioavailability because the entire dose of the drug is immediately in the circulatory system. When a drug is administered by a route other

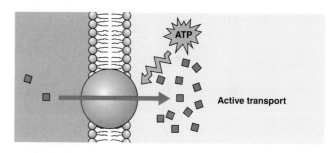

FIGURE 7-4 Active Transport

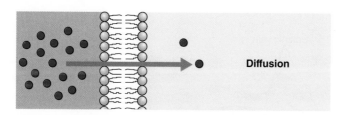

FIGURE 7-2 Passive Transport (Diffusion)

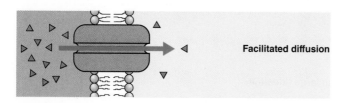

FIGURE 7-3 Facilitated Diffusion (Transport)

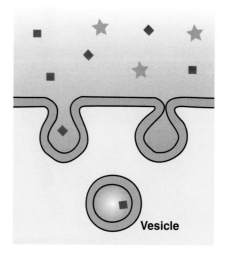

FIGURE 7-5 Pinocytosis

than intravenous, a smaller percentage of the drug enters the circulatory system initially because the entire dose of the drug is not immediately absorbed or metabolism of the drug begins before it can enter systemic circulation because of the hepatic portal system.

The term *absolute bioavailability* is used when comparing the availability of the same drug administered intravenously or by another route, such as ingestion. The term *relative bioavailability* is used when comparing the availability of the same drug that has been manufactured differently, such as the brand name drug versus the generic version of the same drug. Algebraic equations are used to calculate bioavailability; however, because the surgical technologist is not responsible for calculating dosages of a drug to be ordered for patient use, the equations are not provided.

Distribution

Once the drug enters the blood stream, whether by direct administration or absorption, the term *distribution* is used to describe delivery of the drug to the target cells by the circulatory system. The circulatory system also distributes the drug to the site of metabolism and the site of excretion. **Pharmacodynamics**, which is the interaction of the drug molecules with the target receptor, membrane, cell, tissue, organ, or whole body, is described in Chapter Eight. Keep in mind that the drug is delivered not only to the target cells but also to the entire body, which can lead to undesirable effects (refer to Chapter Eight).

Metabolism (Biotransformation)

In pharmacology, the terms *biotransformation* and *metabolism* are synonymous and the word *biodegradation* also has the same meaning. The term *metabolism* usually refers to the chemical changes that a drug substance undergoes as it is being broken down (**catabolism**) within the body in preparation for excretion. Biotransformation is usually an enzymatic process that most often takes place in the liver but may also occur in the blood plasma, the mucosa of the intestine (inner layer), the lungs, and the kidneys. The breakdown products of metabolism (biotransformation) are called **metabolites**, which are smaller than the original drug molecule and less active or inactive substances, which are more easily excreted. The term *half-life* is used to describe the amount of time necessary for the concentration of the drug in the plasma to be reduced by 50% (one-half). The half-life of the drug is used to calculate administration of future doses of the drug. Note that in a few instances, the liver may play a role in building up (**anabolism**) a drug or the drug may be activated in the liver.

Hepatic Portal System

The **hepatic portal system** is a key factor in biotransformation of drugs that are ingested. The hepatic portal system is a venous return system that sends blood from various abdominal organs (such as the stomach, spleen, pancreas, and intestine) directly to the liver (Figure 7-6).

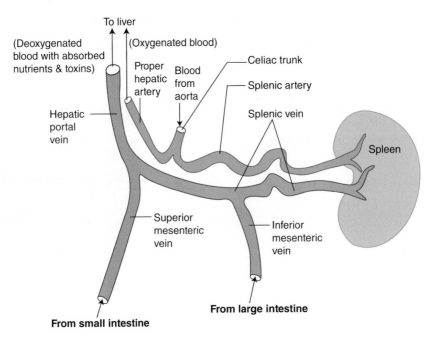

FIGURE 7-6 Hepatic Portal System

Hepatic First Pass Effect   Because of the hepatic portal system, the portion of the drug that is first sent to the liver in the blood via the hepatic vein is biotransformed before it gets into general circulation and can be distributed to the target tissue cells. As a result, the patient does not receive the benefit of the full dose of the drug and the dosages must be calculated (usually increased) to compensate because the bioavailability is reduced. This process is referred to as the **hepatic first pass effect**. Refer to an **anatomy** and **physiology** book for more information concerning the hepatic portal system.

Excretion

The term *excretion* refers to elimination of the drug from the body. Most drugs are **fat soluble** (capable of being dissolved or liquefied in lipids) so that they may be easily taken in through the target cell's membrane, which consists mainly of lipids. Part of the biotransformation process involves changing the fat-soluble drug molecules into metabolites, which are **water soluble** (capable of being dissolved or liquefied in water) and can easily be filtered out of the blood and excreted by the kidneys in the urine. Most drugs are excreted in the urine; however, a small number of drugs are excreted by exhalation or in the feces, saliva, and sweat. Additionally, some drugs are excreted in the breast milk and may cause a hazard for the breast-fed baby, therefore, the lactating mother must pump and discard the affected breast milk and the baby will be given formula as a temporary substitute. Once the drug is eliminated from the mother's body, breastfeeding may continue. The term *clearance* is used to describe removal of a drug from a specified volume of blood plasma. Note: Few drugs are eliminated in their active state without undergoing biotransformation.

Factors That Affect Pharmacokinetics

Numerous factors can enhance or impede movement of the drug through the body, which in turn speed or slow the pharmacokinetics of a particular drug. These same factors may also affect the interaction of the drug with the target receptor, membrane, cell, tissue, organ, or whole body (pharmacodynamics). The following is a partial list generalizing some of the more common factors affecting pharmacokinetics.

- Drug form—The way that the drug is manufactured may affect the rate of absorption. For example, a drug in tablet form may take a few minutes to dissolve while the liquid form of the same drug will begin to be absorbed immediately. Additionally, if a drug must be liberated additional time will be required prior to absorption.

- Route of administration—The way that the drug is given to the patient may also affect the rate of absorption or bypass the process altogether. For example, a drug that is given intravenously will be distributed immediately while the same drug given intramuscularly must be absorbed first.

- Dose—The amount of the drug administered may affect the rate of absorption. For example, a drug administered in a higher concentration is more likely to be absorbed faster than the same drug administered in a lower concentration.

- Interaction with other drugs (including illicit drugs, nicotine, alcohol, over the counter medications such as antacids, vitamins, herbal remedies, nutritional supplements, and prescription medicines)—Presence of other drugs may speed or slow absorption of the drug and may counteract the intended effect of the drug with the target cells.

- NPO status—Presence or absence of food in the stomach may speed or slow absorption. Additionally, certain foods may interrupt pharmacodynamics.

- Patient's age—As a general rule, pediatric and geriatric patient's general metabolism is typically slower than the rest of the population thereby slowing all four processes of pharmacokinetics.

- Comorbid conditions—A **comorbid condition** is a disease or condition that exists in addition to the patient's primary problem. The comorbid disease may exacerbate the primary problem or make treatment of the primary problem difficult. Some examples of comorbid conditions include problems with cardiac function, general circulation, circulation to the target cells, liver function, kidney function, respiratory function, endocrine function (such as thyroid disorders and diabetes), and gastrointestinal tract function (including gastric emptying rate). Depending upon the effects of an individual's comorbid condition(s) all pharmacokinetic processes as well as pharmacodynamics may be disrupted.

- Circadian differences—**Circadian rhythm** is the sleep, wake, and activity pattern that occurs within a 24-hour period. Circadian rhythm is sometimes referred to as the internal or biological clock. Circadian patterns vary between individuals (everyone's clock is different) and within an individual from day to day according to their stress, activity, and wellness levels. During the 24-hour cycle, natural variations in metabolism, hormone activity, and vital signs may affect absorption and distribution of the drug as well as pharmacodynamics. Disruptions in the usual circadian rhythm may further interfere with pharmacokinetics and pharmacodynamics.

- Plasma protein binding—Some drugs bind to plasma proteins (such as albumin) to allow for transport and to protect them from being metabolized by various enzymes. Unfortunately, the bound portion of the drug is not available to the target cells leaving only the free molecules to be delivered to the target cells to accomplish the desired action.

- Tissue binding—**Tissue binding** is a concept that is related to **plasma protein binding**. Instead of binding with a plasma protein, the drug has an affinity for a certain type of tissue such as muscle or fat and is bound there instead making a portion of the drug unavailable to the target cells. However, when the drug is released from the tissue a lingering effect of the drug may be noted. Tissue binding is sometimes referred to as depot storage.

- Pregnancy—Changes in physiology and anatomy during pregnancy can affect all four processes of pharmacokinetics. Absorption may be affected by slower gastric emptying and peristalsis rates and gastric acid production may be inconsistent. Distribution may be affected due to **hemodynamic changes** (which include blood volume, blood pressure, and heart rate fluctuations). Pregnancy typically does not affect metabolism. Excretion is generally increased during pregnancy due to increases in blood flow to the kidneys as well as increased filtration and reabsorption rates.

- Barriers (blood-brain, blood-placenta, blood-testes)—Some membranes, especially in the brain, placenta, and testes are selective and will not allow passage of

TABLE 7-2 Factors That Affect Pharmacokinetics

Factor	Process(es) Affected
Drug form	Absorption—may be sped or slowed (also consider liberation, if applicable)
Route of administration	Absorption—may be sped or slowed (or bypassed altogether)
Dose	Absorption—may be sped or slowed according to the concentration of the drug
Interaction with other drugs	Absorption—may be sped or slowed according to the actions of the other drugs Pharmacodynamics—may be disrupted
NPO status	Absorption—may be sped or slowed according to the presence or absence of food Pharmacodynamics—may be disrupted
Patient's age (pediatric/geriatric)	Absorption—may be slowed Distribution—may be slowed Metabolism—may be slowed Excretion—may be slowed Pharmacodynamics—may be disrupted
Comorbid conditions	Absorption—may be sped or slowed Distribution—may be sped or slowed Metabolism—may be sped or slowed Excretion—may be sped or slowed Pharmacodynamics—may be disrupted
Circadian differences	Absorption—may be sped or slowed Distribution—may be sped or slowed Pharmacodynamics—may be disrupted
Plasma protein binding	Distribution—may be slowed Pharmacodynamics—may be disrupted
Tissue binding	Distribution—may be slowed Pharmacodynamics—may be disrupted
Pregnancy	Absorption—typically slower Distribution—may be sped or slowed Metabolism—not affected Excretion—may be sped
Barriers (blood-brain, blood-placenta, blood-testes)	Distribution—may not be possible Pharmacodynamics—may be disrupted
Physical properties of the drug (drug form, pH, solubility, baricity, ionization state)	Absorption—may be sped or slowed Pharmacodynamics—may be disrupted
Availability of transporters	Distribution—may be sped, slowed, or impossible Pharmacodynamics—may be disrupted

certain drugs from the blood to the target cells while allowing passage of other drugs. The ability of the drug to be available to the target cells must be considered when drugs destined for the brain, placenta, and testes are prescribed.

- Physical properties of the drug—Factors such as drug form, pH, solubility (**hydrophilicity**—ability to be attracted to and dissolved in water and **lipophilicity**—ability to be attracted to and dissolved in fat), **baricity** (**molecular weight**—combined weight of all atoms in the molecule), and the **ionization state** (determination of the drug molecule's charge—may be positive or negative) affect the ability of the drug to be absorbed for distribution and to be absorbed at the site of the target cells.

- Availability of transporters—In some instances, **transporters** such as proteins are needed to bind with the drug to allow distribution of the drug to the target cells and excretion of the drug. Without transporters some drugs would be rendered useless. More research is needed to fully understand this mechanism.

Table 7-2 summarizes the common factors affecting pharmacokinetics and lists the pharmacokinetic process(es) that are affected.

Summary

I. Pharmacokinetics—Movement of the drug through the body.
   a. Liberation—Freeing of a drug from the administration form.
      i. Immediate-release system—Used to describe drug forms that are easily broken down allowing the active ingredient to be available for absorption without delay.
      ii. Modified-release system—Designed to delay or extend liberation of the drug.
         1. Delayed-release—Drug is liberated at a time other than when administered.
         2. Extended-release—Drug is liberated over a prolonged period for the purpose of maintaining the peak effect; thereby reducing the number of doses needed.
            a. Sustained-release—maintains steady liberation of the drug for a prolonged period.
               i. Controlled-release—a form of sustained-release that is designed to maintain a steady concentration of the drug within the body.
   b. Absorption—Taking in the drug molecules via the capillaries to the circulatory system.
      i. Passive transport—Movement of drug molecules from an area of high concentration across a semipermeable membrane to an area of low concentration by osmosis (diffusion) until the concentration on both sides of the membrane is equal. No energy is expended during passive transport.
         1. Facilitated passive diffusion (transport)—Moves the drug molecules from an area of high concentration to an area of low concentration and uses no energy. However proteins are used to develop a pathway (called a protein channel) to help transport the drug molecule across the semipermeable membrane.
      ii. Active transport—Drug molecules (in solution) move from an area of low concentration across a semipermeable membrane to an area of high concentration. Energy, usually in the form of adenosine triphosphate (ATP), is expended during passive transport.
         1. Pinocytosis—A small amount of fluid containing the drug molecule(s) called a vesicle is formed. The entire vesicle is drawn through the cell membrane. Pinocytosis is a form of active transport that is used in very specific circumstances such as absorption of fat-soluble vitamins.
   c. Bioavailability—Describes the amount of a drug that enters the circulatory system and is available to the target tissue cells.
   d. Distribution—Delivery of the drug to the target cells, site of metabolism, and the site of excretion by the circulatory system.
   e. Metabolism (biotransformation)—Chemical changes that a drug substance undergoes as it is being broken down (catabolism) within the body in preparation for excretion.
   f. Hepatic portal system—Venous return system that sends blood from various abdominal organs (such as the stomach, spleen, pancreas, and intestine) directly to the liver.
      i. Hepatic First Pass Effect—Because of the hepatic portal system, a portion of the drug is first sent to the liver in the blood via the hepatic vein where it is biotransformed before it gets into general circulation and can be distributed to the target tissue cells. As a result, the patient does not receive the benefit of the full dose of the drug and the dosages must be calculated (usually increased) to compensate because the bioavailability is reduced.

g. Excretion—Elimination of the drug from the body.

h. Factors that affect pharmacokinetics—Factors that can enhance or impede movement of the drug through the body, which in turn speed or slow the pharmacokinetics of a particular drug. The same factors may also affect pharmacodynamics.

Critical Thinking Review

1. Explain how the term *pharmacokinetics* differs from the term *pharmacodynamics*.
2. Describe the difference between absolute and relative bioavailability.
3. Which route of administration eliminates the need for the drug to be absorbed?
4. Which route of administration allows for 100% bioavailability?
5. The hepatic first pass effect affects drugs given only by one route of administration. Which route is affected? Explain.
6. Give two examples of comorbid conditions that may affect the process of pharmacokinetics.
7. How is facilitated passive diffusion (transport) similar and dissimilar to passive transport?
8. Are metabolism and biotransformation the same thing? Explain.
9. By which process do most drugs enter the circulatory system?
10. What is a metabolite?

References

Biotransformation. (n.d.). *The American heritage® Stedman's medical dictionary*. Retrieved from http:// dictionary.reference.com/browse/biotransformation

Burton, M., Shaw, L., & Schentag, J. (2005). *Applied pharmacokinetics and pharmacodynamics* (4th ed.). Philadelphia, PA: Wolters Kluwer Health.

Circadian rhythm. (n.d.). *The American heritage® Stedman's medical dictionary*. Retrieved from http:// dictionary.reference.com/browse/circadian%20 Rhythm

Copeland, R. (n.d.). *Routes of Administration*. Retrieved from http://www.med.howard.edu/pharmacology/ handouts/Routes05a.ppt

Frey, K., et al. (2008). *Surgical technology for the surgical technologist: A positive care approach* (3rd ed.). Clifton Park, NY: Delmar Cengage Learning.

Grogan, F. (2001). *Pharmacy simplified: A glossary of terms*. Clifton Park, NY: Delmar.

Hopper, T. (2007). *Mosby's pharmacy technician principles & practice* (2nd ed.). St. Louis: Saunders Elsevier.

Kopacek, K. (2007). *Pharmacokinetics*. Retrieved from http://www.merck.com/mmpe/sec20/ch303/ch303a .html#CHDHHHAD

Kwon, Y. (2001). *Handbook of essential pharmacokinetics, pharmacodynamics, and drug metabolism for industrial scientists*. New York: Springer.

Lindup, W. & L'Eorme, M. (n.d.). *Clinical pharmacology: Plasma protein binding of drugs*. Retrieved from http://www.pubmedcentral.nih.gov/pagerender.fcgi?artid=1503970&pageindex=1

Metabolite. (n.d.). *The American Heritage® Stedman's Medical Dictionary*. Retrieved from http:// dictionary.reference.com/browse/metabolite

Moini, J. (2009). *Fundamental pharmacology for pharmacy technicians*. Clifton Park, NY: Delmar Cengage Learning.

Olson, J. (2006). *Clinical pharmacology made ridiculously simple*. Miami: MedMaster, Inc.

Perrie, Y. & Rades, T. (2012). *Pharmaceutics: Drug delivery and targeting*. United States: Pharmaceutical Press.

Pinocytosis. (n.d.). *Merriam-Webster's medical dictionary*. Retrieved from http://dictionary.reference.com/ browse/pinocytosis

Porter, R. et al. (2007). *The Merck manual for healthcare professionals*. Retrieved from http:// www.merck.com/mmpe/index.html

Wharrad, H. (2004). *Pharmacology: Half-life of drugs*. Retrieved from http://www.nottingham.ac.uk/nmp/ sonet/rlos/bioproc/halflife/index.html

Woodrow, R. (2007). *Essentials of pharmacology for health occupations* (5th ed.). Clifton Park, NY: Thomson Delmar Learning.

Chapter
EIGHT

PHARMACODYNAMICS

Student Learning Outcomes

After studying this chapter, the reader should be able to:

- Define the term *pharmacodynamics*.
- Describe the three aspects of pharmacodynamics.

Key Terms

Acid
Addiction
Additive
Adverse effects
Affinity
Agonist
Alopecia
Anaphylaxis
Antagonism by neutralization
Antagonist
Base
Behavioral tolerance
Buffer
Catalyst
Cell membrane

Cellular tolerance
Chemical interactions
Competitive antagonism
Contraindications
Cytoplasm
Detoxification
Drug enzyme interactions
Drug interactions
Drug receptor interactions
Drug theories
Duration of action
Enzyme
Excipient
Homeostasis
Iatrogenic response

Indications
Irreversible antagonism
Metabolic tolerance
Noncompetitive antagonism
Nonspecific responses
Onset of action
Organelle
Partial agonist
Peak effect
pH
pH scale
Pharmacodynamics
Physiological
Physiological antagonism
Physiology

Plasma membrane
Plasmalemma
Primary effect
Psychological
Secondary effects
Side effects
Strong agonist
Synergist
Teratogenic effects
Therapeutic effect
Tolerance
Toxic effects
Weak agonist
Withdrawal

PHARMACODYNAMICS

Pharmacodynamics is the term used to describe the way a drug interacts with the body, specifically the target receptor, membrane, cell, tissue, organ, or whole body. The term *dynamic* refers to an interaction or process. A drug is given because it is known that a specific action will occur, which is intended to cause a change in the function (**physiology**) of the target. The intended drug action is referred to as the **primary or therapeutic effect**.

Remember that there is a link between pharmacodynamics and pharmacokinetics (refer to Chapter Seven). Pharmacokinetic processes occur in a specific order and more than one process may take place at the same time. Also keep in mind that numerous factors can enhance or impede movement of the drug through the body, which in turn speed or slow the pharmacokinetics of a particular drug and the same factors may also affect pharmacodynamics. Timing of future doses of the drug is influenced not only by the pharmacodynamics of the drug but also by the pharmacokinetics as well.

Three Aspects of Pharmacodynamics

There are three aspects related to the pharmacodynamics of a drug. All three relate to a specified time frame and the therapeutic effect. The three aspects are onset of action, peak effect, and duration of action (Figure 8-1).

Onset of Action

The time that elapses from administration of the drug until the therapeutic effect of the drug is noted is referred to as **onset of action**. The pharmacokinetic processes that occur prior to the onset of action include liberation (if necessary), absorption (if necessary), and distribution of the drug to the target cells.

Peak Effect

The time that elapses when the drug is most effective is called the **peak effect**. The pharmacokinetic processes that occur to maintain the peak effect include ongoing liberation (if necessary), absorption (if necessary), and distribution.

Duration of Action

The time that elapses from onset of action to termination of action is referred to as the **duration of action**. The pharmacokinetic processes that cause the drug action to cease are metabolism and excretion. Table 8-1 presents an example in the form of a timeline of the three aspects of pharmacodynamics.

Medication Actions

A drug is given to produce the desired effect by causing a reaction to occur that facilitates a change in the physiology of the target cell. Drugs can change the function of a cell, but they are incapable of initiating new cellular functions.

Drugs that are absorbed from the blood into the target cells do so by the same mechanisms that allowed them to be taken in to the blood for distribution at the site of absorption. Refer to Chapter Seven to review the processes related to active and passive transport.

Drug Theories

There are four methods by which drugs are thought to elicit their responses. The four methods are **drug receptor interactions, drug enzyme interactions, nonspecific responses,** and **chemical interactions**.

Drug Receptor Interactions   Various cells have receptors (usually proteins or glycoproteins) on the **plasmalemma** (also known as the **cell membrane** or the **plasma membrane**), on an **organelle**, or within the **cytoplasm** that fit the molecular structure of a drug exactly. When the drug attaches to the receptor, the process is referred to as a drug receptor interaction. Most drugs have an **affinity** (attraction) to the target cells. This affinity is compared to the way that a key must fit into a lock in order to

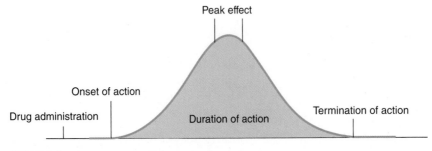

FIGURE 8-1 Three Aspects of Pharmacodynamics

TABLE 8-1 Timeline Representing the Three Aspects of Pharmacodynamics

Time	Response
12:55 PM	Patient complains of postoperative pain and requests medication
1:00 PM	Patient is given a tablet that contains acetaminophen with codeine (which is a narcotic analgesic) to ingest
1:30 PM	Patient notices some relief from the pain (onset of action)
2:30-4:30 PM	Patient receives maximum pain relief (peak effect)
4:30 PM	Patient notices that the level of pain is increasing
5:00 PM	Patient notices that level of pain has returned to the intensity noted prior to administration of the previous dose of the medication (duration of action)

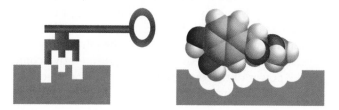

FIGURE 8-2A Drug Receptor Interaction—Lock/Key Analogy

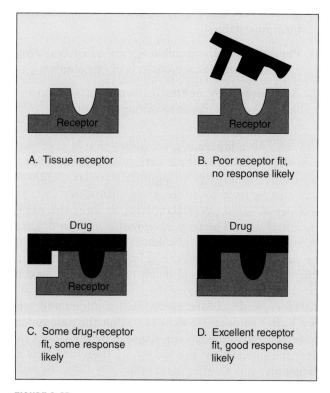

A. Tissue receptor

B. Poor receptor fit, no response likely

C. Some drug-receptor fit, some response likely

D. Excellent receptor fit, good response likely

FIGURE 8-2B Drug Receptor Interaction—Site Specific Binding

Drug Enzyme Interactions   An **enzyme** is a substance that initiates or increases the speed (in other words—acts as a **catalyst**) of a chemical reaction. The enzyme itself is not expended nor does it undergo any lasting change during the reaction. Drug enzyme interactions occur when a drug speeds or inhibits the action of an enzyme or changes the response of the cells affected by the enzyme.

Nonspecific Responses   Drugs that do not seem to act as a result of a drug receptor interaction or a drug enzyme interaction are referred to as having nonspecific responses. These drugs are thought to congregate and act on the plasmalemma or infiltrate the plasmalemma and act on the contents of the cell.

Chemical Interactions   The effects of some drugs are evident without any alteration of cellular function. The result is a simple chemical interaction. For example, sodium bicarbonate (a **base**, commonly known as baking soda $NaHCO_3$ has a **pH** of 8.4), which has many uses, may be used as an antacid because it is known to neutralize hydrochloric **acid** (HCl) (HCl has a pH of approximately 1.5) found in the stomach by producing salt (sodium chloride—NaCL), carbon dioxide, and water (H_2O), which are substances that are more neutral on the **pH scale**. Refer to a general science book for more information concerning the pH scale and acid–base balance.

Drug Interactions

Two or more drugs may be combined intentionally to produce a desired result. Drug combinations that produce desired interactions include synergists, agonists, antagonists, and additives. Unfortunately, some drugs that are prescribed produce an unintentional harmful response when combined with another drug. It is important that healthcare workers (physicians, pharmacists, etc.) have access to current, accurate, and complete information concerning all of the medications that an individual has been prescribed. Computer software that identifies potential harmful drug combinations is available allowing the healthcare provider to avoid unwanted responses.

operate the lock (Figure 8-2 A). If the drug molecule does not fit the receptor at all, no reaction is expected. If the drug molecule partially fits the receptor, a partial reaction may occur. If the drug molecule perfectly fits the receptor, a full reaction is expected (Figure 8-2 B).

Synergist   A **synergist** is a drug that works together with one or more other drugs to produce an enhanced effect making the cumulative effect of the combined drugs greater than the effect of each drug individually. For example, the drug acetaminophen (Tylenol®), which is an analgesic (pain reliever) and antipyretic (fever reducer), may be combined with codeine, which is a Schedule III narcotic analgesic and cough suppressant. When the two drugs are combined the newly formed drug is called acetaminophen with codeine (Tylenol #3®). Acetaminophen with codeine generates a greater analgesic effect than either of the drugs individually.

Agonist   In pharmacology, an agonist is a drug that simulates or prolongs the action of another drug or naturally occurring body substance but may not have an action of its own. The word *agonist* is the opposite of the word *antagonist*. Drugs that are synergists are examples of agonists as are certain drug additives (sometimes called adjunctive agents). For example, hyaluronidase (Amphadase®), which is an enzyme, is often added to a local anesthetic such as lidocaine hydrochloride (Xylocaine®) to promote diffusion of the lidocaine into the tissues. Better diffusion into the tissues means that the onset of the effect of the lidocaine is faster, the drug is more evenly distributed throughout the tissue providing more reliable nerve conduction blockade, and that the effect of the lidocaine is prolonged.

Agonists are identified in three categories:

1. **Strong agonists** produce the greatest effect even though only a small percentage of the available receptors on the plasmalemma may be occupied by the drug.

2. **Weak agonists** produce approximately the same effect as a strong agonist, but must occupy a greater percentage of the cell's receptors.

3. **Partial agonists** produce a weak effect even though all of the available receptors are occupied by the drug.

   Note: The term *agonist* is also used in pharmacology when describing a drug receptor interaction to indicate the presence and potential action of the initial drug. To avoid confusion, the term *initial drug* is used in this textbook in place of the term *agonist* when referring to drug receptor interactions.

Antagonist   In pharmacology, an antagonist is a drug that prevents or reverses the effect of another drug or naturally occurring body substance. The word *antagonist* is the opposite of the word *agonist*. For example, the drug naloxone hydrochloride (Narcan®), which is a narcotic antagonist, is used to reverse the sedative,

hypotensive, and respiratory depressive effects of narcotics. Antagonistic drugs generally do not produce an effect of their own.

Antagonists are identified in five categories:

1. **Competitive antagonism** occurs when the antagonist competes for and binds to the receptor that would normally be occupied by the initial drug (agonist) preventing that drug from acting. Because high doses of the initial drug may overcome the power of the antagonist, this type of antagonism is said to be surmountable.

2. **Noncompetitive antagonism** occurs when the antagonist binds to a receptor site that would not normally be occupied by the initial drug causing a change in the initial drug's receptor site rendering it unrecognizable and unusable by the initial drug. Because high doses of the initial drug cannot overcome the power of the antagonist, this type of antagonism is said to be insurmountable.

3. **Irreversible antagonism**, also called nonequilibrium competitive antagonism, is similar to competitive antagonism; however, the effect is permanent. This type of antagonism is also said to be insurmountable.

4. **Physiological antagonism** occurs when two drugs are given that cancel the effects of one another.

5. **Antagonism by neutralization** occurs when two drugs bind together inactivating one another.

Additive   An **additive** is a substance that is combined with the initial drug for a variety of reasons such as to produce synergistic or agonistic effects. Additives may also be used to dilute, reconstitute, activate, act as a preservative, give flavor to, or alter the pH of the initial drug. The term *excipient* is used to describe an additive that does not affect the performance of the drug. For example, the pH of the drug naloxone (Narcan®) is a base and if left unaltered it would be irritating to the tissue at the site of administration; therefore, hydrochloric acid (HCl) is added and used as a **buffer** to decrease the pH so that the naloxone is more compatible with the tissue. The HCl does not alter the function of the naloxone; therefore, it is an excipient.

Indications

Indications are the reasons why a drug is prescribed. The determination to prescribe a drug is made according to the current medical condition, circumstances of the patient, and the known therapeutic effect of the drug. Factors that affect pharmacokinetics and pharmacodynamics (refer to Chapter Seven) must also be considered. As noted in Chapter One, drugs are given for prophylactic reasons or to diagnose, treat, cure, or mitigate a disease or condition.

Contraindications

Contraindications are the reasons why a drug should be avoided. The determination is made according to other medical conditions and circumstances of the patient as well as the known therapeutic effects, side effects, or adverse effects of the drug. Common problems that contraindicate the use of certain drugs include the age and size of the patient as well as a number of comorbid conditions including pregnancy and impaired function of the cardiovascular, hepatobiliary, renal, respiratory, endocrine, and gastrointestinal systems.

Side Effects

Side effects are expected but undesirable, generally mild, and often tolerable or manageable effects of a drug that are not therapeutic. Examples of side effects include but are not limited to skin irritation, nausea, vomiting, constipation, diarrhea, dry mouth, dizziness, and drowsiness. Occasionally, known side effects of a drug have prompted use of the drug for additional purposes. These are known as **secondary effects**. For example, an antihistamine such as diphenhydramine hydrochloride (Benadryl®) may also be used for its sedative effect.

Adverse Effects

Adverse effects are more serious (than side effects) undesirable effects and may cause harm to the patient. Some adverse effects are predictable and others are unexpected. Treatments are available for some adverse effects, but not all. Examples of adverse effects include but are not limited to mild to severe allergic reactions (including **anaphylaxis**), hair loss (**alopecia**), bone marrow depression, damage to or failure of vital organs such as the heart, liver, lungs, kidneys, and brain.

Toxic Effects

The word *toxin* refers to a poison that is capable of causing injury or death. **Toxic effects** of a drug are usually related to overdosing; however, a toxic effect may also be seen when metabolism or excretion of the drug is impeded. The toxicity level of a new drug is studied carefully during the discovery, development process, and approval processes; therefore, in most situations the toxic level and its effects are known.

Teratogenic Effects

Teratogenic effects are those that cause malformations that affect an embryo or fetus resulting in a congenital defect. Drugs are not the only agents that interfere with embryonic and fetal development—for example, exposure to viruses and radiation may also produce abnormalities that are present at birth.

The Food and Drug Administration (FDA) is the Federal regulatory agency with responsibility for drug safety. The FDA has a classification system for drugs safety that relates to the pregnant woman in an effort to reduce the incidence of congenital defects that result from pharmacologic agents. The classification system is as follows:

- Category A—Controlled human studies of the drug have shown that there is no risk to the human embryo/fetus during any trimester of the pregnancy. The drug is safe to use during pregnancy.

- Category B—Controlled human studies of the drug have shown that there is no risk to the human embryo/fetus even though animal studies have shown risk to the animal embryo/fetus or human studies are lacking. The drug carries a slight risk for use during pregnancy.

- Category C—Controlled human studies of the drug are lacking and animal studies have shown risk to the animal embryo/fetus or animal studies are lacking. The drug carries risk for use during pregnancy, but the potential benefits may outweigh the risk.

- Category D—Controlled human studies and other data have shown that there is risk to the human embryo/fetus. The benefits of the drug may outweigh the risk when the drug is used in life threatening situations or when serious disease is present.

- Category X—Controlled human studies and other data have shown that the drug is contraindicated during pregnancy. The risk of embryologic/fetal harm will not outweigh the benefits of the drug.

Iatrogenic Response

The term *iatrogenic* is used to describe a complication that is inadvertently induced in the patient by a healthcare provider or as a result of medical treatment (including diagnostic procedures). Side effects, adverse effects, toxic effects, and teratogenic effects are all examples of iatrogenic responses that relate to pharmacology. However, iatrogenic responses are not limited to pharmacology. For example, a nosocomial infection is also an example of an iatrogenic response.

Tolerance

Drug tolerance is a result of a decreased response to the same dose of a particular drug over an extended period of time. As a result, the dosage must be increased to produce the desired response. **Tolerance** may be physiological or **psychological** and is usually seen with narcotic analgesics, alcohol, and benzodiazepines as well as other psychotropic drugs. Tolerance is described in three categories:

1. **Metabolic tolerance** (also known as dispositional tolerance)—metabolism of the drug occurs more rapidly.

2. **Cellular tolerance** (also known as reduced responsiveness or downregulation)—the number of receptors that bind to the drug are decreased.

3. **Behavioral tolerance**—the individual learns to conceal the effects of the drug.

Addiction

Addiction results when a drug is needed for the individual to function in a seemingly normal fashion. Like tolerance, addiction may be physiological (chemical) or psychological and is usually seen with narcotic analgesics, alcohol, and benzodiazepines as well as other psychotropic drugs. However, one may also become addicted to caffeine, laxatives, nasal sprays, and the like. Addiction is also called dependence.

Anyone with an addiction is urged to seek assistance. Information concerning treatment options may be obtained by calling 2-1-1 or accessing the **http://www.211.org** web site. 2-1-1 is a confidential and free national information and referral service that is sponsored by the United Way. In addition to receiving information concerning treatment for various addictions, callers may also obtain referrals to low cost or no cost services including healthcare, food, housing, childcare, eldercare, and employment.

Withdrawal

Withdrawal, which is sometimes called **detoxification**, occurs when an individual who is addicted to a drug discontinues use of the drug. Withdrawal may occur suddenly or gradually. Physical and psychological manifestations of withdrawal can vary in intensity and severity from very mild to extremely serious, and in some situations may be deadly. Symptoms of withdrawal can last from as little as a few hours to as long as several weeks. Examples of withdrawal symptoms include nausea, vomiting, diarrhea, constipation, sweating, and tremors. Some individuals experience a rebound effect in which the problem for which the drug was initially administered returns in a seemingly more severe fashion until **homeostasis** is reestablished.

Summary

I. Pharmacodynamics—Term used to describe the way that the drug interacts with the body; specifically the target receptor, membrane, cell, tissue, organ, or whole body.

a. Three aspects of pharmacodynamics—Time and action relationship to the effect of the drug.

   i. Onset of action—Time that elapses from administration of the drug until the therapeutic effect of the drug is noted.

   ii. Peak effect—Time that elapses when the drug is most effective.

   iii. Duration of action—Time that elapses from onset of action to termination of action.

b. Medication actions—Desired effect is produced by due to a reaction that occurs to facilitate a change in the physiology of the target cell. Drugs can change the function of a cell, but they are incapable of initiating new cellular functions.

   i. **Drug theories**—Four methods by which drugs are thought to elicit their responses.

      1. Drug receptor interactions—Occur when a drug molecule attaches to a receptor that is usually a protein or glycoprotein located on the plasmalemma, on an organelle, or within the cytoplasm of the target cell. Most drugs have an affinity (attraction) to the target cells.

      2. Drug enzyme interactions—Occur when a drug speeds or inhibits the action of an enzyme or changes the response of the cells affected by the enzyme.

      3. Nonspecific responses—Type of **drug interaction** that occurs when a drug does not seem to act as a result of a drug receptor interaction or a drug enzyme interaction. The drug is thought to congregate and act on the plasmalemma or infiltrate the plasmalemma and act on the contents of the cell.

      4. Chemical interactions—Effects of some drugs that are evident without any alteration of cellular function, such as neutralization of stomach acid.

   ii. Drug interactions—Two or more drugs are combined to intentionally produce a desired effect or unintentionally that produce an undesirable effect.

      1. Synergist—A drug that works together with one or more other drugs to produce an enhanced effect making the cumulative effect of the combined drugs greater than the effect of one drug alone.

2. Agonist—1. A drug simulates or prolongs the action of another drug or naturally occurring body substance but may not have an action of its own. 2. The term *agonist* is also used in pharmacology when describing a drug receptor interaction to indicate the presence and potential action of the initial drug. To avoid confusion, the term *initial drug* will be used in this textbook in place of the term *agonist* used in this context.

3. Antagonist—A drug that prevents or reverses the effect of another drug or naturally occurring body substance.

4. Additive—Substance that is combined with the initial drug for a variety of reasons such as to produce synergistic or agonistic effects. Additives may also be used to dilute, reconstitute, activate, act as a preservative, give flavor to, or alter the pH of the initial drug.

c. Indications—Reasons why a drug is prescribed.

d. Contraindications—Reasons why a drug should be avoided.

e. Side effects—Expected but undesirable, generally mild, and often tolerable or manageable effects of a drug that are not therapeutic. Examples of side effects include but are not limited to skin irritation, nausea, vomiting, constipation, diarrhea, dry mouth, dizziness, and drowsiness.

f. Adverse effects—Effects that are undesirable and may cause harm to the patient. Some adverse effects are predictable and others are unexpected. Treatments are available for some adverse effects, but not all.

g. Toxic effects—Poisonous effects of a drug that are capable of causing injury or death and are usually related to overdosing however a toxic effect may also be seen when metabolism or excretion of the drug is impeded.

h. Teratogenic effects—Drug effects that cause malformations, which affect an embryo or fetus resulting in a congenital defect.

i. Iatrogenic response—A complication that is inadvertently induced in the patient by a healthcare provider or as a result of medical treatment (including diagnostic procedures). Side effects, adverse effects, toxic effects, and teratogenic effects are all examples of iatrogenic responses that relate to pharmacology.

j. Tolerance—A result of a decreased response to the same dose of a particular drug over an extended period of time. As a result, the dosage must be increased to produce the desired response. Tolerance may be physiological or psychological and is usually seen with narcotic analgesics, alcohol, and benzodiazepine as well as other psychotropic drugs. Tolerance is described in three categories: metabolic, cellular, and behavioral.

k. Addiction—Occurs when a drug is needed for the individual to function in a seemingly normal fashion. Addiction may be physiological (chemical) or psychological and is usually seen with narcotic analgesics, alcohol, and benzodiazepine as well as other psychotropic drugs. However, one may also become addicted to caffeine, laxatives, nasal sprays, and so on. Addiction is also called dependence.

l. Withdrawal—Also known as detoxification. Occurs when an individual who is addicted to a drug discontinues use of the drug. Withdrawal may occur suddenly or gradually. Physical and psychological manifestations of withdrawal can vary in intensity and severity from very mild to extremely serious and in some situations may be deadly. Symptoms of withdrawal can last from as little as a few hours to as long as several weeks. Examples of withdrawal symptoms include nausea, vomiting, diarrhea, constipation, sweating, and tremors. Some individuals experience a rebound effect in which the problem for which the drug was initially administered returns in a seemingly more severe fashion until homeostasis is reestablished.

Critical Thinking Review

1. Describe the link between pharmacokinetics and pharmacodynamics.
2. What are the three aspects of pharmacodynamics and how are they interrelated?
3. Briefly describe the mechanism by which each of the four drug theories are thought to elicit their responses.
4. What is the main benefit of using a synergist?
5. What is an agonist? Briefly describe the three categories of agonists.
6. What is an antagonist? Briefly describe the five categories of antagonists.
7. List eight reasons why an additive may be used.
8. Define the term *prophylactic* and give an indication of why a prophylactic drug may be used.
9. Differentiate between a side effect and an adverse effect.
10. Explain the difference between physiological and psychological addiction.

References

Agonist. (n.d.). *American heritage® Stedman's medical dictionary*. Retrieved from http://dictionary.reference.com/browse/agonist

American Pregnancy Association (2006). *FDA drug category ratings*. Retrieved from http://www.american-pregnancy.org/pregnancyhealth/fdadrugratings.html

Antagonist. (n.d.). *American heritage® Stedman's medical dictionary*. Retrieved from http://dictionary.reference.com/browse/antagonist

Catalyst. (n.d.). *The American heritage® Stedman's medical dictionary*. Retrieved from http://dictionary.reference.com/browse/catalyst

Cohen, B. (2005). *Memmler's the human body in health and disease* (10th ed.). Philadelphia, PA: Lippincott Williams & Wilkins.

Dreyer, M. (1996). *Pharmacology for nurses and other health workers* (2nd ed.). New York, NY: Pearson Education.

Drugs.com (n.d.). *Hyaluronidase*. Retrieved from http://www.drugs.com/ppa/hyaluronidase.html

Drugs.com (n.d.). *Naloxone*. Retrieved from http://www.drugs.com/pro/narcan.html

Dynamics (n.d.). *The American heritage® dictionary of the English language* (4th ed.). Retrieved from http://dictionary.reference.com/browse/dynamics

Enzyme. (n.d.). *The American heritage® Stedman's medical dictionary*. Retrieved from http://dictionary.reference.com/browse/enzyme

Frey, K., et al. (2008). *Surgical technology for the surgical technologist: A positive care approach* (3rd ed.). Clifton Park, NY: Delmar Cengage Learning.

Grogan, J. (2001). *Pharmacy simplified a glossary of terms*. Clifton Park, NY: Delmar Thomson Learning.

Iatrogenic. (n.d.). *The American heritage® Stedman's medical dictionary*. Retrieved from http://dictionary.reference.com/browse/iatrogenic

Junge, T. (January, 2009). "Drug discovery, development and approval processes." *The Surgical Technologist* vol. 41 no. 1: 13-23. Association of Surgical Technologists.

Moini, J. (2009). *Fundamental pharmacology for pharmacy technicians*. Clifton Park, NY: Delmar Cengage Learning.

Moroney, A. (2007). *Pharmacodynamics*. Retrieved from http://www.merck.com/mmpe/sec20/ch304/ch304a.html

Nema, S., Brendel, R., & Washkuhn, R. (2006). *Encyclopedia of pharmaceutical technology* (3rd ed.). New York, NY: Informa Healthcare.

Olson, J. (2006). *Clinical pharmacology made ridiculously simple*. Miami: MedMaster, Inc.

Porter, R. et al. (2007). *The Merck manual for healthcare professionals*. Retrieved from http://www.merck.com/mmpe/index.html

RxList (n.d). *Sodium bicarbonate*. Retrieved from http://www.google.com/search?q=antacid+sodium+bicarbonate&rls=com.microsoft:en-us:IE-SearchBox&ie=UTF-8&oe=UTF-8&sourceid=ie7&rlz=1I7ADBF_en

Rx-s.net. (n.d.). *Acetaminophen; codeine*. Retrieved from http://rx-s.net/weblog/more/acetaminophen-codeine

Synergist. (n.d.). *The American heritage® Stedman's medical dictionary*. Retrieved from http://dictionary.reference.com/browse/synergist

Teratogenic. (n.d.). *The American heritage® Stedman's medical dictionary*. Retrieved from http://dictionary.reference.com/browse/teratogenic

Toxic. (n.d.). *The American heritage® Stedman's medical dictionary*. Retrieved from http://dictionary.reference.com/browse/toxic

United Way. (n.d.). *National 211 collaborative*. Retrieved from http://www.211.org

Chapter
NINE

DRUG HANDLING

Student Learning Outcomes

After studying this chapter, the reader should be able to:

- Describe safe medication practices including the six rights of medication administration and the three verification process and explain the importance of each.
- List several drug dispensing systems regularly utilized in the surgical setting.
- Distinguish drug packaging materials commonly utilized in the surgical setting.
- List the importance of information contained within a drug label.
- Identify drug handling supplies frequently employed in the surgical setting.
- Explain medication preparation in a nonsterile area.
- Demonstrate the process for transfer of medication to the sterile field including labeling and identification to other team members.

Key Terms

Administration set	Dilution	Indication	Six rights
Ampule	Dispense	Infusion	Slip tip
Arthroscopy	Documentation	Leach	Sorbitol
Aspirate	Dose	Medicine cup	Sterile technique
Biohazardous material	Dropper	Meniscus	Syringe
Bulb syringe	Drug label	Needle	Three verification process
Carpule	Eccentric tip	Neonate	Toomey syringe
Cartridge	eMAR	Package insert	Trade name
Catheter tip	Express	Packet	Transfer device
Collar	Flange	Peritoneal fluid	Tube
Compounding	Foley catheter	Pharmacy	Twist tip
Concentration	Glycine	Photochemical reaction	Urologic
Contraindication	Graduated pitcher	Policy	Verification
Control syringe	Hermetic	Principles of asepsis	Vial
Cylinder	Hilt	Procedure	Wound
Cystoscopy	Hub	Reconstitution	
Degradation	Hypodermic	Scored	

DRUG HANDLING

Numerous drug handling techniques are employed to ensure safe medication practices. Various drug dispensing systems, drug packaging, drug labeling, drug handling supplies, and specific techniques are designed to promote patient safety in the surgical environment.

Safe Medication Practices

In addition to the federal and state laws mentioned in Chapter One, numerous organizations including the Association of Surgical Technologists, The Joint Commission, the Centers for Medicare and Medicaid Services, the Institute of Medicine, the Association of periOperative Registered Nurses, and the American Society for Healthcare Risk Managers have all published guidelines that relate to safe medication practices and labeling of medications. In addition to adhering to the policies and **procedures** of the individual facility, that are based on the law and the guidelines offered by the related professional organizations, several additional factors must be considered to ensure safe handling of drugs that are used in the operating room.

Six Rights

Several models or memory tools are available to help ensure that a drug is handled and administered correctly. One such model is called the **six rights** of medication administration. The six rights should be followed exactly for every patient.

1. Right patient
   - For the surgical patient, identity is usually determined in the preoperative holding area and again in the operating room during the time out
   - Any drug or food allergies should be noted during the time out

2. Right drug
   - Drug orders in the operating room are often in the form of standing orders on the surgeon's preference card or are given to the team members verbally; if the verbal order is not understood—ask for clarification
   - Verify the drug name three times

3. Right dose
   - Be sure the **dose** is understood and calculated accurately (e.g., decimal point in the correct location)
   - If **reconstitution** (addition of a liquid to a dried or concentrated substance to return it to its former condition and/or strength) of the drug is necessary, be sure that it is done correctly
     - Follow the manufacturer's instructions

   - Verify the dosage three times
     - Also consider if the dosage is consistent with the age/size, diagnosis, and gender of the patient

4. Right route of administration
   - Be sure that the route of administration is appropriate for the surgical patient
     - As explained in Chapter Six, not all routes of administration are appropriate for use in the surgical environment

5. Right time and frequency
   - In the surgical environment, drugs are generally given when ordered and frequency is usually not a concern unless the procedure is lengthy

6. Right documentation/labeling
   - Information documented in the patient's chart should include (at minimum) the name of the drug, dose, route of administration, time that the medication was given, and any unusual responses
   - **Documentation** should occur as soon as possible following administration of the drug but never prior to the drug actually being given
   - Within the sterile field, all storage locations of the drug must be labeled (e.g., the medicine cup and the syringe)

Other models concerning medication rights consist of a greater number of rights; however, the additional steps (such as the right education or the right to refuse) do not integrate well into the surgical environment especially when the patient is under general anesthesia therefore the six right model is most often used.

Three Verifications

Another safe medication practice involves checking each medication three times. The policies and procedures of the facility may require use of the three **verification** system. In the surgical environment, the verifications generally take place when the following events occur.

1. First verification—Takes place when the medication is removed from the storage location or when the items on the procedure cart are checked for accuracy according to the surgeon's preference card.

2. Second verification—Occurs just prior to removal of the drug from the container (e.g., just prior to drawing up into a syringe or transferring onto the sterile field). The syringe and/or other storage location (such as a medicine cup) are labeled per facility **policy** (usually just prior to or just following transference of the medication onto the sterile field).

3. Third verification—Occurs immediately following removal of the drug from the container.

When a drug is transferred to the sterile field, two individuals (such as the circulator and the surgical technologist) are involved in the transfer and both individuals must be actively involved in the verification, which usually takes place visually and verbally. Information that is verified includes (at minimum) the name of the drug, the strength of the drug, the expiration date and any other pertinent facts. If the drug is passed to another surgical team member, the drug information is verbalized again as the drug is transferred (and each time thereafter). For each drug used, the entire **three verification process** is employed.

Drug Dispensing Systems

Several methods for dispensing drugs are available. In the hospital setting, one or more of these systems may be in use. Some require the presence of a pharmacist while others may be simply convenient storage locations or automated systems.

Pharmacy

The main hospital **pharmacy** is typically open 24 hours a day and seven days a week. One or more pharmacists are present at all times to meet the drug needs of all hospital departments. In addition to the pharmacist(s), pharmacy technicians and transportation aides may also be employed in supportive roles. Responsibilities of the pharmacy staff include ordering and stocking medications, preparing fluids for **infusion**, **compounding**, accounting for controlled substances (narcotics), generating patient charges, and dispensing drugs among other tasks

including implementation and enforcement of safe drug handling and administration techniques. Access to the pharmacy is limited and transactions are typically handled via a service window or the medications are delivered to the patient care area. In addition to the main pharmacy, the facility may have an outpatient (retail) pharmacy as well as satellite pharmacies in various departments such the chemotherapy unit or the surgical suite.

Satellite Pharmacy (OR)

A satellite pharmacy is set up as a convenience for the physicians, staff, and patients in the surgical suite. The satellite pharmacy may not only serve the medication needs that relate to the patient in surgery but may also provide drugs for use in the preoperative holding area, the postanesthesia care unit, and possibly the endoscopy suite. The satellite pharmacy may simply be a limited access storage location that is more readily accessible to surgical personnel or it may be staffed by pharmacy personnel during certain hours to enhance the functionality.

Automated Dispensing Systems

Automated dispensing systems are available for use throughout the hospital setting. The automated devices (machines) are stocked with medications or supplies commonly used in the area of need (such as the surgical unit) and staff members are granted varying levels of access with the use of identification badge scanning technology, by entering a password, or through fingerprint analysis (Figure 9-1A). Automated dispensing systems provide a method for inventory control, charging the patient for items used during their care, and tracking

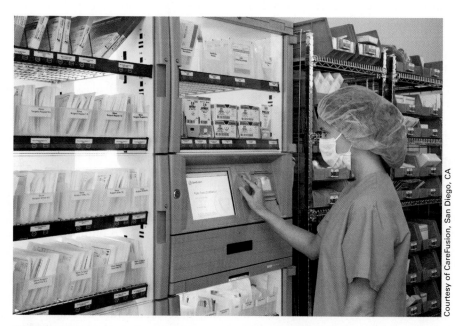

FIGURE 9-1A Pyxis Procedure Station™ System — Capable of Dispensing a Variety of Supplies

Courtesy of CareFusion, San Diego, CA

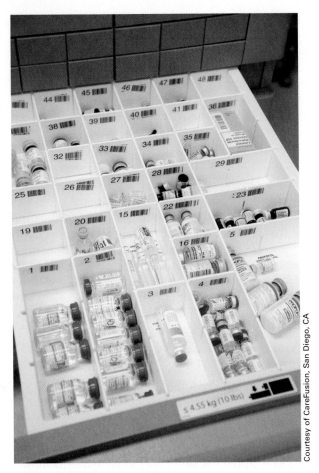

Courtesy of CareFusion, San Diego, CA

FIGURE 9-1B Pyxis® Anesthesia System — Secure Drug Inventory Management

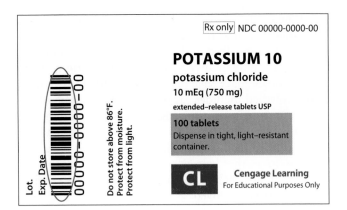

Rx only   NDC 00000-0000-00

POTASSIUM 10

potassium chloride

10 mEq (750 mg)

extended–release tablets USP

100 tablets
Dispense in tight, light–resistant container.

CL   Cengage Learning
For Educational Purposes Only

Lot.
Exp. Date
00000-0000-00

Do not store above 86°F.
Protect from moisture.
Protect from light.

FIGURE 9-2 Manufacturer's Drug Label Identifying Bar Code Technology

access to secured controlled substances (Figure 9-1B). Unopened non-narcotics and unused supplies may be returned to the machine, and the charge is removed from the patient's bill. Unopened or unused narcotics are generally returned to the pharmacy for reconciliation. Automated dispensing systems may provide access to more than one type of medication or supply item.

Electronic Medication Administration Record Keeping System

An electronic medication administration record (**eMAR**) keeping system that employs barcode technology on drug packages and labels and may be used for inventory control and generating patient charges (Figure 9-2). Use of the eMAR may also help reduce human errors related to administration of a drug to the wrong patient, administration of the wrong drug, or administration of the wrong dose. Additionally, use of an electronic system can help to identify potential drug interactions and **contraindications**, propose a dosing schedule, as well as notify the user of any patient

allergies, alternative drugs that could be available at a reduced cost (such as a generic), and of any follow-up lab screenings that should be scheduled.

Drug Packaging

Various techniques are used for packaging drugs. Most medications used in the surgical environment are intended for single patient use and packaged in appropriate quantities. If a drug is opened for a patient and all or part of the quantity is not used, the drug (or remainder of the drug) is usually discarded. In limited circumstances, the unused portion of the drug may be sent to the patient care area for future use. Usually, the contents of the drug container are sterile; however, in most circumstances the outside of the container is not. Certain containers may be packaged sterilely by the manufacturer or sterilized at the facility to allow them to be placed on the sterile field. Only packaging types commonly utilized in the surgical environment are described in this chapter.

Ampule

An **ampule** is a small glass tube that contains a solution, usually a sterile pharmaceutical (Figure 9-3). The ampule is heat sealed to make it **hermetic** (air tight). The narrow portion (neck) of the ampule is **scored** (score line may be highlighted with a colored band applied by the manufacturer) so that the glass can be broken open easily to allow the solution to be removed for use. Some ampules are clear and others are made of tinted (often amber or brown) glass to protect the contents from **degradation** due to **photochemical reactions** that may occur if the drug is exposed to light. The ampule is appropriately labeled at the manufacturing plant with all necessary information concerning the enclosed drug. In addition, the label may be printed in distinctive colors to help differentiate various drugs.

Prior to opening an ampule, be sure that all of the solution is in the bottom (larger) portion of the ampule.

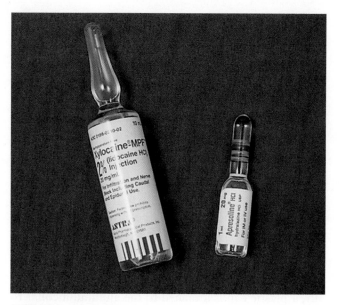

FIGURE 9-3 Ampules

piped to the point of use and delivered via an outlet or a smaller portable cylinder may be employed. Outlets are color coded and as an added safety measure, the configuration of the matching color coded connectors are not interchangeable (e.g., the configuration of the oxygen outlet/connector system is different than that of the nitrous oxide outlet/connector system). Cylinders are pressurized and must be stored, transported, and handled with care. Information concerning cylinder safety is found in the facility policy and procedure manual. A regulator (valve) is attached to the pressurized cylinder to allow controlled release of the necessary amount of the gas for patient use. Each cylinder is labeled and color coded for identification purposes. Table 9-1 lists some of the common medical gases and the related identifying color used in the United States. Additional information about gases is found in Chapter Five, along with a photo of oxygen cylinders with regulators attached.

Gently tap the ampule while holding it in an upright position to allow air to displace any solution that may have become trapped in the upper portion of the ampule. Prior to opening an ampule, the upper portion of the ampule may be wrapped in gauze or a safety device may be used to reduce the risk of injury to the hands. The hands are pushed away from the body as the neck of the ampule is snapped open at the scored line and the hands are separated to avert possible injury to the hands from broken glass. When removing the solution from the ampule (usually with a syringe and needle), use of a filter needle may be recommended to remove any particulate matter (such as glass).

Cylinder

Pressurized **cylinders** (also called tanks) are used to store gases. Medical gases, such as oxygen and nitrous oxide, are often stored in a large tank in a central location and

Preloaded Syringe/Cartridge

Some liquid drugs intended for parenteral use are preloaded directly into a sterile syringe at the manufacturing plant. Each syringe contains a premeasured dose of the prescribed medication and is labeled and color coded (if necessary) accordingly. The syringe may have a sterile **hypodermic** needle pre-attached; otherwise the user will remove the sterile cap and attach the appropriate sized **needle** at the point of use, if needed.

Some medications are prepared in a sterile cartridge. In some regions, a cartridge may also be known as a **carpule** (Carpuject™/Tubex™). The cartridge is essentially the barrel portion of the syringe that is later inserted into a reusable holder/plunger mechanism at the time of use (Figure 9-4). The cartridge may have a sterile hypodermic needle attached; otherwise the user will remove the sterile cap and attach the appropriate sized needle at the point of use.

TABLE 9-1 Color Coding of Common Medical Gases in the United States

Name of Gas	Outlet or Cylinder Color
Carbon Dioxide (CO_2)	Gray
Helium (He)	Brown
Medical Air (a mixture of oxygen, nitrogen, carbon dioxide, and argon)	Yellow
Nitrogen (N_2)	Black
Nitrous Oxide (N_2O)	Blue
Oxygen (O_2)	Green (international, white)
Suction (not a medical gas; however, the vacuum outlet/connector system is similar in configuration to the medical gas outlet/connectors; therefore, they are often grouped together for logistical reasons)	White

A.

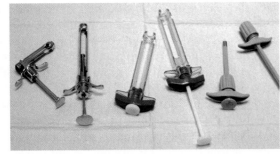

B.

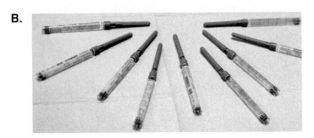

FIGURE 9-4 A. Variety of Reusable and Disposable Holder/Plunger Mechanisms. B. Prefilled Cartridges

Tube

Semisolids, such as creams, gels (includes lubricants), and ointments are often supplied in a **tube** (Figure 9-5). Some tubes are sealed with foil, metal, or plastic. A broken seal could be an indication of tampering or that the contents have been previously used for another patient; therefore, the tube should be discarded. If the seal is intact, it must be punctured prior to expressing (squeezing out) the contents. If the tube is sealed, the outer side of the protective cap will likely contain a pointed piercing mechanism that can be used to puncture the seal. Keep in mind that the piercing mechanism may not be sterile and when it is inserted into the tube it will render

the contents of the tube near the cap nonsterile. In this situation, a nonsterile team member will discard a small amount of the semisolid prior to placing the required quantity of the drug on the sterile field.

In order to transfer the contents of the tube to the sterile field, a nonsterile team member will remove the cap from the tube, puncture the seal (if necessary), and **express** the desired amount of the medication onto a designated area of the sterile field.

Vial

A **vial** is a small plastic or glass bottle that contains a sterile medication, which may be either in the solution or powder form (Figure 9-6). Vials are sealed with a sterile stopper (sometimes referred to as a septum), which is manufactured from rubber or another suitable substance that is held in place with an aluminum **collar**. Additionally, a plastic cap is attached to the aluminum collar to protect the sterility of and allow easy access to the stopper. The vial (clear or tinted) is appropriately labeled and color coded (if necessary) at the manufacturing plant with all essential information concerning the contents.

Medication may be removed from a vial using one of three methods:

1. The plastic cap is removed without touching the sterile stopper, the stopper is disinfected with an alcohol swab (if necessary), and a needle with a syringe attached is inserted through the stopper and used to extract the liquid medication. If the medication is in powder form, it will most likely be reconstituted by injecting the appropriate type and amount of liquid into the vial containing the powder and then the resultant solution is extracted for use.

Note: Because the stopper creates an airtight seal; it may be necessary to inject air into the vial to equalize the pressure within the vial to make extraction of the contents easier.

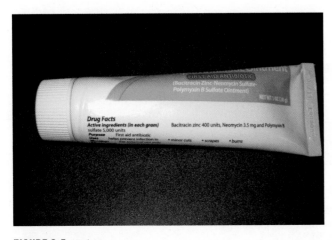

FIGURE 9-5 Tube

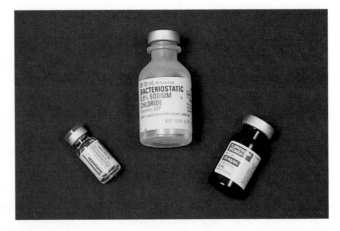

FIGURE 9-6 Vials

2. The plastic cap is removed without touching the sterile stopper, the stopper is disinfected with an alcohol swab (if necessary), and a sterile transfer device is used to convey the contents of the vial to a syringe or to pour the medication into a container (such as a medicine cup) on the sterile field.

3. The plastic cap and/or aluminum collar as well as the stopper are removed utilizing appropriate technique and the medication is poured into a container (such as a medicine cup) on the sterile field. When pouring, be sure to protect the integrity of the label from damage that may be caused by dripped or spilled medication.

Packet

A **packet** resembles miniature envelope and typically contains a small amount (single dose) of a sterile product. Packets may be manufactured of foil, plastic, and/or paper (Figure 9-7). One end of the packet may be notched to allow the end of the packet to be removed (torn away) or packet may be designed to allow the edges to be peeled apart to expose the contents. Prep pads (alcohol or povidone-iodine), suppositories, and semisolids are examples of products that are often contained within a packet.

When transferring the contents of a packet to the sterile field, a nonsterile team member will open the packet and express the contents (such as a semisolid) onto a designated area of the sterile field. Alternatively, the sterile team member may carefully grasp the contents of the packet (such as an alcohol saturated prep pad) and place it on the sterile field.

Solution Bag

Sterile fluids for injection, infusion, and irrigation may be contained within a solution bag, often referred to as IV (intravenous) bags (Figure 9-8). Solution bags

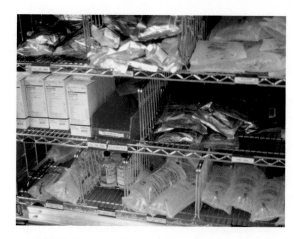

FIGURE 9-8 There Are Many Types of Prepackaged IV Solutions

range in size from 50 milliliters to 5 liters. More than 200 commercially prepared solutions are available and various electrolytes, medications, and nutrients may be added to the solution via an injection prior to administration to the patient. In some cases, a glass bottle must be substituted for a solution bag because the solution contained within may cause the bag (made of a soft polyvinyl chloride—PVC/vinyl) to degrade, causing a component of the vinyl to **leach** into the solution. Nitroglycerin is an example of a medication that when added to sterile fluid for intravenous administration must be placed in a glass bottle (and the administration set may not contain PVC). Solution bags are often packaged

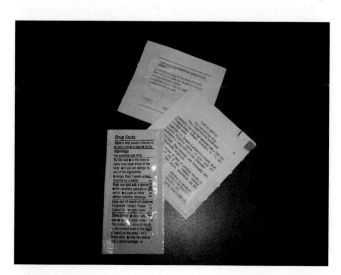

FIGURE 9-7 Packets

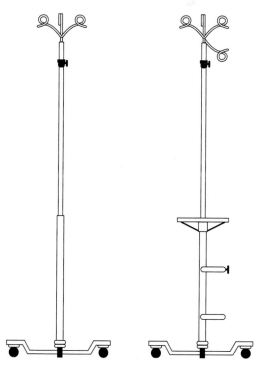

FIGURE 9-9 IV Stand

within a protective cover that must be removed prior to use. Additionally, the administration port is covered with a protective cap that is removed immediately prior to use. An administration set or a transfer device must be connected to the sterile administration port (following removal of the protective cap) on the solution bag or bottle to convey the solution to the patient or to the sterile field. Solution bags are typically hung from an adjustable height intravenous standard (IV stand/IV pole) and empty by gravity (Figure 9-9). As the height of the bag is increased, the effect of gravity is also increased causing the solution to drain from the bag faster.

Administration Set/Transfer Device   Intravenous **administration** sets (sometimes referred to as IV tubing or an infusion set) allow a sterile pathway for fluid from an IV bag and are available in numerous configurations, but all have similar features (Figure 9-10). Typically, the outside of the administration set is not sterile, but the inside (fluid pathways and areas under the protective caps) is sterile; however, in some cases both the inside and the outside of the administration set may be sterile. Sterility conditions are noted on the packaging. If connected to an IV bag, a non-vented administration set is used and the IV bag collapses as the fluid flows out of the bag. If connected to a glass bottle, a vented administration set is needed so that air will displace the solution in the bottle to allow the solution to flow from the bottle. There is a spike at one end of the administration set that connects to an administration port on the solution bag or bottle. The spike and the administration port are both sterile and both have protective caps that must be removed prior to inserting into the spike into the administration port using sterile technique. Prior to inserting the bag spike into the administration port, it is important to ensure that the roller clamp on the administration set is closed to prevent the solution from flowing out of the bag prematurely. Once the administration set is connected to the solution bag, the drip chamber is filled to approximately half of its capacity. Filling the drip chamber half-full allows the user to monitor the flow rate (speed at which the solution is progressing) through the tubing (by counting the number of drops per minute) and also prevents air from entering and moving through

the tubing. Next, the administration set is primed by slowly releasing the roller clamp to allow the fluid from the solution bag to displace any air in the tubing. When priming the administration set, it may be helpful to invert the injection ports to prevent air bubbles from becoming trapped. Once the solution reaches the end of the administration set, the roller clamp is closed to prevent leakage. The solution bag and administration set are then ready for use and may be connected to an intravascular catheter allowing infusion into the patient. In the surgical environment, the flow rate is typically controlled by the anesthesia provider and/or the circulator. In the preoperative holding area and postanesthesia care unit, monitoring fluid administration is the responsibility of the nursing personnel.

A **transfer device** is a rigid spout that is attached to a vial or a solution bag using the same technique described for attaching the administration set. When the transfer device is attached, the protective cap is removed, and the solution can be transferred to another vial or solution bag or poured into a container on the sterile field.

Solution Bottle

Sterile fluids for irrigation may be contained within a solution bottle. Solution bottles range in size from 50 milliliters to 4 liters. Examples of sterile fluids for irrigation include normal saline, water, **glycine**, and **sorbitol**. Solution bottles are firm plastic containers (manufactured from a compound of ethylene and propylene) that do not leach or allow vapor transmission. Each solution bottle is double sealed to protect the sterility of the contents. If the outer seal is broken, the contents of the bottle should not be used.

Sterile fluid for irrigation may be removed from a bottle using one of two methods:

1. The outer seal may be removed and a vented irrigation set is attached to the bottle by piercing the inner seal with the spiked end of the tubing. Irrigation sets are frequently used during endoscopic (**cystoscopy** and **arthroscopy**) procedures. Due to the volume of solution that may be needed, the irrigation set may be capable of connecting one to four bottles to the tubing with the use of a Y-type device.

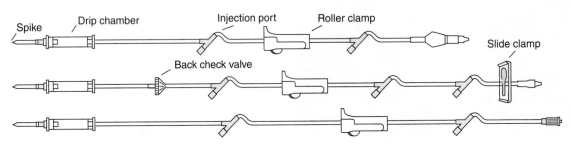

FIGURE 9-10 Basic Administration Set

2. Both the outer and inner seals are removed and the solution is poured into a container on the sterile field. When pouring solution into a container, the label is held in the palm of the hand or turned away from the lip of the bottle where the solution will exit to preserve the integrity of the label in case any fluid were to drip or spill. Additionally, the lip of the bottle is considered sterile and is the only portion of the bottle that may extend over the sterile field during transfer of the liquid from the bottle to the sterile container. When pouring, a minimum of 12 inches should be maintained between the lip of the bottle and the sterile container. Bottles should never be recapped for later use as recapping could render the remaining contents of the bottle nonsterile. Larger solution bottles may have a ring incorporated in the bottom of the bottle. The user has the option to insert his or her index or middle finger in the ring to prevent accidental dropping of the bottle.

Drug Labels and Package Inserts

Drug labeling is regulated by the United States Food and Drug Administration (USFDA or more commonly FDA), which is a division of the United States Department of Health and Human Services. FDA regulations affecting drug labeling extend beyond the label affixed to the medication container, but to the packaging material as well as the package insert. The **package insert** is a printed detailed description of the drug containing in-depth information that is too extensive to fit on the drug label.

When a medication is removed from its original container, it will be necessary for a surgical team member to label each location of the drug (such as a medication cup or a syringe). Information concerning subsequent drug labeling in the surgical environment is presented later in this chapter.

Necessary Information

The FDA mandates that the labeling information provided contain the 17 items listed:

1. Indications and Usage
   - **Indications** are the reason(s) why a drug may be used. A drug may have more than one indication, meaning that it may be used to treat more than one problem.
   - Usage refers to the action of the drug or how it acts to treat the indicated problem.

2. Dosage and Administration
   - Dosage refers to the amount of the drug needed to treat the indicated problem as well as the interval of time between doses.
   - Administration is the route by which the drug is given. The drug may be administered by more than one route. Routes of administration appropriate for use in the surgical environment are presented in Chapter Six.

3. Dosage Forms and Strengths
   - The dosage form refers to the way the drug is prepared for use (gas, liquid, solid). The drug may be manufactured in more than one form to allow administration by more than one route. Drug forms are presented in Chapter Five.
   - Strength refers to the amount of the main (active) ingredient(s) in the designated unit of measure (such as the number of milligrams per milliliter). Strength is sometimes referred to as the **concentration**.

4. Contraindications
   - Contraindications are the reasons why a drug should not be given (such as during pregnancy). The hazards of the drug outweigh the benefits in the given situation.

5. Warnings and Precautions
   - All known risks or hazards of the drug are listed and any known preventive measures are provided.

6. Adverse Reactions
   - All undesirable effects are listed. The undesirable effects may be predictable (nausea, hair loss, sensitivity to sunlight, etc.) or may be unpredictable (such as an allergic reaction).

7. Drug Interactions
   - Any known alteration of the action of a drug when taken in combination with another drug (prescription or over-the-counter) or food (including nutritional supplements) is listed along with methods for preventing or managing the alteration, if known.
   - Also included in this section are any known alterations to laboratory tests that might occur during administration of the drug.

8. Use in Specific Populations
   - The term *specific populations* refers to special circumstances that relate to the patient's gender, pregnancy, lactation status, age (pediatric/geriatric), as well as to those with comorbid conditions (diabetes, kidney disease, liver disease, etc.).

9. Overdosage
   - Must include dosage amounts, signs, symptoms, and laboratory findings that indicate overdosage as well as recommended treatments, such as administration of an antidote, gastric lavage, and hemodialysis.

10. Drug Abuse and Dependence
    - If the drug is a controlled substance, the schedule (class) must be listed.
    - The types of abuse including the physical and psychological signs of abuse are described and include the possible dosage amount and length of time of exposure that can lead to tolerance and/or dependence.
    - Methods of diagnosis of dependence, the effects of prolonged abuse and withdrawal, and options for treatment of dependence are described.

11. Description
    - Proprietary, generic, and chemical names of the drug (refer to Chapter Three for additional information concerning drug nomenclature).
    - Dosage forms and routes of administration.
    - Listing of all ingredients (active and inactive, such as coloring or flavoring).
    - Sterility.
    - Radioactivity (and any data related to radioactivity).
    - Pharmacologic (therapeutic) classification.
    - Physical or chemical characteristics (such as pH).
    - Lot number.
    - Expiration date.

12. Clinical Pharmacology
    - Pharmacodynamics—Interaction of the drug molecule with the target (receptor, membrane, cell, tissue, organ, or whole body) is described.
    - Pharmacokinetics—Movement of the drug within the body is described. The four main processes involved in pharmacokinetics are absorption, distribution, biotransformation (metabolism), and excretion.

13. Nonclinical Toxicology
    - Capability of the drug to cause cancer (carcinogenesis), birth defects (mutagenesis), or damage to the reproductive system.

14. Clinical Studies
    - All clinical studies related to use of the drug must be cited.

15. References
    - All scientific authorities related to this drug are listed.

16. How Supplied/Storage and Handling
    - Forms in which the drug is available are listed and include identifiers such as color, shape, imprinting, and so on.
    - Any special storage (such as refrigeration requirements, protection from light, etc.) or handling information (such as instructions for reconstitution, **dilution**, etc.) is described.

17. Patient Counseling Information
    - All information for safe and effective patient use is listed. Examples include driving, eating, and sun exposure restrictions, as well as the best time of day to administer the medication.

Items on the label must be presented in the order listed and the FDA also regulates the content of each section. Information contained within the label is intended to benefit not only the patient but the individual prescribing the medication as well as those preparing and administering the drug.

Drug Handling Supplies

Numerous supplies are employed in the surgical environment to handle drugs. The term *drug handling* refers to storing, measuring, transferring, administering, and conveying drugs to the sterile field.

Syringes

Syringes are usually transparent to allow the user to view the volume of the contents and range in capacity from 0.5 milliliter (ml) to 60 ml. Markings (calibrations) on the syringe indicate the capacity. The term *cubic centimeter* (cc) may be used interchangeably with the term *ml* to measure volume, but according to the Institute for Safe Medication Practices (refer to Chapter Three) the term *ml* is preferred to reduce the risk of interpretation errors.

This type of syringe is often used in conjunction with a needle. In addition to being used to transfer medications from their storage container to the patient, syringes are also used to transfer medications to another location (such as the sterile field), for irrigation, to withdraw fluid or air from the body (e.g., during a thoracentesis), or to insert fluid or air into the body or a medical device (such as sterile water into the balloon of a **Foley catheter** or air into the cuff of an endotracheal tube). Syringes are sterile (packaged in a plastic container or a peel/blister package), come in a variety of configurations, have several hub/tip options available, and may be disposable (usually made of nontoxic, biocompatible plastic with a stopper on the end of the plunger) or reusable (usually made of glass). Occasionally, stainless steel may be used on the hub and/or finger controls of a reusable syringe.

Components of a syringe are identified in Figure 9-11. The barrel is a tube-like structure designed to contain the material to be drawn into or ejected from the syringe. The length and circumference of the barrel vary according to the manufacturer and the intended use of the syringe. The tapered end of the barrel is called the **hub** or the tip. A sterile needle or cap may be attached to the hub or the hub may be connected to another medical device, such as IV tubing or a catheter. A **flange** (rim) on

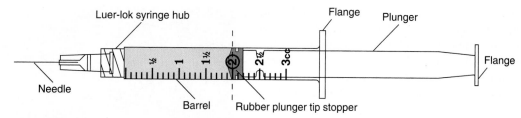

FIGURE 9-11 Components of a Syringe

the opposite end of the barrel provides support for the user's index and middle fingers when ejecting the contents of the syringe. The plunger fits into the barrel of the syringe and can be pulled away from the hub to create a vacuum to draw in the desired contents or pushed toward the hub to eject the contents. The stopper on the plunger creates a seal that reduces the risk of the contents of the syringe from squirting retrograde out of the barrel when pressure is applied to the plunger. A flange on the opposite end of the plunger serves as a support for the user's thumb when ejecting the contents of the syringe as well as a place to grasp the plunger when drawing in the contents.

Slip Tip   One of the hub/tip syringe options is called a **slip tip**. The slip tip is tapered to fit inside of a needle hub and the needle remains in position via friction. In most situations the friction connection is stable; however, if the needle is not securely attached, incorrectly attached, or excessive pressure is applied to a slip-tip syringe, the needle may dislodge from the syringe.

Twist Tip (Luer-lok®)   Another hub/tip syringe option is the **twist tip** or Luer-lok®. The twist tip syringe is threaded, consisting of a collar with grooves inside that allow the needle to be twisted (screwed) into place. If the needle is applied correctly to the twist-tip mechanism, this type of connection is the most stable even when excessive pressure is applied to the syringe.

Eccentric Tip   The **eccentric hub/tip** option is an off-center tip that is used when the syringe must remain nearly parallel to the injection site (such as during an intradermal injection).

Control Syringe   A **control syringe**, also called a ring syringe, has three finger rings instead of flanges. Two of the rings are attached to the barrel and one is attached to the plunger. The rings provide increased stability (control) of the syringe in the hand of the user and allow additional pressure to be applied to eject the contents if resistance occurs. Typically, the user inserts the thumb into the plunger ring and the index and ring fingers into the barrel rings freeing the middle finger to stabilize the syringe barrel.

Irrigating   Syringes for irrigation are sterile, disposable (made of specialized plastic that is biocompatible and nontoxic), and available in several configurations and sizes. In addition to being used to irrigate **wounds**, they are also used to **aspirate** (withdraw by suction) fluid from the body or to insert fluid or air into a body cavity through a medical device (such as into the stomach via a nasogastric tube). Many irrigating syringes (large bulb, small bulb, Toomey) incorporate a catheter tip.

Catheter Tip   The **catheter tip** is a large blunt tapered tip (similar to but larger than a slip tip) that can be inserted into a medical device (such as a Foley catheter) to allow air or fluid to be inserted or withdrawn. Catheter tip syringes can also be used without being connected to a medical device. Catheter adaptors, sometimes called Christmas tree adaptors, can be attached to the hub of a regular syringe to transform it to a catheter tip syringe.

Large Bulb Syringe (Asepto)   **Bulb syringes** are used to wash, insert, or withdraw fluids from large surgical or traumatic wounds and body orifices. A large bulb syringe (sometimes referred to as an asepto syringe) employs a catheter tip and has two components: the barrel, which is usually transparent and the bulb. The end of the barrel near the bulb is flanged to provide finger rests for the user when compressing the bulb, and markings (calibrations) on the barrel indicate the capacity of the syringe. The bulb fits snugly into the barrel creating a seal and the bulb is pliable to allow the user to compress and release it easily. With use, the bulb may become loose or dislodged from the barrel and the user may need to tighten or reinsert the bulb into the barrel of the syringe.

When filling the bulb syringe (with 0.9% sodium chloride for irrigation, for example) the tip is exposed to the atmosphere, the bulb is compressed to expel the air and held in the compressed position, the tip is inserted into the solution to be drawn in, and the compression on the bulb is released allowing the syringe to fill by negative pressure. Be sure that the tip of the syringe is not obstructed by the bottom or sides of the solution container because the obstruction will prevent the syringe from filling. If additional solution is to be drawn into the syringe, the tip is pointed upward to allow the solution already in the syringe to flow into the bulb, any air remaining in the syringe is expelled by gently compressing the bulb, and with the bulb still compressed the tip is reinserted into the solution and the bulb is released to allow additional solution to enter the syringe. If desired, the previous step may be repeated as needed until the syringe is completely full. Use caution to avoid accidentally expressing any of the solution when expelling the air because it could create a hazard (slippery surface, medication exposure, exposure to **biohazardous material**) for the user or other surgical team members, splashing of fluid could contaminate the sterile field, and it is wasteful.

Keep in mind that if both the barrel and the bulb are filled with fluid, the syringe will likely hold an additional one to two times the volume marked on the barrel depending on the size of the bulb. For example, if the barrel is expected to hold 50 ml and the bulb is also filled, the total capacity may be 100–150 ml. This is important to remember when estimating the amount of irrigation fluid used during the surgical procedure.

Ear Syringe Ear syringes are also called small bulb syringes, nasal syringes, and ulcer syringes. The ear syringe is a sterile disposable item, which is constructed as a single unit of soft plastic that has a bulb on one end and a tapered opening on the other end. The ear syringe is used for irrigation and aspiration of small surgical and traumatic wounds and body orifices (such as the airway of a **neonate**). The same technique that is used to fill the large bulb syringe is used to fill the ear syringe. However, it is more difficult to know when the ear syringe is full or how much irrigation fluid was used because it is not transparent.

Toomey Syringe **Toomey syringes** are also known as piston syringes and are most commonly used during **urologic** surgical procedures. The Toomey syringe consists of a transparent barrel with markings to indicate the capacity and a plunger. The tip of the Toomey syringe may be removable and is similar in configuration to a catheter tip, but the design is slightly smaller to allow the syringe to be attached to standard urology instruments (such as a cystoscope to allow irrigation of the bladder). The Toomey syringe may also be equipped with a catheter tip (to allow bladder irrigation following Foley catheter placement) and a slip tip or twist tip (that can be used to inflate the balloon of a Foley catheter). Double flanges on the end of the barrel near the plunger provide a secure place for the user to grasp. The plunger has a stopper on the barrel end and a large thumb ring that allows the user to draw in the desired contents or eject the contents under pressure while maintaining control of the syringe on the opposite end.

Needles

Needles are hollow tubes made of stainless steel that have been beveled and sharpened at one end to form a point. The body of the needle is called the shaft and

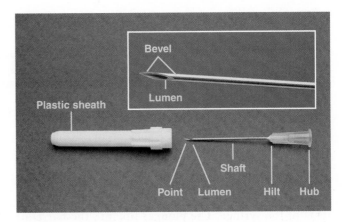

FIGURE 9-12 **Components of a Needle**

the transition of the shaft to the flanged hub is called the **hilt**. The hub may be constructed of stainless steel, aluminum, or plastic. The hollow space inside of the body of the needle is called the lumen. Protective covers, sometimes called sheaths, are available to maintain the sterility of the needle and reduce the risk of accidental injury. Plastic needle hubs, sheaths, and packaging materials may be color coded to indicate the needle gauge. Needle components are identified in Figure 9-12.

Needles are most often used with syringes by attaching the hub of the needle to a slip tip or a twist tip syringe. Needle length is measured from the tip to the hilt and can range from 3/8 of an inch to several inches, according to the intended use. Needle diameter is measured using the Stubs gauge (g) system. Low gauge numbers represent large diameter needles and high gauge numbers represent small diameter needles. Needle gauges range from an outside diameter of 10 g (approximately 3.4 millimeters or 0.13 inches), which is the largest to 33 g (approximately 0.2 millimeters or 0.008 inches), which is the smallest. The corresponding inside diameters (measurement of the lumen) are 2.69 millimeters or 0.11 inches for the 10 g needle and 0.09 millimeters or 0.0035 inches for the 33 g needle. Each gauge size needle is available in several lengths and specialty needles are available in a broader range of sizes. Typically, a larger gauge needle is used to draw solutions into a syringe because it is faster and causes less turbulence, thereby reducing the amount of air dispersed in the solution. Prior to injecting the solution into the patient, the larger needle may be replaced with a smaller gauge needle to reduce the amount of pain and tissue damage associated with the injection and to help retain the solution at the injection site.

Several types of needles are used in the surgical setting. Needles for injection, also referred to as hypodermic needles, are the most common. Intravascular needles (with or without a catheter) and spinal needles are frequently used as well. Blunt needles may occasionally be used when filling a syringe (from an ampule, for example) or for irrigating a small wound.

Safe handling of sharps, including needles, is paramount in preventing the spread of infection from bloodborne (and other) pathogens. A bloodborne pathogen is an infectious organism found in human blood that can be transferred from one individual to another via blood to blood contact (such as would occur if a healthcare worker was to receive a needlestick injury with a hypodermic needle, or other sharp item [scalpel, endoscopic trocar, suture needle, etc.] that has already been used on the patient or vice versa). Refer to a microbiology textbook for more information concerning pathogens and prevention of the spread of disease and a surgical technology textbook for information concerning personal protective attire, the **principles** of asepsis, and the related sterile and safety practices that will be employed in the surgical environment.

Several regulatory agencies, state and federal laws, and facility policies and procedures are in place to protect the surgical team members from harm in the surgical environment. Typically, an individual facility's policies and procedures reflect agency regulations as well as the state and federal laws and in some instances the facility policies may be stricter. If there is a conflict between federal law, state law, or facility policy, the stricter rule must be applied. The surgical technologist must be aware of and follow all regulations that pertain, not only to sharps safety, but to all aspects of surgical practice in their locale.

The Needlestick Safety and Prevention Act of 2000 was implemented to help prevent sharps injuries to healthcare workers and states that a written exposure control plan must be in place that includes the following:

- Identification of at risk employees.

- Communication of hazards to employees and providing training to prevent injury.

- Provision for hepatitis B prophylaxis.

- Implementation of precautionary measures including the use of personal protective attire, appropriate housekeeping measures, and engineering and work practice controls.

Engineering controls involve the use of safe medical devices in two categories: automatically activated protection and user-activated protection

that must be used whenever possible. Examples of safety engineered medical devices include syringes with needles that automatically retract following use (automatically activated protection) and syringes with needles that the user must manually activate following use (user-activated protection). Safety engineered scalpels and other medical devices used in the surgical environment are also available.

Examples of work practice controls include implementation of policies and procedures that comply with or exceed the standards and regulations set forth by the United States Department of Labor Occupational Safety and Health Administration (OSHA) that relate to handling contaminated sharps. In a 2011 document entitled, *OSHA Fact Sheet: Protecting Yourself When Handling Contaminated Sharps*, OSHA defines contaminated sharps as "objects that can penetrate a worker's skin, such as needles, scalpels, broken glass, capillary tubes and the exposed ends of dental wires." The document goes on to say that cuts or needlesticks from contaminated sharps place the worker at risk for exposure to and contraction of bloodborne pathogens, including but not limited to, hepatitis B and C viruses (HBV/HCV) and human immunodeficiency virus (HIV)—the virus that leads to acquired immune deficiency syndrome (AIDS). Additionally, the OSHA document states that "Contaminated sharps must never be sheared or broken. Recapping, bending, or removing needles is permissible only if there is no feasible alternative or if such actions are required for a specific medical or dental procedure. If recapping, bending, or removal is necessary, employers must ensure that workers use either a mechanical device or a one-handed technique." When using the one-handed technique (Figure 9-13), the user places the cap on a flat surface and then scoops the needle into the cap using one hand. The opposite hand may not be used to steady the cap. If working within the sterile field, caution must be exercised to ensure that the needle does not inadvertently puncture the sterile drape causing a breach in **sterile technique**. Once the needle is loosely covered with the cap, the

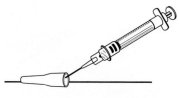

1. Scoop into cap using one hand. Do not touch the cap with the other hand.

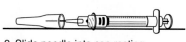

2. Slide needle into cap resting on table.

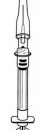

3. Holding the barrel of the syringe in one hand, carry to the sharps container. Do not push the cap onto the syringe.

FIGURE 9-13 One Handed Scoop Technique for Recapping a Needle

syringe is held upright (to keep the cap in position) and the entire unit is discarded into the biohazardous waste (sharps) container.

Containers for disposal of contaminated sharps must be closable, leak proof (bottom and sides), puncture resistant, labeled as hazardous and/or colored red, and be kept in an upright position to prevent spillage (Figure 9-14). Do not overfill the sharps container and ensure that it is replaced routinely. Special sharps containers designed specifically for use within the sterile field during a surgical procedure are also available (Figure 9-15). When the surgical procedure is complete, the sharps container from the sterile field (that may contain scalpel blades, suture needles, hypodermic needles, and other sharp objects) is carefully closed and discarded into a larger sharps container located elsewhere in the operating room.

- Records of all sharps injuries must be maintained (usually in the form of an incident report). The record must include a detailed explanation of how the injury

occurred, the body part affected, where the injury occurred (department/work area), and the device (type and brand, if known) involved in the injury. Information about the injured employee is confidential. In some states, all sharps injuries must be reported to the appropriate state agency for investigation.

- All exposure incidents must be evaluated (usually by members of the safety committee or risk management team). The goal of the evaluation is to reduce the risk of future incidents in an effort to protect not only the staff, but patients and visitors as well.

Dropper

A **dropper** is used to instill liquid medication into the nose, eyes, or ears. Droppers may also be used to measure a small amount of medication that is to be added to another liquid or to insert medication into the mouth of an infant. A similar technique is used to fill a dropper as is used to fill a bulb syringe. A dropper consists of a plastic or glass barrel that is tapered at one end. The barrel may have calibrations to indicate the volume. A pliable bulb is attached to the opposite end that is squeezed to fill the dropper and to **dispense** the medication. The bulb of the dropper may be controlled to allow release of one drop at a time or the entire contents of the dropper may be ejected. A dropper may be incorporated in the cap of a medication bottle or may be available separately (Figure 9-16).

Metal, Plastic, and Glass Containers

Within the sterile field, containers for solutions range in size from large basins, which are capable of holding approximately 6 to 10 liters of fluid to smaller containers that will only store 30 ml of fluid. The large basins typically contain sterile water, the medium basins are frequently used for irrigation fluid such as normal

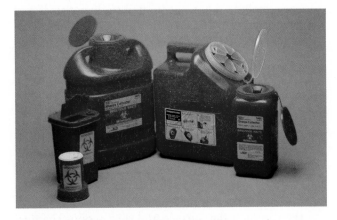

FIGURE 9-14 Biohazardous Sharps Containers

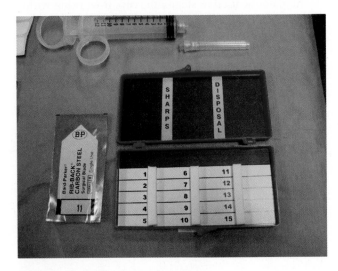

FIGURE 9-15 Sterile Sharps Container

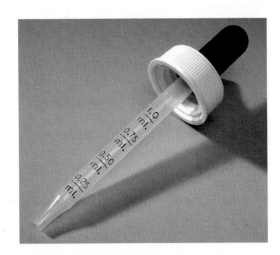

FIGURE 9-16 Calibrated Dropper

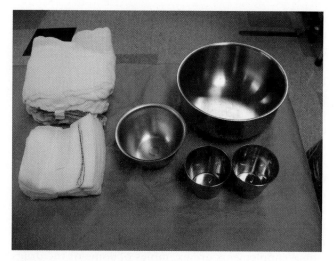

FIGURE 9-17 Metal Containers

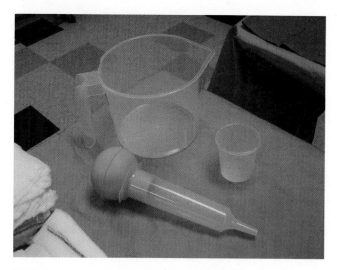

FIGURE 9-19 Graduated Pitcher and Bulb Syringe

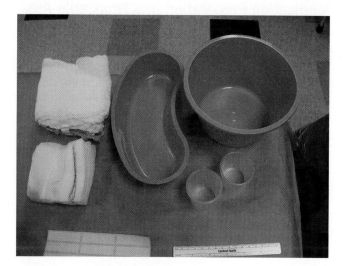

FIGURE 9-18 Plastic Containers

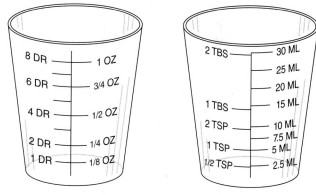

FIGURE 9-20 Plastic Medicine Cup

saline, and the smaller units are often used for medications. These containers may be manufactured of metal (Figure 9-17), plastic (Figure 9-18), or glass.

When measuring liquid medications in a container, the most accurate method is to view the calibrations at eye level, although this method may not be practical within the sterile field. Another consideration when measuring liquids is the **meniscus**, which is the convex or concave crescent that forms at the upper surface of a liquid. When measuring a liquid in which a meniscus has formed, measure from the center of the meniscus.

Graduated Pitcher   Use of the term *graduated* is another way of saying that the container is marked with calibrations to indicate the volume. Because of the handle and spout, pitchers allow the user to pour the contents into a surgical wound, such as the abdominal cavity,

rather than utilizing a bulb syringe to irrigate the wound (Figure 9-19). **Graduated pitchers** are routinely designed to hold one liter of solution.

Medicine Cup   The **medicine cup** is used to store small amounts of fluid (Figure 9-20). Calibrations found on the medicine cup can be in drams, ounces, tablespoons, or milliliters. The type of measurement most commonly used in the surgical environment is milliliters; however, because medicine cups are used in settings other than surgery, other types of measurements may also be present. For example, packaging for a bottle of cough syrup may include a medicine cup that is marked in tablespoons because it is intended for household use.

Infusion Pumps

A variety of infusion/volumetric pumps are available that can be programmed to deliver solutions at an established flow rate (Figure 9-21). Some infusion pumps are designed to administer a controlled amount of a fluid from a solution bag and some are designed to administer fluid from a

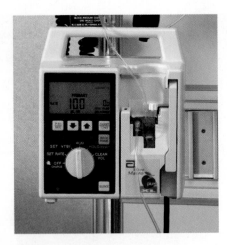

FIGURE 9-21 Infusion Pump

syringe. An optional feature available with some volumetric pump/infusion systems is the ability to control the temperature (warm or cool) of the fluid being administered. A patient controlled analgesia (PCA) device that is used to allow the patient to self-administer pain medication within set parameters is another example of a volumetric pump.

Intrathecal   The term *intrathecal* means within a sheath. In the case of an intrathecal infusion pump, the sheath is the dura mater. Intrathecal infusion pumps are used to deliver analgesics, local anesthetics, clonidine, and antispasmodics to the spinal cord via the cerebrospinal fluid. A catheter is surgically inserted into the subarachnoid space and connected to a pump that is implanted in the subcutaneous tissue of the abdomen. The pump is prefilled with the prescribed medication and can be refilled by injecting

more of the drug through the patient's skin into an injection port on the pump. The pump is battery operated and the battery is expected to last three to five years.

Other   Several additional types of infusion pumps are available. In some cases a catheter is implanted and connected to an external pump and other situations the complete unit is implanted (in a similar fashion to the intrathecal pump). The catheter may be inserted into an artery, body cavity, epidural space, organ, subcutaneous tissue, vein, ventricle, or other location—as needed. The device may be programmed to deliver a bolus of the prescribed medication at scheduled intervals or to deliver a continuous dose. Analgesics, antibiotics, antispasmodic drugs, chemotherapy agents, heparin, insulin, and nutritional supplements are examples of some of the drugs that can be given with the use of an infusion pump.

Medication Preparation in a Nonsterile Area

Sometimes medications must be prepared by a nonsterile team member outside of the sterile field using sterile technique. Examples of medication preparation in a nonsterile area include preparation of local anesthetics that may be injected prior to performance of the skin prep, reconstitution of a medication, medication that will be used by the anesthesia provider, and medication that will later be transferred to the sterile field.

Drawing Medication into a Syringe

Table 9-2 provides an example of the procedural steps and patient care considerations related to drawing medication into a syringe off the sterile field. This is a sterile

TABLE 9-2 Drawing Medication into a Syringe (Off the Sterile Field)

Procedural Steps	Patient Care Considerations
1. Obtain information about the needed medication(s) from the surgeon's preference card (Figure 9-22), written order, or verbal order: • Name • Strength • Amount 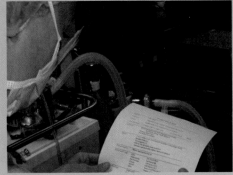 Figure 9-22 Obtain Information from the Surgeon's Preference Card	In addition to knowing the name, strength, and amount of the drug ordered, the team members may need to be familiar with: • Indications • Drug classification • Action of the drug • Route of administration • Possible reactions to the drug • Contraindications • Special storage or administration instructions • Antagonist, if one is available • Usual dosages • Action times • Possible drug interactions • Symptoms of overdose • Overdose management

2. Gather supplies from their storage location(s) (Figure 9-23)

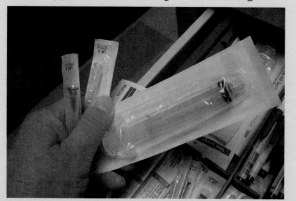

Figure 9-23 Gather Supplies from Their Storage Location

- Alcohol wipe, if necessary
- Correct style(s) and size(s) of syringe(s)
- Correct needle gauge(s) and length(s)
- Items for labeling

3. Select the drug from its storage location

Note: If more than one drug is ordered, gather all supplies and drugs simultaneously to save time

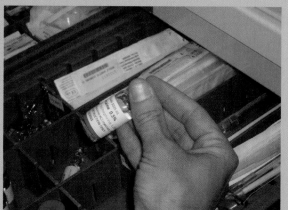

Figure 9-24 Select the Drug from the Storage Location and Perform the First Verification

Implement safe medication practices:
- Ensure that the six rights of medication administration are employed (right patient, right drug, right dose, right route of administration, right time and frequency, and right documentation/labeling)
- The first verification of the three verification process takes place as the drug is removed from its storage location or from the case cart—medication label is checked (at minimum) for drug name, strength, and expiration date (Figure 9-24)

4. Verify the patient's allergy status

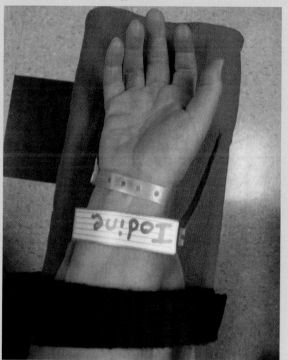

Figure 9-25 Verify the Patient's Allergy Status

Allergy information is obtained:
- Ask the patient, if possible
- Read the patient's chart
- Check to see if the patient is wearing an identification band (usually colored red) that lists the known allergies (Figure 9-25)
- Ask another surgical team member, such as the circulator or anesthesia provider
- Participate in the time out

5. Prepare supplies for withdrawal of the medication

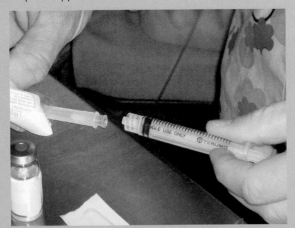

Figure 9-26 Assemble the Appropriate Size Syringe and Needle

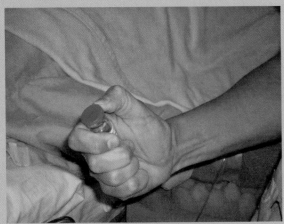

Figure 9-27 Open the Medication Container (Vial)

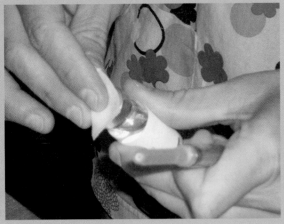

Figure 9-28 Disinfect the Stopper

- The principles of asepsis must be applied and sterile technique must be practiced
- Appropriate size syringe and needle are removed from their packaging and assembled (Figure 9-26) using sterile technique
- The second verification of the three verification process takes place just prior to removal of the drug from the container—medication label is checked (at minimum) for drug name, strength, and expiration date
- Medication container (usually an ampule or a vial) is opened using sterile technique (Figure 9-27) and/or if necessary, the stopper is disinfected with an alcohol swab or other approved disinfectant (Figure 9-28)

6. Medication is withdrawn from the container (Figure 9-29)

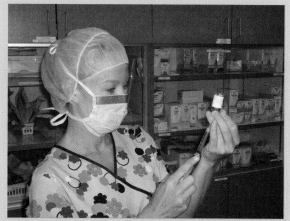

Figure 9-29 Withdraw Medication from the Container

- Needle is inserted into medication container using sterile technique and correct amount of the medication is drawn into the syringe
- If a vial is used, it may be necessary to invert the vial and use the air displacement technique
- Do not touch the plunger of the syringe because it must remain sterile
- Express any air contained within the syringe
- Ensure that the correct amount of medication remains in the syringe

7. Medication label information is rechecked for accuracy

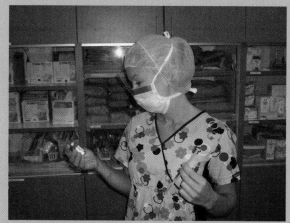

Figure 9-30 Perform the Third Verification

- The third verification of the three verification process takes place immediately following removal of the drug from the container—medication label is checked (at minimum) for drug name, strength, amount, and expiration date (Figure 9-30)

8. Needle for injection is applied to the syringe

- NO recapping of needles (unless absolutely necessary, then use the one-handed technique)!
  - If necessary, the needle used to withdraw the medication from the container is removed and the correct needle for injection is applied to syringe using sterile technique

9. Label according to facility policy

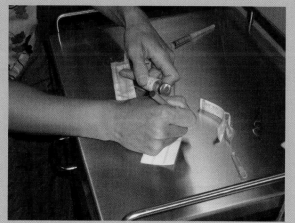

Figure 9-31 Create a Label

- The syringe is labeled as needed by creating a label (Figure 9-31) or by applying a preprinted label
- Use caution not to obscure calibrations on syringe with label

Note: Keep the original medication container as a reference until the procedure is complete for documentation and verification purposes.

task performed by a nonsterile team member. Federal law, state law, or facility policy and procedure may require variances in the way that the skill is performed. Remember, the stricter regulation must be applied.

Transfer to the Sterile Field

Medications that will be used within the sterile field must be transferred from the nonsterile area to the sterile area. Transfer of medications to the sterile field requires participation by two surgical team members. One team member, usually the circulator, performs the nonsterile functions and a second team member, usually the surgical technologist (who is scrubbed in) performs the sterile functions. Each team member has specific duties and responsibilities during transfer of medications to the sterile field.

Circulator's Duties and Responsibilities

The duties and responsibilities of the nonsterile team member, usually the circulator, during transfer of medications to the sterile field include:

- Obtaining the drug (and any necessary related supplies, such as a syringe and needles) from its storage location (based on the written, verbal, or standing order of the physician)

- Performing the first verification of the drug label (name, strength, amount, and expiration date)

- Preparing the drug for transfer to the sterile field
  - Reconstituting the drug, if necessary
  - Preparing and/or opening the container
  - Drawing the drug into a syringe using the technique described in Table 9-2

- Approaching the sterile field with the drug (and other supplies, if needed)

- Performing the second verification of the drug label (name, strength, amount, and expiration date) with the sterile team member

- Transferring the drug (and other supplies, if needed) to the sterile field
  - Opening a sterile package (such as a peel pack) containing the drug (ampule, vial, carpule, etc.) for placement onto the sterile field
  - Pouring the drug into a sterile receptacle (from a solution bottle or bag using a transfer device or from a vial)
  - Ejecting the drug from a syringe into a sterile receptacle
  - Allowing the sterile team member to receive the drug into the sterile field with the use of a syringe and needle
  - Expressing the drug from a tube or packet

- Performing the third verification of the drug label (name, strength, amount, and expiration date) with the sterile team member

- Keeping the original medication container as a reference until the procedure is complete

- Monitoring the patient for any unexpected reactions to the drug

- Recording the amount of the drug used on the patient's operative record

Surgical Technologist's Duties and Responsibilities

The duties and responsibilities of the sterile team member, usually the surgical technologist, during transfer of medications to the sterile field include:

- Requesting the drug (and any necessary related supplies) from the circulator (based on the written, verbal, or standing order of the physician) in advance of anticipated use within the sterile field

- The sterile team member may not be directly involved with performance of the first verification of the drug label every time; however, if the drug was ordered in advance the sterile team member could perform the first verification (when obtaining the drug from its storage location or when verifying that all necessary items are on the case cart) prior to scrubbing in

- Observing for any breach of sterile technique as the nonsterile team member prepares the drug and approaches the sterile field with the drug (and other supplies, if needed)

- Preparing the drug receptacle within the sterile field
  - Positioning a basin or medicine cup near the edge of the sterile field to allow the nonsterile team member easy access to the container when transferring (pouring, ejecting from a syringe, etc.) the drug
  - Assembling the correct syringe and needle combination to receive the drug into the sterile field

- Performing the second verification of the drug label (name, strength, amount, and expiration date) with the nonsterile team member

- Receiving the drug (and other supplies, if needed) into the sterile field
  - Removing the drug from a sterile package
  - Steadying the sterile container (if necessary) while the drug is ejected from a syringe or poured
  - Aspirating the drug into a syringe
  - Identifying the location for placement of drug expressed from a tube or a packet

- Performing the third verification of the drug label (name, strength, amount, and expiration date) with the nonsterile team member

- Accurately labeling all locations of the drug within the sterile field

- Announcing the name and strength of the medication each time it is passed to the sterile team member who will be responsible for administering the drug

- Monitoring the patient for any unexpected reactions to the drug

- Keeping track of and reporting the total amount of the drug that was used to the circulator and/or anesthesia provider for inclusion on the patient's operative record

- Discarding any unused portions of the drug
  - Disposal of unused narcotics (sometimes referred to as wasting of narcotics) will likely require witnessing by a licensed team member and completion of additional documentation

Drug Labeling on the Sterile Field   Anytime a drug or solution is removed from its original container, the subsequent location(s) of the drug or solution must be labeled (even if only one drug is used). For example, a drug may be poured from the original container into a medicine cup within the sterile field and then a portion of the drug from the medicine cup may be drawn into a syringe; both the medicine cup and the syringe must be labeled (Figure 9-32). Several devices are available for use when labeling medications on and off the sterile field.

Labeling Devices   Items used for labeling may be supplies commonly found within the sterile field or may be

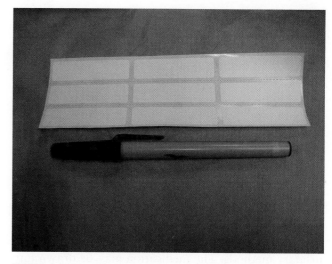

FIGURE 9-33 Sterile Marking Pen and Blank Labels

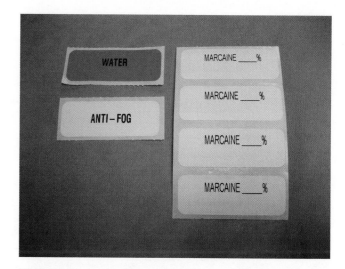

FIGURE 9-34 Customized Preprinted Sterile Labels

devices manufactured specifically for labeling of medications. A simple method that may be used to label medication within the sterile field involves the use of a sterile marking pen and blank labels with an adhesive backing (Figure 9-33). If blank labels are not available, skin closure strips may be substituted. Customized preprinted sterile labels (Figure 9-34) are available for order and may be included in specialty back table packs or basin sets. Additionally, medication labeling kits are available from several manufacturers.

Containers on the Sterile Field   Most medications and solutions utilized within the sterile field are clear liquids that can easily be confused. The surgical technologist is responsible for ensuring that all containers within the sterile field are appropriately labeled, including those containing sterile water and 0.9% (normal) saline. Facility policies and procedures that include best practices such as

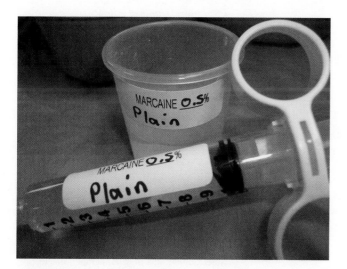

FIGURE 9-32 Labeled Medication Cup and Syringe

avoiding the use of certain error-prone abbreviations and the use of appropriate dose designations are employed. Information concerning the Institute for Safe Medication Practices List of Error-Prone Abbreviations, Symbols, and Dose Designations is found in Chapter Three.

Identifying to Other Team Members Each time that a drug is passed to another surgical team member, the name and strength of the medication is verbally identified to the individual who will be responsible for administration of the drug. Although the drug container is labeled, the drug name and strength are always announced.

Methods of Transfer

Medications are transferred to the sterile field via three primary methods. The medication may be drawn into a syringe (from an ampule or a vial), accepted into a sterile container (poured directly from a vial or a bottle, conveyed from a vial or solution bag with the use of a transfer device, or by ejecting it from a syringe), or expressed from a tube or packet. Examples of medications that would be used frequently within the sterile field include local anesthetics, hemostatic agents, antimicrobial agents, anticoagulants, antispasmodics, dyes, contrast media, sterile water, and 0.9% (normal) saline.

Table 9-3 provides an example of the team member involvement, procedural steps, and patient care considerations related to transferring medication to the sterile field. Performance of this task requires teamwork between a nonsterile team member (usually the circulator) and a sterile team member (usually the surgical technologist). Federal law, state law, or facility policy and procedure may require variances in the way that the skill is performed. Remember, the stricter regulation must be applied.

TABLE 9-3 Transferring Medication to the Sterile Field

Team Member Involvement	Procedural Steps	Patient Care Considerations
Preliminary Actions (regardless of method of transfer used)		
Circulator and Surgical Technologist May also involve other surgical team members including the surgeon, surgical assistant, and anesthesia provider	Patient's allergy status is known to all surgical team members	Obtain allergy information by: • Asking the patient, if possible • Reading the patient's chart • Checking to see if the patient is wearing an identification band (usually colored red) that lists the known allergies • Asking another surgical team member • Participating in the time out
Circulator and Surgical Technologist	Gather information about the needed medication from the surgeon's preference card, other written order, or verbal order; necessary information includes: • Name • Strength • Amount	In addition to knowing the name, strength, and amount of the drug ordered, the team members may need to be familiar with: • Indications • Drug classification • Action of the drug • Route of administration • Possible reactions to the drug • Contraindications • Special storage or administration instructions • Antagonist, if one is available • Usual dosages • Action times • Possible drug interactions • Symptoms of overdose • Overdose management
Circulator and/or Surgical Technologist Shared responsibility unless the medication order is received after the surgical technologist has scrubbed in, then the circulator will gather the supplies and bring them to the operating room	Gather supplies from their storage locations or verify that correct supplies have been placed in/on the case cart	Necessary supplies may include: • Alcohol wipe • Correct style(s) and size(s) of syringe(s) • Correct needle gauge(s) and length(s) • Items for labeling Note: Some items may be included in the back table pack or basin set and it may not be necessary to gather them from other storage locations

Circulator and/or Surgical Technologist	Obtain the drug from its storage location	Implement safe medication practices:
Shared responsibility (according to regulations) unless the medication order is received after the surgical technologist has scrubbed in, then the circulator will obtain the drug and bring it to the operating room	Note: If more than one drug is ordered, all supplies and drugs are gathered simultaneously to save time	• Ensure that the six rights of medication administration are employed (right patient, right drug, right dose, right route of administration, right time and frequency, and right documentation/ labeling) • The first verification of the three verification process takes place as the drug is removed from its storage location or from the case cart—medication label is checked (at minimum) for drug name, strength, amount, and expiration date
Circulator and/or Surgical Technologist Shared responsibility unless the medication order is received after the surgical technologist has scrubbed in, then the circulator will transfer the supplies to the sterile field or provide them to the surgical technologist	Necessary supplies are conveyed to the sterile field or to the surgical technologist (Figure 9-35) 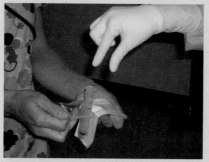 Figure 9-35 Syringe Is Conveyed to the Surgical Technologist	The principles of asepsis must be applied and sterile technique must be practiced

Transferring Medication from a Vial to a Syringe

Circulator	Prepares the vial for withdrawal of the medication and approaches the sterile field with the medication	Vial is opened and/or if necessary, the stopper is cleaned with an alcohol swab or other approved disinfectant
Circulator and Surgical Technologist	Circulator holds the vial in a way that allows both team members to visually and verbally identify the pertinent information on the medication label (Figure 9-36) 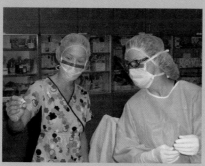 Figure 9-36 Vial Label Is Visible to Both Team Members (Second Verification)	The second verification of the three verification process takes place just prior to removal of the drug from the vial—medication label is checked (at minimum) for drug name, strength, amount, and expiration date

Circulator and Surgical Technologist	Medication is withdrawn from the vial (Figure 9-37)	Surgical technologist prepares the syringe and needle
		Circulator inverts and stabilizes the vial
	 Figure 9-37 Team Members Collaborate to Transfer Medication from a Vial to a Syringe	Surgical technologist inserts the needle into the center of the stopper and draws correct amount of the medication into the syringe using the air displacement technique, if necessary
		Surgical technologist expresses any air contained within the syringe by gently tapping on the barrel and ensures that the correct amount of medication remains in the syringe
Circulator and Surgical Technologist	Circulator holds the vial in a way that allows both team members to recheck the medication label for accuracy (Figure 9-38) 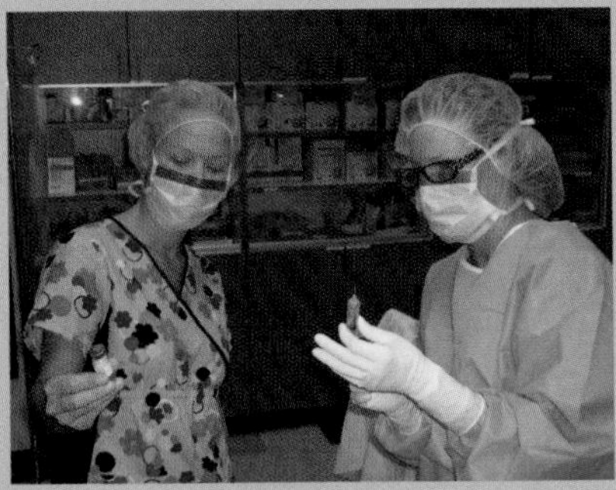 Figure 9-38 Vial Label Is Reviewed by Both Team Members Following Withdrawal of the Medication (Third Verification)	The third verification of the three verification process takes place just immediately following removal of the drug from the vial—medication label is checked (at minimum) for drug name, strength, amount, and expiration date
Surgical Technologist	Needle for injection is applied to the syringe	If necessary, the needle used to withdraw the medication from the container is removed and the correct needle for injection is applied to syringe
		Recapping of needles is NOT allowed (unless absolutely necessary, then the one-handed technique is used)!
Surgical Technologist	Label according to facility policy 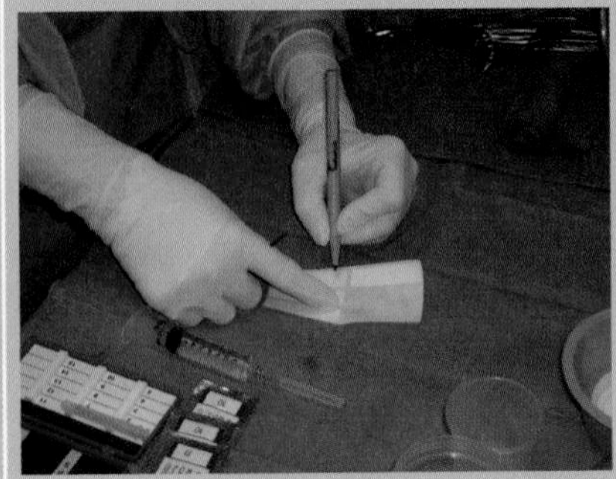 Figure 9-39 A Sterile Label Is Created	The syringe is labeled as needed by creating a label (Figure 9-39) or using a preprinted label using caution not to obscure calibrations on syringe with label
Circulator	Vial is kept in the operating room until the procedure is complete	For documentation and verification purposes

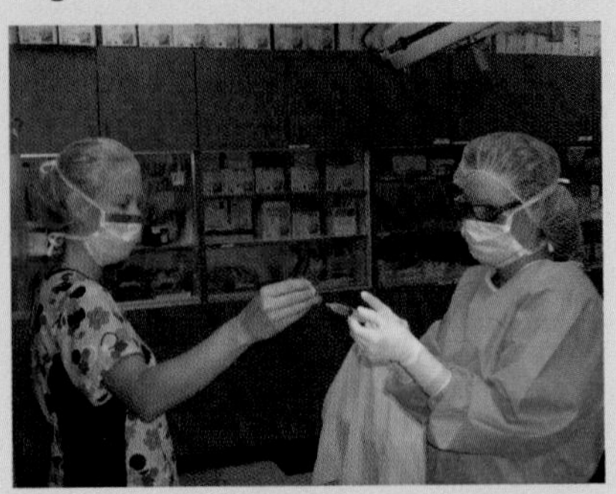

Transferring Medication from an Ampule to a Syringe

Circulator	Prepares the ampule for withdrawal of the medication and approaches the sterile field with the medication	Ensures that all of the solution is in the bottom portion of the ampule by gently tapping the ampule to allow air to displace any solution that may be trapped in the upper portion of the ampule (Figure 9-40)

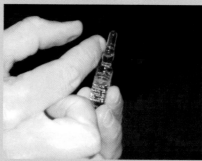

Figure 9-40 Displace Solution in the Upper Chamber of the Ampule by Gently Tapping

Snaps ampule open at the scored area on the neck (Figure 9-41) by pushing the hands away from the body (Figure 9-42)

Uses approved safety devices, as needed

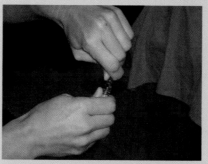

Figure 9-41 Snap Scored Neck of Ampule to Open

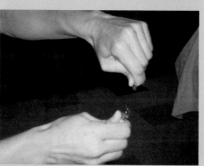

Figure 9-42 Push Hands Away from Body When Opening an Ampule

Circulator and Surgical Technologist	Circulator approaches the sterile field and holds the ampule in a way that allows both team members to visually and verbally identify the pertinent information on the medication label	The second verification of the three verification process takes place just prior to removal of the drug from the ampule—medication label is checked (at minimum) for drug name, strength, amount, and expiration date

Circulator and Surgical Technologist	Medication is withdrawn from the ampule 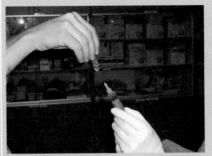 Figure 9-43 Medication Is Removed from an Inverted Vial 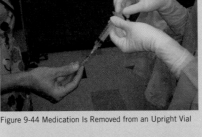 Figure 9-44 Medication Is Removed from an Upright Vial 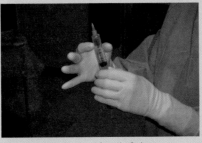 Figure 9-45 Air Is Expressed from the Syringe	Surgical technologist prepares the syringe and needle (use of a filter needle may be indicated) Circulator stabilizes the ampule in an inverted (Figure 9-43) or upright (Figure 9-44) position, as needed while the surgical technologist inserts the needle into the ampule and draws the correct amount of the medication into the syringe. Surgical technologist expresses any air contained within the syringe (Figure 9-45) and ensures that the correct amount of medication remains in the syringe
Circulator and Surgical Technologist	Circulator holds the ampule in a way that allows both team members to recheck the medication label for accuracy	The third verification of the three verification process takes place just immediately following removal of the drug from the ampule—medication label is checked (at minimum) for drug name, strength, amount, and expiration date
Surgical Technologist	Needle for injection is applied to the syringe (Figure 9-46) 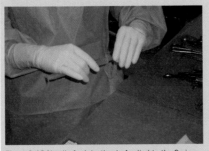 Figure 9-46 Needle for Injection Is Applied to the Syringe	If necessary, the needle used to withdraw the medication from the container is removed and the correct needle for injection is applied to syringe Recapping of needles is NOT allowed (unless absolutely necessary, then the one-handed technique is used)!
Surgical Technologist	Label according to facility policy	The syringe is labeled as needed by creating a label or using a preprinted label using caution not to obscure calibrations on syringe with label
Circulator	Ampule is kept in the operating room until the procedure is complete	For documentation and verification purposes

Transferring Medication to a Container on the Sterile Field (From a Vial, Syringe, or Solution Bottle)		
Circulator	Prepares the vial, syringe, or solution bottle for transfer of the medication and approaches the sterile field with the medication or solution

Note: The syringe technique is another method of transferring a medication from a vial or an ampule to the sterile field—it is often used to transfer medications that have been reconstituted | If using a vial, the stopper is removed ensuring that the contents of the vial remain sterile

If using a syringe, the medication is drawn into the syringe using sterile technique and labeled, if necessary

If using a solution bottle, both caps are removed ensuring that the contents of the bottle remain sterile |
| Circulator and Surgical Technologist | Circulator approaches the sterile field and holds the vial, syringe, or solution bottle in a way that allows both team members to visually and verbally identify the pertinent information on the medication label | The second verification of the three verification process takes place just prior to transfer of the drug from the vial, syringe, or solution bottle to the sterile field—medication label is checked (at minimum) for drug name, strength, amount, and expiration date |
| Surgical Technologist | Prepares the container to receive the medication | Container is placed near the edge of the sterile field where it is easily accessible to the circulator or is held in a mutually convenient location by the surgical technologist |
| Circulator and Surgical Technologist | Medication is conveyed to the sterile field
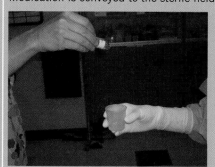
Figure 9-47 Medication Is Poured from a Vial
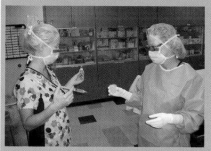
Figure 9-48 Medication Is Ejected from a Syringe
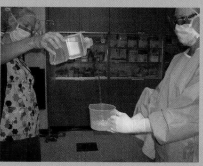
Figure 9-49 Solution Is Poured from a Bottle | Surgical technologist holds or stabilizes the container, if necessary

If using a vial, the circulator pours the contents into the container using sterile technique ensuring that the integrity of the medication label is preserved (Figure 9-47)

If using a syringe, the circulator ejects the medication into the container using sterile technique (Figure 9-48)

If using a solution bottle, the circulator pours the contents into the container using sterile technique ensuring that the integrity of the label is preserved (Figure 9-49) |

Circulator and Surgical Technologist	Circulator holds the vial, syringe, or solution bottle in a way that allows both team members to recheck the medication label for accuracy	The third verification of the three verification process takes place just immediately following transfer of the drug from the vial, syringe, or solution bottle to the sterile field—medication label is checked (at minimum) for drug name, strength, amount, and expiration date
Surgical Technologist	Label according to facility policy	The container is labeled as needed by creating a label or using a preprinted label using caution not to obscure calibrations on the container
Surgical Technologist	Prepare medication or solution for use 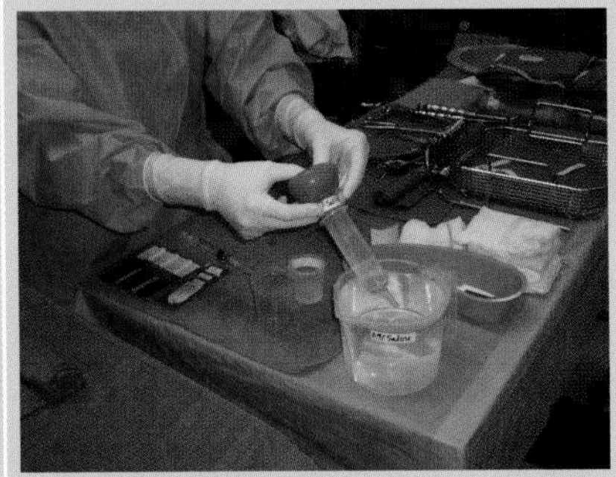 Figure 9-50 Solution Is Aspirated into a Bulb Syringe	Medication or solution may be drawn into a syringe (additionally, use of a needle may be indicated) Medication or solution may be aspirated into a bulb syringe (Figure 9-50) All locations of the medication or solution are labeled, as needed
Circulator	Original medication or solution container is kept in the operating room until the procedure is complete	For documentation and verification purposes
Transferring Medication from a Tube to the Sterile Field		
Circulator	Prepares the tube for expression of the medication and approaches the sterile field with the medication 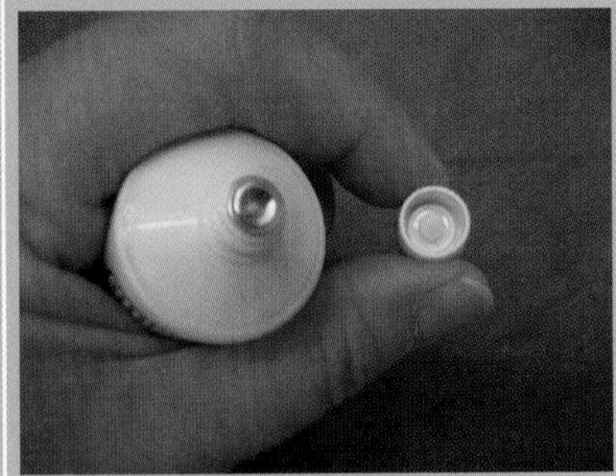 Figure 9-51 Preparation of a Tube	Removes the cap from the tube and punctures the seal, if necessary (Figure 9-51)
Circulator and Surgical Technologist	Circulator approaches the sterile field and holds the tube in a way that allows both team members to visually and verbally identify the pertinent information on the medication label	The second verification of the three verification process takes place just prior to removal of the drug from the tube—medication label is checked (at minimum) for drug name, strength, amount, and expiration date

Circulator and Surgical Technologist	Medication is conveyed to the sterile field	Surgical technologist determines where the medication will be placed on the sterile field
	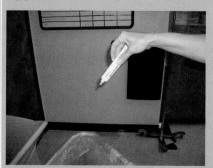 Figure 9-52 A Small Amount of the Medication Is Discarded 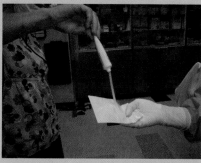 Figure 9-53 Medication Is Expressed onto the Sterile Field	If necessary, the circulator discards a small amount of the medication (Figure 9-52) Circulator expresses the desired amount of the medication onto a designated area of the sterile field (Figure 9-53)
Circulator and Surgical Technologist	Circulator holds the tube in a way that allows both team members to recheck the medication label for accuracy (Figure 9-54) 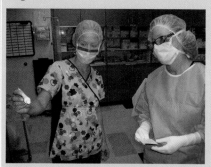 Figure 9-54 Team Members Recheck Label for Accuracy	The third verification of the three verification process takes place just immediately following removal of the drug from the tube—medication label is checked (at minimum) for drug name, strength, amount, and expiration date
Surgical Technologist	Prepare medication for use	As needed
Surgical Technologist	Label according to facility policy	If the medication is used immediately, labeling may not be necessary (e.g., ointment applied to the wound at the end of the procedure)
Circulator	Tube is kept in the operating room until the procedure is complete	For documentation and verification purposes

Summary

I. Safe medication practices—Must follow federal and state law as well as facility policies and procedures
   a. Six rights—Memory tool to ensure that drugs are handled and administered correctly
      i. Right patient—Identify patient and note any food or drug allergies
      ii. Right drug—According to physician's order, verify drug name three times
      iii. Right dose—Understand and calculate correctly; reconstitute according to manufacturer's instructions; verify dose three times; ensure that dose is consistent with age, size, diagnosis, and gender of patient
      iv. Right route of administration—Appropriate for surgical patient
      v. Right time and frequency—Usually given when ordered; frequency is a concern during lengthy procedures
      vi. Right documentation labeling—Document in patient's chart as soon as possible following administration; label all storage locations of the drug within the sterile field
   b. Three verifications—Check (at minimum) name of drug, strength of drug, expiration date, and any other pertinent facts.
      i. First verification—When drug is removed from storage location or when procedure cart is checked for accuracy
      ii. Second verification—Just prior to removal of drug from storage container
      iii. Third verification—Immediately following removal of drug from storage container

II. Drug dispensing systems
   a. Pharmacy—Available at all times in the hospital setting; staffed by a pharmacist; centrally located
   b. Satellite pharmacy (OR)—Located in patient care area; may have limited hours/access
   c. Automated dispensing systems—Machine stocked with drugs and other supplies; varying levels of protected access; useful in inventory control and generating patient charges

III. Electronic medication administration record keeping system—Employs bar code technology on drug packages; useful in inventory control and generating patient charges

IV. Drug Packaging—Contents of package are sterile but outside is usually not sterile
   a. Ampule—Small airtight glass tube containing a liquid medication
   b. Cylinder—Pressurized tank used to store gases
   c. Preloaded syringe/cartridge—Syringe or barrel portion of a syringe that is preloaded with a specified dose of a liquid medication
   d. Tube—Soft cylindrical container designed to store semisolids
   e. Vial—Small glass or plastic bottle that may contain a liquid or powdered medication; sealed with a stopper (sometimes referred to as a septum) held in place with an aluminum collar
   f. Packet—Resembles a miniature envelope; typically contains a small amount (single dose) of a sterile product (prep pad, suppository, semisolid)
   g. Solution bags—Glass or polyvinyl chloride; range in size from 50 milliliters to 5 liters; more than 200 commercially prepared solutions available; used in conjunction with an administration set or a transfer device
      i. Administration/transfer device—Provides a sterile pathway for fluid from a solution bag to the patient or to the sterile field
   h. Solution bottles—Firm plastic bottles containing sterile fluids for irrigation

V. Drug labels and package inserts—Regulated by FDA
   a. Necessary information—Must contain all 17 items; information pertains to patient, individual prescribing, and those preparing and administering the drug
      i. Indications and Usage
      ii. Dosage and Administration
      iii. Dosage Forms and Strengths
      iv. Contraindications
      v. Warnings and Precautions
      vi. Adverse Reactions
      vii. Drug Interactions
      viii. Use in Specific Populations
      ix. Overdosage
      x. Drug Abuse and Dependence
      xi. Description
      xii. Clinical Pharmacology
      xiii. Nonclinical Toxicology
      xiv. Clinical Studies
      xv. References
      xvi. How Supplied/Storage and Handling
      xvii. Patient Counseling Information

VI. Drug handling supplies—Supplies for storing, measuring, transferring, administering, and conveying drugs to the sterile field
   a. Syringes—Cylindrical device with either a plunger or a bulb attachment that is used to inject fluids into or withdraw fluids from the body; manufactured from glass, metal, plastic, and/or rubber.
      i. Slip tip—Tapered syringe tip; fits inside of a needle; secures needle via friction
      ii. Twist tip (Luer-lok®)—Threaded syringe tip; allows needle to be twisted (screwed) securely in place

      iii. Eccentric tip—Off-center syringe tip; used when syringe must remain parallel to injection site

      iv. Control syringe—Syringe that employs three finger rings instead of flanges; rings provide increased stability (control) of syringe

      v. Irrigating—Syringe used to irrigate wounds and to aspirate fluid from the body or to insert fluid or air into a body cavity through a medical device

         1. Catheter tip—Blunt tapered syringe tip that can be inserted into a medical device (such as a Foley catheter) to allow air or fluid to be inserted or withdrawn

         2. Large bulb syringe (asepto)—Two-piece bulb syringe for irrigation and aspiration of large surgical or traumatic wounds and body orifices

         3. Ear syringe—One-piece bulb syringe for irrigation and aspiration of small wounds or body orifices

         4. Toomey syringe—Specialty syringe typically used during urologic procedures

  b. Needles—Slender, hollow, pointed instrument that typically fits onto the end of a syringe; used to pierce body tissue to allow for injection or withdrawal of fluids

  c. Dropper—Plastic or glass barrel that is tapered at one end with a pliable bulb/stopper attached to the opposite end; used to instill liquid medication into the nose, eyes, or ears

  d. Metal, plastic, and glass containers—For use within the sterile field

      i. Graduated pitcher—Container constructed with a handle and a spout that is marked with calibrations to indicate the volume; allow the user to pour irrigation fluid into a surgical wound; typically hold one liter of solution

      ii. Medicine cup—Container used to store small amounts of fluid; calibrations in drams, ounces, tablespoons, or milliliters

  e. Infusion pumps—Programmable device used to deliver solutions at an established flow rate from a solution bag or from a syringe

      i. Intrathecal—Infusion pumps used to deliver analgesics, local anesthetics, clonidine, and antispasmodics to the spinal cord via the cerebrospinal fluid; used in conjunction with a catheter that is surgically inserted into the subarachnoid space and connected to a pump that is implanted in the subcutaneous tissue of the abdomen

      ii. Other—Additional types of infusion pumps are available; catheter is implanted and connected to an external pump or the complete unit is implanted; used to administer analgesics, antibiotics, antispasmodic drugs, chemotherapy agents, heparin, insulin, and nutritional supplements

VII. Medication preparation in a nonsterile area—Prepared by a nonsterile team member outside of the sterile field; technique used to prepare local anesthetics that may be injected prior to performance of the skin prep, reconstitution of a medication, medication that will be used by the anesthesia provider, and medication that will later be transferred to the sterile field

  a. Drawing Medication into a syringe—Procedural steps and patient care considerations

VIII. Transfer to the sterile field—Transfer from the nonsterile area to the sterile area; requires participation by two surgical team members

  a. Circulator's duties/responsibilities—Nonsterile team member role defined

  b. Surgical technologist's duties/responsibilities—Sterile team member role defined

      i. Drug labeling on the sterile field—All locations of the drug or solution must be labeled

         1. Labeling devices—Devices include sterile marking pen and blank adhesive labels, customized preprinted labels, labeling kits

         2. Containers on the sterile field—All containers must be labeled according to facility policy and procedure

         3. Identifying to other team members—verbally identify to individual who will administer the drug

  c. Methods of transfer—Three primary methods: draw into a syringe, accept into a sterile container, or express from a tube or packet

Critical Thinking Review

1. List the six rights of medication administration and explain the importance of each. Be sure to describe how the six rights apply to care of the surgical patient.
2. Give an overview of the three verification process and provide a description of when each verification occurs in the surgical setting.
3. Differentiate between a vial and an ampule.
4. Why are some ampules manufactured from tinted glass?
5. List the color outlet or tank color that matches the gasses named.

Name of Gas	Outlet or Cylinder Color
Carbon Dioxide (CO_2)	
Helium (He)	
Medical Air (a mixture of oxygen, nitrogen, carbon dioxide, and argon)	
Nitrogen (N_2)	
Nitrous Oxide (N_2O)	
Oxygen (O_2)	
Suction (not a medical gas; however, the vacuum outlet/connector system is similar in configuration to the medical gas outlet/connectors, therefore, they are often grouped together for logistical reasons)	

6. What types of medications are packaged in tubes?
7. What does the term *contraindication* mean? Provide two examples of situations in which a drug may be contraindicated.
8. Identify five situations in which use of a syringe may be indicated.
9. In which situation is a Toomey syringe most commonly used? Why?
10. Which has a larger diameter, a 10 gauge needle or a 33 gauge needle? Defend your answer.

References

Advanced Precautions for Today's OR. (n.d.). *2000 federal needlestick safety and prevention act*. Retrieved from http://www.orprecautions.com/needlestickact.html

Ahn, W., Bahk, J., & Lim, Y. (2012). *The "gauge" system for the medical use*. Retrieved from http://www.anesthesia-analgesia.org/content/95/4/1125.1.full

Ampule. (n.d.). *Merriam-Webster's medical dictionary*. Retrieved from http://dictionary.reference.com/browse/ampule

Anthem. (2012). *Implantable infusion pumps*. Retrieved from http://www.anthem.com/medicalpolicies/policies/mp_pw_a053366.htm

Anthony, P. (2004). *Delmar learning's pharmacy technician certification exam review* (2nd ed.). Clifton Park, NY: Thomson Delmar Learning.

Association of periOperative Registered Nurses. (2006). *AORN guidance statement: Safe medication practices in perioperative settings across the life span*. AORN Journal August 2006: 276+. Retrieved from http://lirnproxy.museglobal.com/MuseSessionID=c

a2d863d0b5dd1d0b17e9e8583726/MuseHost=go.galegroup.com/MusePath/ps/i.do?action=interpret&id=GALE%7CA150862618&v=2.1&u=lirn_main&it=r&p=HRCA&password=ip&sw=w&authCount=1

Association of Surgical Technologists. (2005). *Guideline statement for safe medication practices in the perioperative area*. Retrieved from http://www.ast.org/pdf/Standards_of_Practice/Guideline_Safe_Medication_Practices.pdf

Bennington, L. (2002). *Gale encyclopedia of nursing and allied health*. Retrieved from http://www.healthline.com/galecontent/medical-gases

Broyles, B., Reiss, B., & Evans, M. (2007). *Pharmacological aspects of nursing care* (7th ed.). Clifton Park, NY: Thomson Delmar Learning.

Centers for Medicare and Medicaid Services (2006). *CMS regulations and guidance manual*. Retrieved from http://www.cms.gov/Regulations-and-Guidance/Guidance/Transmittals/downloads//R22SOMA.pdf

Curren, A. M. (2010). *Dimensional analysis for meds* (4th ed.). Clifton Park, NY: Delmar Cengage Learning.

Dartmouth-Hitchcock. (2012). *Intrathecal infusion pump*. Retrieved from http://patients.dartmouth-hitchcock.org/pain_mgt/intrathecal_infusion_pump.html

Drugs.com (n.d.). *Sterile water for irrigation*. Retrieved from http://www.drugs.com/pro/sterile-water-for-irrigation.html

Flange. (n.d.). *The American heritage® Stedman's medical dictionary*. Retrieved from http://dictionary.reference.com/browse/flange

Food and Drug Administration (2006). *Final rule on prescription drug labeling*. Retrieved from http://www.ncsl.org/default.aspx?tabid=14757

Frey, K., et al. (2008). *Surgical technology for the surgical technologist: A positive care approach* (3rd ed.). Clifton Park, NY: Delmar Cengage Learning.

Galan, N. (2009). *How to select the correct needle size for an injection*. Retrieved from http://pcos.about.com/od/medication1/qt/needlesize.htm

Health Care Without Harm (n.d.). *Vinyl IV bags leach toxic chemicals*. Retrieved from http://www.bbraunusa.com/images/bbraun_usa/IValert.pdf

Institute for Safe Medication Practices (2010). *Frequently asked questions*. Retrieved from http://www.ismp.org/faq.asp

Lal, R. & Kremzner, M. (December 1, 2007). "Introduction to the new prescription drug labeling by the Food and Drug Administration." *American Journal of Health System Pharmacy* vol 64, no. 23, pp. 2488–2494. Retrieved from http://www.medscape.com/viewarticle/566885_2

LoCicero, C. (2006). *Labeling for human prescription drug and biological products—implementing the new content and format requirements.* Retrieved from http://www.fda.gov/downloads/AboutFDA/CentersOffices/CDER/ucm119349.pdf

Lumen. (n.d.). *The American heritage® Stedman's medical dictionary.* Retrieved from http://dictionary.reference.com/browse/lumen

Moini, J. (2009). *Fundamental pharmacology for pharmacy technicians.* Clifton Park, NY: Delmar Cengage Learning.

Stein, H. G. (October 2006). *Glass ampules and filter needles: An example of implementing the sixth 'R' in medication administration.* MedSurg Nursing. Retrieved from http://findarticles.com/p/articles/mi_m0FSS/is_5_15/ai_n17215448

Strategic Applications Incorporated Infusion Technologies. (2011). *Needle gauge chart.* Retrieved from http://www.sai-infusion.com/files/ConversionTable.pdf

Strength. (n.d.). *Drugs@FDA glossary of terms.* Retrieved from http://www.fda.gov/Drugs/informationondrugs/ucm079436.htm#S

The Joint Commission. (2011). *National patient safety goals.* Retrieved from http://www.jointcommission.org/standards_information/npsgs.aspx

Uhle, E. I., Becker, R., Gatscher, S., Bertalanffy, H. (2000). "Continuous intrathecal clonidine administration for the treatment of neuropathic pain." *Journal of Stereotactic and Functional Neurosurgery* vol 75, no. 4, pp. 167-175 (DOI: 10.1159/000048402). Retrieved from http://content.karger.com/ProdukteDB/produkte.asp?Doi=48402

United States Department of Health and Human Services Food and Drug Administration Center for Drug Evaluation and Research (CDER)/Center for Biologics Evaluation and Research (CBER). (2006). *Guidance for industry warnings and precautions, contraindications, and boxed warning sections of labeling for human prescription drug and biological products—content and format.* Retrieved from http://www.fda.gov/downloads/Drugs/GuidanceComplianceRegulatoryInformation/Guidances/ucm075096.pdf

United States Department of Labor Occupational Health and Safety Administration. (2011). *OSHA fact sheet: Protecting yourself when handling contaminated sharps.* Retrieved from http://www.osha.gov/OshDoc/data_BloodborneFacts/bbfact02.pdf

United States Department of Labor Occupational Health and Safety Administration. (2002). *Model plans and programs for the OSHA bloodborne pathogens and hazard communication standards.* Retrieved from http://www.osha.gov/Publications/osha3186.pdf

Unites States Department of Labor Occupational Health and Safety Administration. (n.d.). *Bloodborne pathogens and needlestick prevention.* Retrieved from http://www.osha.gov/SLTC/bloodbornepathogens

United States National Library of Medicine. (2011). *AIDS: Acquired immune deficiency syndrome.* Retrieved from http://www.ncbi.nlm.nih.gov/pubmedhealth/PMH0001620

University of North Carolina Eshelman School of Pharmacy. (2011). *Syringes and needles.* Retrieved from http://pharmlabs.unc.edu/labs/parenterals/syringes.htm

Vree, P. (2005). *The challenge of health care developments for hospital pharmacy.* Pharmacy World & Science. Retrieved from http://www.springerlink.com/content/p6442828218g3u89/fulltext.pdf?page=1

Wisconsin Department of Health Services (n.d.). *Six rights of medication administration.* Retrieved from http://dhs.wisconsin.gov/rl_dsl/MedManagement/sixRghtsMedAdm.pdf

Woodrow, R. (2007). *Essentials of pharmacology for health occupations* (5th ed.). Clifton Park, NY: Thomson Delmar Learning.

Chapter
TEN

MEDICATIONS COMMONLY USED IN THE SURGICAL ENVIRONMENT

Student Learning Outcomes

After studying this chapter, the reader should be able to:

- List and describe various medication types commonly used for surgical patients.
- Predict the type of situations in which each medication type would be prescribed.
- Provide at least one example of a medication in each category.

Key Terms

Adrenergic
Amnesia
Analeptic
Analgesic
Antibiotic
Anticholinergic
Anticoagulant
Anticonvulsant
Antiemetic
Antihistamine
Antihypertensive
Antimuscarinic
Antimycotic
Antineoplastic
Antipyretic
Antiseptic
Barbiturate
Benzodiazepine
Beta-adrenergic blocker

Beta-blocker
Beta-lactam
Biological response modifier
Cholinergic
Cholinergic blocker
Coagulant
Colloid plasma expander
Crystalloid
Cycloplegic
Disinfectant
Dye
Emetic
Fibrinolysis
H_1 receptor antagonist
H_2 antagonist
Hemolytic
Hemostatic
Hypnotic
Inotropic effect

Insulin
Irrigate
Isotonic
Loop diuretic
Lubricant
Methicillin-resistant
  Staphylococcus aureus
  (MRSA)
Mydriasis
Miotic
Mitotic inhibitor
Mydriatic
Negative contrast media
Nerve conduction blocking
  agent
Neuroleptic
Neuromuscular blocker
Osmotic diuretic
Oxytocic

Paradoxical
Positive contrast media
Procoagulant
Sedative
Soporific
Stain
Sterilant
Tamponade
Tensile strength
Thrombolytic
Tranquilizer
Vasoconstrictor
Vasodilator
Zonulysis

MEDICATIONS COMMONLY USED IN THE SURGICAL ENVIRONMENT

Chapter Three provides information concerning the three types of drug nomenclature as well as an introduction to the many ways that drugs are classified. To review, the main classifications are:

- Principal Action—Main action determined by the type of chemical used in preparing the drug. Principal action is sometimes referred to as chemical action.

- Body System Affected—Many drugs are classified according to the body system that is affected by the action of the drug.

- Physiological Action—Drugs that change the function of the body (physiologic action) are placed in this category.

- Therapeutic Action—Drugs are also classified according to the benefits they provide.

In this chapter, the focus is on describing the action(s) of the drugs within each classification and subclassification and the emphasis is on medications commonly used during the three phases of surgical case management. To review from Chapter One, drugs are given for prophylactic reasons or to diagnose, treat, cure, or mitigate a disease or condition. Keep in mind that a drug may be assigned more than one classification.

Amnesics

The term *amnesia* refers to loss of memory. Amnesic drugs are given to the patient prior to or during a medical or surgical procedure to induce temporary memory loss. Midazolam (Versed®) is a **benzodiazepine** that has amnesic properties.

Analgesics/Antipyretics

The term *analgesia* refers to reduction or elimination of pain and the term *antipyretic* refers to reduction or elimination of fever. Often, a single drug, such as aspirin which is a salicylate, is capable of performing both functions.

Analgesics are available in several strengths (such as over-the-counter, prescription and narcotic) and can be used to treat mild, moderate, or severe pain. The term *analgetic* may also be used to describe analgesic drugs.

Three types of drugs (salicylates, acetaminophen, and nonsteroidal anti-inflammatory drugs) have antipyretic properties. The terms *febrifuge, antithermic,* and *antifebrile* may also be used to describe an antipyretic drug.

Anesthesia Agents

Note: Content of this segment is limited to local and topical anesthesia agents and does not include information concerning general anesthetics or anesthesia administration techniques.

The term *anesthesia* refers to lack of sensation. Drugs in this category are sometimes referred to as **nerve conduction blocking agents** because they prevent conduction of pain sensation impulses initiated in the nerves at the surgical site from reaching the brain. Anesthesia agents are used to manage intraoperative and postoperative pain. Anesthesia agents fall into two subclassifications known as amino amides and amino esters. Drugs in both classifications may be manufactured with or without epinephrine added. If epinephrine is added by the manufacturer, red color coding will be visible on the label. The term *plain* is sometimes used to indicate that epinephrine has not been added to the anesthesia agent.

Amino Amides

Drugs in the amino amide group are biotransformed in the liver and excreted by the kidneys in the urine. Because biotransformation takes place in the liver, amino amides may cause toxicity in individuals with abnormal liver function. Table 10-1 identifies several drugs in the amino amide group and provides information concerning the possible routes of administration, onset of action, duration of action, and the recognized maximum/toxic adult dose.

Amino Esters

Drugs in the amino ester group are biotransformed in the blood plasma by pseudocholinesterase, which is an enzyme produced in the liver. Table 10-2 identifies several drugs in the amino ester group and provides information concerning the possible routes of administration, onset of action, duration of action, and the recognized maximum/toxic adult dose.

Agonistic Anesthetic Agents

Two medications are often used in conjunction with local anesthesia agents to enhance and/or prolong their effects. The two medications that act as agonists to anesthetic agents are epinephrine (adrenaline) and hyaluronidase (Amphadase®, Hylenex®, and Vitrase®). One or both agents are added to an anesthetic agent and administered parenterally.

Epinephrine is a vasoconstrictor that not only helps reduce the risk of bleeding at the surgical site, but also helps to retain the anesthetic agent in the area of infiltration for a prolonged period of time. Due to its vasoconstrictive properties, epinephrine use should be restricted in small children and in individuals who experience

TABLE 10-1 Amino Amides

Name of Drug	Type of Nerve Conduction Blockade	Onset of Action	Duration of Action	Maximum/Toxic Dose (Adult)
bupivacaine hydrochloride (Marcaine® and Sensorcaine®)	Local Regional	Slow	Long (2–5 hours)	2.5–3 mg per kg 400 mg per 24-hour period
etidocaine (Duranest®)	Topical Local Regional	Slow	Long (3–12 hours)	300–400 mg
lidocaine hydrochloride (Xylocaine® and Lignocaine®)	Topical Local Regional	Rapid	Intermediate (1–3 hours)	7 mg per kg 400–500 mg
mepivacaine hydrochloride (Carbocaine®)	Local Regional	Rapid	Intermediate (1–3 hours)	5–6 mg per kg 400–500 mg

Notes: Lidocaine is also classified as an antidysrhythmic and etidocaine is contraindicated in children under the age of 12.

TABLE 10-2 Amino Esters

Name of Drug	Type of Nerve Conduction Blockade	Onset of Action	Duration of Action	Maximum/Toxic Dose (Adult)
benzocaine (Americaine® and Anbesol®)	Topical	Slow	Short	200–300 mg
Chloroprocaine (Nesacaine®)	Local Regional	Rapid	Short	800–1,000 mg
cocaine hydrochloride	Topical	Slow	Short	4 mg per kg 200 mg
procaine hydrochloride (Novocaine®)	Local Regional	Slow	Short	1,000 mg
tetracaine hydrochloride (Pontocaine®)	Topical Regional	Slow	Long	2 mg per kg 120 mg

Notes: Cocaine is also classified as a narcotic; because cocaine is a narcotic it is metabolized differently than the other amino esters (cocaine is biotransformed in the liver and excreted by the kidneys in the urine).

hypertension, coronary artery disease, or vascular compromise at the planned surgical site. For the same reason, epinephrine is not recommended for use in body regions served by small blood vessels such as the ears, digits of the hands and feet, nose, and penis. The rhyme, "ears – fingers, toes, penis, nose" may serve as a useful reminder of the restricted areas.

Hyaluronidase is an enzyme that allows the anesthetic agent to penetrate the connective tissue more readily and, therefore, enhances and prolongs the effect of the anesthetic agent.

Anticoagulants/Fibrinolytics

The term *anticoagulant* refers to interference with or prevention of the blood clotting (coagulation) process and the term *fibrinolytic* refers to destruction of fibrin, which is a major component of a blood clot. Anticoagulants, such as heparin and warfarin (Coumadin®) act to deter blood clots from forming and fibrinolytics, such as tissue plasminogen activator (tPA) and reteplase (Retavase®) act to break apart blood clots that have already formed. The terms *fibrinolytic* and ***thrombolytic*** may be used interchangeably.

Anticonvulsants

The term ***anticonvulsant*** refers to prevention of or reducing the effects of a seizure. A seizure is caused when there is abnormal electrical activity in the brain. Seizures can range in severity from mild to serious. A patient experiencing a seizure may exhibit changes in consciousness, emotion, sensation, vision, and taste as well as changes in muscle tone including loss of muscle control or muscle twitching and tightening that cause spasmodic movements. Anticonvulsants are also referred to as antiepileptics because epilepsy is a common seizure disorder. Examples of anticonvulsant drugs include phenytoin (Dilantin®) and midazolam (Versed®).

Antiemetics

The term *antiemetic* refers to reduction or elimination of nausea and vomiting (emesis). Antiemetic drugs are used to treat the side effects of general anesthetics, opiate/opioid analgesics, and chemotherapy agents as well as motion sickness and nausea/emesis gravidarum (morning sickness) related to pregnancy. Antiemetic drugs are actually a collection of drugs from several other drug classifications. Table 10-3 provides an abbreviated listing of antiemetic drugs and their classifications. The table also includes examples of naturopathic and alternative antiemetic treatments.

Antihistamines

Histamines are amine compounds (organic compounds containing ammonia) that are released by the mast cells (type of cell found in connective tissue) during an allergic reaction. Common allergens include pollens, foods, medications, and venom related to snake and insect bites. Release of histamines causes dilation and increased permeability of blood vessels, which leads to common allergy symptoms such as sneezing, allergic rhinitis (runny nose), itching, swelling (of the eyelids, lips, tongue, throat, etc.), increased production of gastric acid, smooth muscle contraction, and urticaria (hives) as well as more severe symptoms such a hypotension and anaphylaxis. The prefix anti- means against. Therefore, **antihistamines** are drugs used to reduce or counteract the effects of histamines during an allergic reaction. Antihistamines are also known as H_1 **receptor antagonists**. An example of an antihistamine is diphenhydramine (Benadryl®).

Anti-Infective Agents

The term *anti-infective* agent is used to identify a broad range of chemicals that are capable of killing pathogens or hindering their growth. Pathogens are substances, which are capable of causing disease such as bacteria, fungi, and viruses. Antibacterial, antifungal, and antiviral agents are all examples of anti-infective agents. Anti-infective agents are grouped according to their action and use.

Refer to a microbiology book for information concerning the various types of pathogens, classifications, and identification techniques.

Beta-Lactams

Beta-lactams are a group of antibacterial agents that includes penicillins, cephalosporins, and carbapenems (among others). Drugs in the beta-lactam group are not effective against resting bacteria but work by inhibiting the enzymes necessary to manufacture the cell wall as the bacteria reproduces.

Penicillins are natural or semisynthetic substances that are derived from *Penicillium* molds, which are commonly found on the skin of citrus fruits. Penicillins are available in oral or parenteral forms. Drugs in the penicillin group are further divided into four classifications.

TABLE 10-3 Antiemetic Drug Classifications and Examples

Antiemetics	Drug/Therapy Name
Alternative	Acupuncture Hypnosis
Anticholinergics (also known as antimuscarinics, cholinergic blockers, and parasympatholytics)	Scopolamine
Antihistamines (H_1 histamine receptor antagonists)	Diphenhydramine (Benadryl®) Hydroxyzine (Vistaril®) Promethazine (Phenergan®)
Benzodiazepines	Midazolam (Versed®)
Cannabis/Cannabinoids	Cannabis (medical marijuana) Nabilone (Cesamet®)
Dopamine antagonists	Droperidol (Inapsine®) Metoclopramide (Reglan®)
Naturopathic	Peppermint Zingiber officinale (ginger)
Steroids	Dexamethasone (Decadron®)

- Ampicillin-like drugs—Primarily effective against enterococci and some gram-negative bacilli. Examples of ampicillin-like drugs include ampicillin (Omnipen®, Polycillin®, and Principen®) and amoxicillin (Amoxil® and Moxilin®).

- Broad-spectrum penicillins—Also called antipseudomonal penicillins. Primarily effective against many strains of *Pseudomonas aeruginosa*. Examples of broad-spectrum penicillins include carbenicillin (Geocillin®), piperacillin (Pipracil®), and ticarcillin (Ticar®).

- Penicillin G-like drugs—Primarily effective against most gram-positive bacteria and a few gram-negative cocci. Examples of penicillin G-like drugs include Penicillin G (Bicillin L-A®) and Penicillin V (V-Cillin® and Beepen-VK®).

- Penicillinase-resistant penicillins—Penicillinase is an enzyme that is produced by certain bacteria that make the bacteria resistant to penicillins. Therefore, penicillinase-resistant penicillins are effective against bacteria such as **methicillin-resistant Staphylococcus aureus** (MRSA) and *Staphylococcus pneumonia*. Examples of penicillinase-resistant penicillins include dicloxacillin (Dycill® and Dynapen®), nafcillin (Nallpen® and Unipen®), and oxacillin (Bactocill®).

Note: Methicillin (Staphcillin®) is a penicillin that was widely used until bacterial resistance rendered it ineffective.

Cephalosporins are substances derived from the *Acremonium* fungus (formerly called *Cephalosporium*) commonly found in soil. Cephalosporins are available in oral or parenteral forms. Drugs in the cephalosporin group are further classified in generations.

- First-generation cephalosporins—Primarily effective against gram-positive cocci. First-generation drugs include cefazolin (Ancef®) and cephalexin (Keflex®).

- Second-generation cephalosporins and cephamycins—Primarily effective against gram-positive cocci and some gram-negative bacilli and cephamycins are effective against *Bacteroides*. Second-generation drugs include cefotetan (Cefotan®) and cefoxitin (Mefoxin®).

- Third-generation cephalosporins—Primarily effective against *Haemophilus influenzae*, some enterobacteriaceae (such as *Escherichia coli*, *Klebsiella pneumonia*), and *Pseudomonas aeruginosa*. Third-generation drugs include cefotaxime (Claforan®) and ceftriaxone (Rocephin®).

- Fourth-generation cephalosporin—Primarily effective against gram-positive cocci and gram-negative bacilli. Currently, the only known fourth-generation drug is cefepime (Maxipime®) that is only available parenterally.

- Fifth-generation cephalosporin—Primarily effective against MRSA. Currently the fifth-generation drug ceftobiprole (Zeftera® and Zevtera®) is in use abroad, but is not currently available in the United States.

Carbapenems originate from thienamycin, which is a product of the *Streptomyces cattleya* bacteria that is found in soil. Carbapenems are primarily effective against *Haemophilus influenza*, anaerobes, most enterobacteriaceae, and methicillin-resistant staphylococci and streptococci. Examples of carbapenems include ertapenem (Invanz®) and imipenem (Primaxin®). Carbapenems are available only parenterally.

Sulfonamides

The sulfonamides, sometimes called sulfa drugs, are synthetic agents that work by disrupting synthesis of folic acid, thereby negatively impacting production of deoxyribonucleic acid (DNA) and purine. Sulfonamides are primarily effective against many gram-positive and gram-negative bacteria and may be administered topically, orally, or parenterally. Allergic reactions to sulfonamides are common and bacterial resistance is extensive. Examples of sulfonamide drugs include sulfacetamide (Klaron®), sulfamethoxazole (Gantanol®), and sulfasalazine (Azulfidine®).

Polypeptides

Drugs in the polypeptide group, sometimes referred to as the polymyxins, are produced by the organism *Bacillus polymyxa* which is a gram-positive bacterium. Polypeptides bind to the bacterial cell membrane disrupting the cell's ability to release toxins. Polypeptides are primarily effective against most gram-negative bacteria and are available for topical and parenteral administration. Examples of polypeptides include bacitracin (Baciguent® and Baci-IM®), polymyxin B (Polytrim®), and polymyxin E (Colistin®).

Aminoglycosides

Drugs in the aminoglycoside group were originally derived from bacteria in two groups: the drugs ending with the suffix -mycin originate from the *Streptomyces* family while the drugs ending with the suffix -micin originate from the *Micromonospora* family. Now, many of the aminoglycosides are synthetic. Aminoglycosides have been proven to interrupt protein synthesis of the ribosomes in the bacterial cell thereby preventing growth of the cell; however, there is evidence that aminoglycosides are also capable of degrading the bacterial cell wall causing destruction of the cell. Aminoglycosides are effective against most gram-negative aerobic bacilli (especially

Pseudomonas aeruginosa) and facultative (able to survive in more than one environment) anaerobic bacilli. Aminoglycosides are available in topical, oral, and parenteral forms. Examples of aminoglycosides include gentamicin (Garamycin®), kanamycin (Kantrex®), neomycin, streptomycin, and tobramycin.

Tetracyclines

Tetracyclines are derived from *Actinobacteria*, which is part of the *Streptomyces* family. Tetracyclines disrupt protein synthesis of the cell rendering the cell incapable of reproduction. Tetracyclines are effective against a wide variety of gram-negative and gram-positive bacteria. Tetracyclines are available for topical, oral, and parenteral administration. Examples of tetracyclines include doxycycline (Monodox® and Vibramycin®), minocycline (Dynacin® and Minocin®), and tetracycline (Tetracon®).

Antifungals

Fungal infections are referred to as mycoses. Mycoses include fungi, molds, and yeasts that can affect the skin, mucous membranes, tissues, and blood. Antifungal drugs, also known as **antimycotics**, are used to inhibit the growth of or kill fungal infections and are made from mold or produced synthetically. Antifungal drugs are available in topical, oral, and parenteral forms. There are three main classifications of antifungal drugs:

- Polyenes—React with substances in the fungal cell membrane to form channels that allow the cell contents to be expelled rendering the cell unable to reproduce. Examples of polyene antifungal drugs include amphotericin B (Amphocin®), nystatin (Mycostatin®), and pimaricin (Natamycin®).

- Azoles—Inhibit an enzyme necessary to the structure of the fungal cell membrane and internal functions of the cell thereby preventing growth of the fungus. Examples of azole antifungal drugs include fluconazole (Diflucan®), itraconazole (Sporanox®), posaconazole (Noxafil®), and voriconazole (Vfend®).

- Echinocandins—Inhibit synthesis of the fungal cell wall disrupting the life cycle of the fungus. Examples of echinocandins include caspofungin (Cancidas®), micafungin (Mycamine®), and anidulafungin (Eraxis®).

Antimicrobials

Broad spectrum antimicrobials are used in the surgical setting as antiseptics, disinfectants, and sterilants. Concentration and exposure time of the agent is determined by the manufacturer in accordance with guidelines issued by the Centers for Disease Control (CDC). Variations in concentration and exposure time allow the same agent to be effective at more than one level.

Antiseptics **Antiseptics** are used on living tissue (during the surgical scrub or the skin prep) to prohibit growth of or destroy microorganisms. The term *biostasis* is used to describe antiseptics that cause inactivity of microbes and the term *biocide* is used to describe agents that kill microbes. Examples of topical antiseptics include alcohol, chlorhexidine, chloroxylenol, and iodine/iodophor.

Disinfectants **Disinfectants** are used on fomites (inanimate objects) to destroy pathogens. Disinfectants are too harsh to use on living tissue. Disinfection occurs on three levels:

- Low-level disinfection kills most bacteria but not bacterial spores and is ineffective against the organism that causes tuberculosis. Low-level disinfectants also kill some viruses and fungi. Low-level disinfectants are used on noncritical items; noncritical items come in contact with only intact skin (e.g., a blood pressure cuff). Examples of low-level disinfectants include isopropyl alcohol (70–90%), sodium hypochlorite, phenol (carbolic acid), iodophor, and quaternary ammonium compounds.

- Intermediate-level disinfection kills most microorganisms (bacteria, fungi, and viruses) including the tuberculosis bacilli and the hepatitis B virus but not bacterial spores. Intermediate-level disinfectants are used on semi-critical items; semi-critical items come in contact with nonintact skin and mucous membranes (e.g., airway maintenance devices). Examples of intermediate-level disinfectants include isopropyl alcohol (70-90%), sodium hypochlorite, phenol (carbolic acid), and iodophor (concentrations and/or exposure times are increased).

- High-level disinfection kills all microorganisms with the exception of bacterial spores and prions. High-level disinfectants are used on critical items; critical items come in contact with sterile tissue (e.g., urinary catheters and surgical instruments). Examples of high-level disinfectants include glutaraldehyde and ortho-phthalaldehyde.

Note: Sterilization is preferred when using most critical items, but some critical items are delicate and cannot withstand the chemical exposure, heat, or pressure associated with certain sterilization techniques.

Sterilants Sterilization is a chemical or physical process by which all microorganisms including bacterial spores are killed. Examples of chemical **sterilants** include ethylene oxide gas (EO or EtO), hydrogen peroxide plasma

(Sterrad®), glutaraldehyde (Cidex®), and peracetic acid (Steris®). Steam is the primary physical process used for sterilization because it is easily accessible and inexpensive.

Antineoplastics (Chemotherapy Agents)

Antineoplastic drugs (also known as chemotherapy agents and anticancer drugs) are used in the treatment of various types of cancer. The term *neoplasm* means new growth and when talking about cancer, the new growth is malignant. Treatments for cancer include surgery, radiation, chemotherapy and/or alternative therapies. There are several classifications of chemotherapeutic drugs and each class has its own mechanism of action. A chemotherapeutic drug may be prescribed alone or a combination with other drugs and therapies. Chemotherapeutic agents are available in topical, oral, and parenteral forms. Because antineoplastic drugs have toxic effects, healthcare workers must adhere to safe handling practices concerning transport, storage, preparation, administration, and disposal of antineoplastic drugs and any related supplies. Table 10-4 identifies some common antineoplastic drug classifications, mechanism of action,

examples of drugs in each class, and the type of cancer affected by each drug.

Autonomic Agents

Autonomic agents affect the autonomic (involuntary) portion of the central nervous system. Organs involved with the autonomic nervous system include the glands, the heart, and the smooth muscles of the blood vessels and hollow viscera. Messages are transmitted between the central nervous system and the autonomic organs via autonomic pathways that involve two motor neurons. For the impulse to be carried across the synapse in the ganglia connecting the two motor neurons, a chemical called a neurotransmitter must be present. The autonomic nervous system has two divisions:

- Sympathetic—The sympathetic portion of the autonomic nervous system provides the fight-or-flight response that is activated when a major stressful incident occurs. The term ***adrenergic*** means activated by adrenaline. The adrenergic neurotransmitter adrenaline (epinephrine) and a related substance called noradrenaline (norepinephrine) activate the sympathetic portion of the nervous system.

TABLE 10-4 Antineoplastic Drugs

Classification	Mechanism of Action	Drug Name (Limited Examples)	Type of Cancer Affected
Alkylating Agents	Modify the DNA base of the cancer cell by adding an alkyl group thereby disrupting transcription and replication of the cell	• carmustine (BCNU® and BiCNU®) • cisplatin (Platin® and Platinol®) • thiotepa (Thioplex®)	• Brain • Leukemia • Lymphoma • Metastatic bladder cancer • Metastatic ovarian cancer • Metastatic testicular cancer • Sarcoma • Bone
Antiandrogen	Block the production of testosterone or the ability of testosterone to bind with cells that depend on testosterone for growth	• leuprolide acetate (Lupron Depot®) • bicalutamide (Casodex®) • flutamide (Drogenil®)	• Prostate cancer
Antibiotic antineoplastics	Bind to DNA interfering with transcription or inhibit enzymes that maintain integrity of DNA	• bleomycin (Blenoxane®) • doxorubicin (Rubex®) • mitomycin (Mutamycin®)	• Breast cancer • Hodgkin's disease • Leukemias • Lymphoma • Sarcoma • Testicular
Antiestrogen	Block the production of estrogen or the ability of estrogen to bind with cells that depend on estrogen for growth	• anastrozole (Arimidex®) • fulvestrant (Faslodex®) • letrozole (Femara®) • tamoxifen (Nolvadex®)	• Breast

Antimetabolites	Interfere with cell metabolism by interrupting production of enzymes that affect DNA structure	• methotrexate (Trexal®) • 5-fluorouracil (Adrucil® and Efudex®) • 6-mercaptopurine (Purinethol®) • Cladribine (Leustatin®)	• Breast • Gastro intestinal • Gestational choriocarcinoma • Leukemias • Leukemic meningitis • Ovarian • Bone
Biological response modifiers	Immune system substances such as antibodies and cytokines that increase the patient's biological response to the tumor	• Interferons • Interleukin-2 • Colony stimulating factors • Tumor necrosis factor Note: This section contains general classifications of biological response modifiers rather than specific drugs	• Lymphocytic leukemia • Melanoma • Colorectal • Neuroblastoma • Renal • Non-Hodgkin's lymphoma
Plant alkaloids (also called **mitotic inhibitors**)	Interrupt various stages of cell division (mitosis) according to the type of drug	• vinblastine (Velban®) • vincristine (Oncovin®) • etoposide (VP-16) • teniposide (VM-26)	• Lung • Breast • Ovarian • Thyroid • Esophageal • Bladder • Head and neck • Kaposi sarcoma • Renal
Steroid hormones (includes antiandrogens and antiestrogens)	Reduce hormone concentration to tumors dependent on hormones for growth	• goserelin (Zoladex®) • degarelix (Firmagon®) • dutasteride (Avodart®) • finasteride (Proscar®) • aminoglutethimide (Cytadren®) • anastrozole (Arimidex®) • letrozole (Femara®) • exemestane (Aromasin®)	• Prednisone-sensitive lymphoma • Androgen-sensitive prostate • Estrogen-sensitive breast

- Parasympathetic—The parasympathetic portion of the autonomic nervous system is the normal operational mode of the body and helps return an individual to homeostasis following a major stressful incident. The term *cholinergic* means activated by acetylcholine. The cholinergic neurotransmitter acetylcholine activates the parasympathetic portion of the nervous system.

Autonomic agents are available in oral and parenteral forms. Refer to an anatomy and physiology book for additional information concerning the divisions of the nervous system, the related structures, and the functions of each.

Adrenergics

Adrenergics (also called sympathomimetics or adrenergic agonists) are used to mimic the effects of the sympathetic nervous system. Adrenergics are capable of causing bronchodilation, stimulation of the heart, increasing blood flow to the voluntary (skeletal) muscles, pupil dilation (**mydriasis**), and constriction of the peripheral blood vessels. Examples of adrenergics include ephedrine, epinephrine (adrenaline), dopamine (Intropin®), isoproterenol (Isuprel®), metaraminol (Aramine®), and norepinephrine (Levophed®).

Adrenergic Blockers (Alpha and Beta)

Adrenergic blockers, also called adrenergic antagonists and sympatholytics, inhibit the effects of the sympathetic nervous system. There are two types of adrenergic blockers; alpha-blockers and beta-blockers.

- Alpha-blockers are capable of relaxation of the smooth muscle found at the bladder neck and in the prostate and reducing hypertension. Examples of alpha-blockers include doxazosin (Cardura®), tamsulosin (Flomax®), and terazosin (Hytrin®).

- **Beta-blockers** are capable of reducing hypertension, resolving cardiac dysrhythmias, lowering intraocular pressure, and relieving angina pectoris as well as migraine headaches. Examples of beta-blockers include atenolol (Tenormin®), metoprolol (Lopressor®), and propranolol (Inderal®).

Cholinergics

Cholinergics, also called parasympathomimetics and muscarinics, are used to mimic the effects of the parasympathetic nervous system. Cholinergics are capable of slowing of the heart, pupil constriction, increased gastrointestinal peristalsis, increased production of secretions (such as gastric juices, mucous, saliva, and sweat), increased contractibility of the urinary bladder, increased strength of the skeletal muscles, pupil constriction (miosis), and decreased intraocular pressure. Examples of cholinergics include bethanechol (Urecholine®), edrophonium (Tensilon®), neostigmine (Prostigmin®), and pilocarpine (Isopto Carpine®).

Cholinergic Blockers

Cholinergic blockers (also called **anticholinergics, antimuscarinics**, and **parasympatholytics**) are used to block the effects of the parasympathetic nervous system. Cholinergic blockers are capable of decreased production of secretions (such as gastric juices, mucous, saliva, and sweat), decreased peristalsis of the gastrointestinal tract, dilation of the pupils, and decreased contractibility of the urinary bladder. Examples of cholinergic blockers include atropine, glycopyrrolate (Robinul®), homatropine (Isopto Homatropine®), propantheline (Pro-Banthine®), and scopolamine (Transderm Scop®).

Blood Replacement Interventions

Blood replacement intervention may be necessary because of disease processes, effects of certain medications, surgery, and trauma. Several options are available when attempting to restore the patient's normal blood volume and blood pressure. Available options include autologous blood, homologous blood, and non-blood replacements such as colloid plasma expanders.

Autologous Blood

Autologous blood (the prefix -auto means self or same) is taken from and reinfused to the same individual. Autologous blood is preferred over donated blood products because the danger of incompatibility and the risk of disease transmission are eliminated. Collection, processing, storage, and return of the blood must take place using sterile technique. Autologous blood cannot be used in some situations; those situations include presence of fever or infection, use of some hemostatic agents and antibiotics, presence of cancer cells, and exposure of the blood to amniotic fluid or gastrointestinal contents. In the surgical setting, a patient may donate his or her own blood for reuse preoperatively, intraoperatively, or postoperatively.

- Preoperatively, autologous blood may be collected from the patient (usually at a blood donation center) in advance of anticipated need, packaged, labeled, stored in the appropriate conditions (usually refrigerated in the blood bank), and returned to the patient as needed.

- Intraoperatively, blood that is lost during surgery is salvaged (suctioned from the surgical wound or extracted from saturated surgical sponges), mixed with an anticoagulant, filtered, and separated to allow only the red blood cells as well as some plasma proteins important to the clotting cascade and platelets to be returned to the patient intravenously. Equipment for processing the blood may be located in the operating room or in the lab. Alternatively, if blood processing equipment is not available, the blood may be salvaged in a collection bag that has been treated with an anticoagulant and returned to the patient intravenously with the use of a specialized blood filter without any additional processing.

- Postoperatively, blood is collected into a specialized wound drainage system. According to the situation, the blood may or may not be processed (anticoagulated, filtered, separated, and/or washed) prior to intravenous reinfusion.

Donated Blood Products

Donated blood products are said to be homologous (the prefix -homo means similar such as from a similar species) or allogeneic (meaning different, but of the same kind). Donated blood products are taken from one individual and infused into someone else. Donated blood products available for transfusion include whole blood, red cells, platelets, and plasma (and fractions thereof) and all blood donors and donated blood products are prescreened to reduce the risk of transmission of disease from the donor to the recipient.

Type and Cross Matching There are four blood types (A, B, AB, and O) plus the Rh factor (also called factor D), which is considered to be present (positive) or absent (negative). Individuals with the blood type O– (Rh negative) are considered to be the universal blood donor because in an emergency situation, O– blood can be received by any individual and individuals with the blood type AB+ (Rh positive) are considered to be the universal blood recipient because in an emergency situation, blood of any type can be received with little risk for occurrence of a transfusion reaction. Certain blood types cannot be mixed because of the risk of an allergic reaction or a **hemolytic** transfusion reaction during which the transfused donor blood cells are destroyed by the recipient's immune system. Initial symptoms of a hemolytic transfusion reaction involve reddening of the skin, back and/or flank pain, fever and/or chills, dizziness and/or fainting, and hematuria (blood in the urine) and more serious complications can include anemia, respiratory distress, kidney failure, and shock. Symptoms of a hemolytic transfusion reaction may appear during or shortly after the blood transfer begins or may be delayed for several days. If any type of reaction is detected in the recipient, the transfusion must be terminated immediately, treatment initiated, and the event documented. To reduce the risk of a hemolytic transfusion reaction, a procedure called a type and cross match is performed on the blood of both the donor and the recipient. The blood is tested to identify not only the blood type and Rh factor but also to determine the presence of any additional antibodies in the donor blood that could be harmful to the recipient.

Standards for blood collection, processing, storage, and transfusion are set forth by the American Association of Blood Banks (AABB). Refer to a hematology book or an anatomy and physiology book for additional information concerning the blood, blood types, and possible transfusion reactions.

Whole Blood Use of whole blood is recommended in situations where significant blood loss occurs (due to surgical intervention or as a result of a traumatic event). Whole blood has not had any portion removed (although an anticoagulant has been added) and quickly restores blood volume and helps to maintain blood pressure while replacing all of the lost blood components.

Component Therapy Instead of transfusing whole blood, specific portions of the blood may be separated and used as needed. One unit (450 milliliters or approximately 474 grams) of whole blood from a single donor may be divided to benefit multiple recipients. Blood components include red blood cells (sometimes called packed cells) and platelet rich plasma which may be further separated into platelet concentrate and plasma. Cryoprecipitate (that contains Factor VIII, fibrinogen, von Willebrand factor, and Factor XIII), plasma proteins, albumin, immunoglobulin, and other clotting factor derivatives are examples of components that can be fractionated from blood plasma.

Colloid Plasma Expanders

A colloid is a large molecular weight insoluble particle such as gelatin or a starch placed in a solution that can be administered as a plasma expander to patients experiencing low blood volume. Plasma proteins (albumin, fibrinogen, globulin, and others in small amounts) are the natural colloids found in blood. Colloids are too large to pass through the capillary membrane and are useful in maintaining colloid osmotic pressure (also called oncotic pressure). Oncotic pressure draws in and retains fluid within the blood vessels helping to maintain blood pressure and circulate remaining red blood cells so that oxygen is provided to the tissues. Colloid solutions are hypertonic. Examples of **colloid plasma expanders**

include albumin (available in 5% and 25% strengths), dextran (available in 6% and 10% strengths), hydroxyethyl starch/hetastarch (Hespan® and Voluven®), pentastarch (Pentaspan®), polygeline (Haemaccel®), and succinylated gelatin (Gelofusine®).

Note: Information concerning crystalloid solutions is found in the IV Fluids segment of this chapter.

Cardiovascular Agents

Cardiovascular agents affect not only the heart but the blood vessels as well. Cardiovascular agents are capable of correcting some heart rhythm abnormalities by changing the speed at which electrical impulse are conducted through the heart muscle (dromotropic effect) and increasing or decreasing the heart rate (chronotropic effect), the force of the contractions of the heart (**inotropic effect**), and the blood pressure. Cardiovascular agents are available in oral and parenteral preparations and some drugs produce more than one effect on the cardiovascular system.

Antidysrhythmics

Heart rhythm abnormalities are called dysrhythmias. Sometimes the term *arrhythmia* is used synonymously with the term *dysrhythmia*. Refer to an anatomy and physiology or a cardiology book for information concerning normal heart rhythm, various types of dysrhythmias, and the causes of each. According to the Vaughan-Williams classification system, there are four main classifications of antidysrhythmic drugs and some miscellaneous drugs that are also used to treat dysrhythmias.

- Class I (Sodium-channel blockers)—Lengthen the amount of time needed for an electrical impulse to move from the sinoatrial node, through the heart, to the Purkinje fibers and stimulate the ventricles to contract which increases the amount of time between heartbeats. Sodium-channel blockers reduce the number of sodium ions available to conduct the impulse; thereby, slowing movement of the impulse. There are three types of sodium-channel blockers:
  - Type IA—Slow the heart rate by delaying the time between heartbeats. Examples of Type IA sodium-channel blockers include disopyramide (Norpace®), procainamide (Pronestyl®), and quinidine (Cardioquin®).
  - Type IB—Slow the heart rate by delaying movement of the electrical impulse as it travels through the cardiac conduction system. Examples of Type IB sodium-channel blockers include lidocaine (Xylocaine®), mexiletine (Mexitil®), and tocainide (Tonocard®).

- Type IC—Significantly slow the heart rate by reducing the speed of movement of the electrical impulse by increasing the time that elapses between the sinoatrial node emitting the impulse until the ventricles contract. Examples of Type IC sodium-channel blockers include flecainide (Tambocor®) and propafenone (Rhythmol®).

- Class II (Beta-blockers—also called **beta-adrenergic blockers**)—Slow the heart rate by reducing the effects of influences from sympathetic nervous system. Beta-blockers block the effects of catecholamines such as epinephrine and norepinephrine at the adrenergic receptors. In addition to correcting dysrhythmias, beta-blockers are also useful in reducing hypertension, relieving angina, and decreasing the metabolic needs of the heart. Examples of beta-blockers include atenolol (Tenormin®), metoprolol (Lopressor®), and propranolol (Inderal®).

- Class III (Potassium-channel blockers)—Slow electrical impulses as they move through the heart and increase the time between heartbeats. Potassium-channel blockers reduce the number of potassium ions available to conduct the impulse; thereby, slowing movement of the impulse.

- Class IV (Calcium-channel blockers)—Reduce the force of each heartbeat. Calcium-channel blockers limit the amount of calcium in the muscle which reduces the contractile force of the muscle and decreases the heart's need for oxygen and nutrients. In addition to correcting dysrhythmias, calcium-channel blockers are also useful in decreasing blood pressure in patients with hypertension, preventing cerebral vasospasm, and reducing chest pain related to angina pectoris. Examples of calcium-channel blockers include diltiazem (Cardizem®) and verapamil (Isoptin® and Calan®).

- Miscellaneous
  - Adenosine (Adenocard®)—Slows the electrical impulse as it passes through the atrioventricular node.
  - Nutritional supplements such as magnesium and potassium promote nerve and muscle function. In addition to their cardiac effects, both magnesium and potassium are essential to many body functions.

Coronary Dilators

Coronary dilators are used to relieve chest pain related to angina. Angina is caused by narrowing of the coronary arteries due to the presence of plaque or vasospasm. Nitrate and non-nitrate drugs are used to cause vasodilation of the coronary arteries, thereby restoring blood flow to the heart. Additionally, coronary dilators are useful in lowering the blood pressure, treatment of heart failure and myocardial infarction, and inhibition of platelet aggregation. Coronary dilators are available in topical (often prescribed sublingually), oral, and parenteral forms. Nitrate coronary dilators affect the large coronary arteries. Examples of nitrate coronary dilators include nitroglycerin (Nitrostat® and Nitrobid®) and pentaerythritol tetranitrate. Non-nitrate coronary dilators affect the small coronary arteries. Examples of non-nitrate coronary dilators include dipyridamole (Permole®), iproveratril (Isoptin®), and papaverine (Pavabid®).

Inotropic Agents

Inotropic agents are used to change the force of a muscle contraction; especially contraction of the heart muscle. Inotropic agents may have a positive (increase) or negative (decrease) impact on the contractile force. Digoxin (Lanoxin®) and digitoxin (Crystodigin® and Digitaline®), which are cardiac glycosides, are examples of positive inotropic agents. Beta blockers (also known as beta adrenergic blocking agents) such as propranolol (Inderal®) and calcium channel blockers such as verapamil (Isoptin® and Calan®) are examples of negative inotropic agents.

Vasopressors and Peripheral Vasodilators

Drugs classified as vasopressors constrict the muscles of the blood vessel wall causing the lumen of the vessel to narrow. As a result, the blood meets more resistance as it moves through the blood vessel and the patient's blood pressure increases. Vasopressors are available in oral and parenteral forms. Examples of vasopressors include metaraminol (Aramine®) and phenylephrine (Neo-Synephrine®).

Drugs classified as vasodilators relax the muscles of the blood vessel wall causing the lumen of the vessel to widen. As a result, the blood meets less resistance as it moves through the blood vessel and the patient's blood pressure decreases. Peripheral vasodilators are available in topical, oral, and parenteral forms. Examples of peripheral vasodilators include cyclandelate (Cyclospasmol®), nylidrin (Arlidin®), and papaverine (Pavabid®).

Antihypertensive Agents

The term *hypertension* is used to describe high blood pressure. According to the National Heart Lung and Blood Institute, blood pressure is considered to be elevated when the systolic pressure is at or above 140 millimeters of mercury (mm Hg) and/or the diastolic pressure is at or above 90 mm Hg. **Antihypertensive** agents are prescribed to lower the blood pressure to within normal limits (120/80 mm Hg or below). Several classifications of drugs are used to treat hypertension. Table 10-5 provides a list of some of the types of drugs used to treat hypertension, the mechanism of action, and examples of drugs in each class.

TABLE 10-5 Antihypertensive Agents

Classification	Mechanism of Action	Example(s)
Alpha-blockers	Slow nerve impulses that control muscles in the blood vessel wall causing dilation of the vessel	doxazosin (Cardura®) prazosin (Minipress®)
Angiotensin antagonists	Prevent angiotensin from causing vasoconstriction	candesartan (Atacand®) losartan (Cozaar®) olmesartan(Benicar®)
Angiotensin converting enzyme (ACE) inhibitors	Block production of angiotensin thereby preventing vasoconstriction	benazepril (Lotensin®) fosinopril (Monopril®) ramipril (Altace®)
Beta-blockers	Reduce the force of the heartbeat	atenolol (Tenormin®) metoprolol (Lopressor®) propranolol (Inderal®)
Calcium channel blockers	Restrict the amount of calcium in the muscle, which in turn reduces the contractile force of the muscle	diltiazem (Cardizem®) verapamil (Isoptin® and Calan®)
Diuretics	Increase the amount of sodium and water excreted by the kidneys	chlorothiazide (Diuril®) furosemide (Lasix®) triamterene (Dyrenium®)
Nervous system inhibitors	Decrease nerve impulses from the central nervous system that control muscles in the blood vessel wall causing dilation of the vessel	clonidine (Catapres®) methyldopa (Aldomet®)
Vasodilators	Relax smooth muscle in the blood vessel wall	hydralazine (Apresoline®) minoxidil (Loniten®)

Central Nervous System Stimulants

Central nervous system stimulants are used to speed physiological processes and increase mental alertness by mimicking the stimulatory effects of the sympathetic nervous system. Amphetamines, analeptics, and emetics are examples of central nervous system stimulants.

Amphetamines

Amphetamines have a high potential for abuse and are classified as narcotics. Methamphetamine is an example of an amphetamine that is a Class I narcotic (no currently accepted medical use) and cocaine, because of its use as a topical anesthetic and vasoconstrictor during nasal surgery, is an example of a Class II (currently accepted medical use) amphetamine. Amphetamines are also used as psychotropic drugs to increase wakefulness, concentration, motivation, and a sense of well-being. Amphetamines called anorexiants such as benzphetamine (Didrex®) and phentermine (Fastin®) are appetite suppressants that promote weight loss. Ephedrine is used as a vasoconstrictor. In individuals diagnosed with attention deficit hyperactivity disorder (ADHD), amphetamines such as methylphenidate (Ritalin®), have a **paradoxical** effect by accelerating the release of dopamine, a neurotransmitter, to stimulate certain underused areas of the brain allowing better mental focus for extended periods.

Analeptics

Analeptic drugs are used following opiate induced respiratory depression (as would be evident during emergence from anesthesia, a drug-induced coma, or a narcotic overdose) to stimulate the respiratory center within the brain stem. Respiratory stimulation is often accompanied by an increase in the patient's state of wakefulness and blood pressure. Analeptic drugs are also used in cases of narcolepsy and neonatal apnea. Analeptic drugs are available in oral, rectal, and parenteral forms. Examples of analeptic drugs include doxapram (Dopram®, Stimulex®, or Respiram®) and aminophylline (Truphylline®).

Coagulants/Hemostatics

Coagulants, also called **hemostatic** agents or **procoagulants**, are drugs or other substances that are used to promote blood clot formation and maintenance. Coagulants are used to treat clotting disorders, as antagonists to anticoagulants, and to help control bleeding induced by trauma or surgery. Coagulants occur naturally in the blood and certain blood products can be administered as coagulants (refer to the Blood Replacement Interventions section of this chapter for additional information concerning blood products that contain fibrinogen and blood clotting factors). Coagulants are available in topical, oral, and parenteral forms. Examples of coagulants include:

- Absorbable gelatin—Does not seem to affect the clotting cascade but rather provides a physical surface that encourages clotting; provides a more stable clot than collagen-based coagulants; may be used alone (in its dry state) or moistened with saline, a vasoconstrictor such as epinephrine, or a coagulant such as topical thrombin.
  - Gelfoam®—Porcine origin; applied topically as a foam sponge or a powder.
  - FloSeal®—Bovine origin; applied topically as a viscous gel with the use of a syringe.
  - Surgifoam®—Porcine origin; applied topically as a paste, sponge, or powder.
- Aluminum sulfate—Also called a styptic; causes vasoconstriction at the capillary level; applied topically in powder or gel form.
- Aminocaproic acid (Amicar®)—Inhibits **fibrinolysis**; often prescribed in conjunction with desmopressin; given systemically to stabilize existing blood clots during periods of excessive bleeding. May be given to hemophiliacs up to 24 hours preoperatively to enhance clotting.
- Aprotinin (Trasylol®)—Inhibits fibrinolysis; given systemically during coronary artery bypass surgery as a prophylactic to reduce blood loss.
- Bone wax—Beeswax origin; use minimum amount necessary; applied topically to seal exposed bone surfaces preventing escape of blood (**tamponade**).
- Chitosan (Chitopack C®, Chito-Seal®, and Trauma DEX®)—Shellfish origin; applied topically as a sponge, gel, or film to stimulate division of fibroblasts increasing the speed of clot formation; promotes sedimentation of collagen fostering an increase in the speed of wound healing; possesses antimicrobial properties.
- Collagen (Avitene®, D-Stat®, Instat®, and Helistat®)—Bovine origin; applied topically as a foam, powder, sheet, sponge, spray to provide a matrix that attracts platelets, which will aggregate and form a platelet plug; use of a coagulant such as topical thrombin may enhance the result.
- Desmopressin acetate (DDAVP®)—Promotes production of clotting factors that occur naturally in the blood; given systemically to individuals with hemophilia or von Willebrand's disease intra- and postoperatively to maintain hemostasis; also prescribed during situations of uncontrolled hemorrhage if the patient does not have a coagulopathy.

- Epinephrine (adrenaline)—Not a coagulant but a vasoconstrictor that is administered topically or systemically to constrict blood vessels, thereby slowing the flow of blood at the site of the injury or surgical incision allowing the clotting mechanism to work more efficiently.
- Fibrin-based glue/sealants (BioGlue®, Tisseel®, Vivostat®)—Derived from albumin and contain fibrin; also used to fortify friable tissue; may be used as a medium to convey antibiotics and coagulants to the surgical site; applied topically with the use of a syringe to create crosslinks that act as a basis for clot formation.
- Oxidized cellulose (Surgicel®, Surgicel Nu-knit®)—has a high **tensile strength**; low pH may promote hemostasis; applied topically as a knitted patch or in fibrillar tufts, rolls, and pads to absorb blood and activate the clotting cascade by interacting with blood proteins and platelets. Two additional cellulose-based agents (ActCel® and Blood-STOP®) are in development and are pending FDA approval.
- Polymers (BioHemostat®, CoSeal®, FocalSeal®, Quick Relief®)—Applied topically as a sponge that expands when exposed to body fluid occluding the wound, thereby exerting pressure on the wound to control bleeding.
- Protamine—Ichthyoid or recombinant DNA origin; given systemically as a heparin antagonist; binds with heparin to form an inactive complex.

  Note: When used alone, protamine has anticoagulant properties.

- Silver nitrate—Protect from light; also has antimicrobial properties; applied topically (with an applicator that has been impregnated with silver nitrate) to superficial wounds and surfaces to sear the tissue by causing a chemical burn.
- Topical thrombin (Evithrom®, Recothrom® and Thrombostat®)—Bovine, human plasma, or recombinant DNA origin; may be added to other products such as absorbable gelatin or collagen products to further support coagulation; applied topically to bleeding tissue to increase the amount of thrombin available to support the transformation of fibrinogen to fibrin initiating a foundation for platelet aggregation and formation of a mature clot.

- Tranexamic acid (Cyklokapron®)—Inhibits fibrinolysis; 10 times more potent than aminocaproic acid; given systemically to individuals with hemophilia undergoing invasive surgical procedures.

- Vitamin K (Mephyton®, Aqui-Mephyton®, and Synkayvite®)—Supplements the vitamin K level in the body (which is necessary to support the normal blood clotting mechanism) and acts as an antagonist to warfarin (Coumadin®); administered systemically.

Contrast Media

Contrast media is used during radiographic (x-ray) studies to enhance visualization by differentiating body structures. Contrast media can be administered locally (into a joint, a cavity, or a lumen), enterally (ingested or via enema) or given systemically (orally or intravenously). The terms *contrast medium* and *dye* are often used interchangeably; however, in actuality, a dye is used to add pigment (coloration) to the tissue.

Positive contrast media (compounds that contain iodine or barium) is radiopaque (absorbs x-rays well) and shows as white or light grey on the x-ray image. Iodinated positive contrast media is used when studying most body systems (biliary, cardiovascular, reproductive, skeletal, and urinary) with the exception of the gastrointestinal tract where barium is utilized. Iodinated positive contrast media is further divided into ionic and nonionic (organic) forms. When using ionic contrast media the risk of side effects is greater and the solution typically has a higher osmolality than the nonionic form. The term *osmolality* pertains to the concentration of the solution; solutions with higher osmolality appear denser on the radiographic image. Often the brand name of the solution can be used as an indicator to which body system the drug is best suited. For example, the term *vaso* means vessel (Vasoray® is used on blood vessels), *uro* means urinary (Urografin® is used on the urinary system), *gastro* means stomach (Gastrografin® is used on the upper digestive tract), and so forth. Sometimes contrast media is used full strength, but often the physician may request that the solution be diluted. The order for dilution may be given as a ratio. A ratio of 50:50 would mean that the contrast media would be diluted in half with another solution such as normal saline; for example, 25 ml of contrast mixed with 25 ml of 0.9% NaCl. Examples of ionic and nonionic iodinated positive contrast media are provided in Table 10-6.

Negative contrast media (gasses such as air, carbon dioxide, metrizamide, and oxygen) is radiolucent (allows x-rays to pass through) and shows as dark gray on the x-ray image.

Radioactive isotopes (also called radionuclides) are also used as contrast media. Radioactive isotopes are used to identify tumors, infections, congenital abnormalities, and the function of various tissues. Different isotopes have an affinity for various types of tissue and converge in the related structure; for example, bone, heart, kidney, lung, and thyroid among others. The isotope is given intravenously, by inhalation, or is ingested and collects in the most active cells of target tissue. The isotopes emit gamma radiation which is detected by a specialized camera, similar to a Geiger counter, called a gamma camera or a scintillation camera. The image (two dimensional or three dimensional) is interpreted by a computer and displayed on a monitor or printed on paper or film where the area of concern appears dark grey or black. A portable gamma camera is available for use in the operating room. Precautionary measures must be implemented when working with radioactive isotopes.

Diuretics

Diuretics increase the amount of urine that is excreted. The amount of water and salt excreted is increased because reabsorption of sodium and chloride are decreased. Diuretics are administered orally or parenterally. In general, diuretics are prescribed to reduce edema, treat

TABLE 10-6 Ionic and Nonionic Iodinated Positive Contrast Media

Iodinated Positive Contrast Media	Generic Name	Brand Name(s)
Ionic	diatrizoate	Angiografin®, Hypaque®, Renografin®, Urografin®
	iothalamate	Conray® and Vasoray®
	ioxaglate	Isopaque® and Gastrografin®
	ioxithalamate	Telebrix®
	metrizoate	Hexabrix®
Nonionic	iodixanol	Visipaque®
	iohexol	Omnipaque®
	ioxilan	Oxilan®
	iopamidol	Isovue®
	iopromide	Ultravist®

congestive heart failure and ascites caused by cirrhosis of the liver or a malignancy, decrease hypertension, and to promote urine production and subsequent elimination (diuresis) in cases of renal insufficiency. There are several types of diuretics that work by various mechanisms. Thiazide and potassium-sparing are used to treat nonsurgical problems while carbonic anhydrase inhibitor, loop, and osmotic diuretics are more frequently utilized in the surgical environment. Situations specific to each type of diuretic are presented in the related segment.

Thiazide diuretics impede absorption of sodium and chloride in the distal portion of the nephron. There is also evidence that thiazide diuretics prevent reabsorption of chloride in the ascending loop of Henle. Thiazide diuretics are useful in reducing the risk of formation of calcium containing kidney stones because they lower calcium excretion in the urine. Examples of thiazide diuretics include chlorothiazide (Diuril®) and indapamide (Lozol®). When sodium is reabsorbed, it is exchanged for potassium which can lead to depletion of potassium in the body. Oral thiazides are relatively inexpensive and are therefore the most widely used diuretic.

Potassium-sparing diuretics block the exchange of sodium for potassium in the distal tubule, thereby retaining potassium. Potassium-sparing diuretics are considered as a replacement for thiazide diuretics when dietary modifications to replace the potassium lost with the use of thiazide diuretics (hypokalemia) are ineffective as well as to treat hypokalemia from other causes. Examples of potassium-sparing diuretics include amiloride (Midamor®) and spironolactone (Aldactone®).

Carbonic Anhydrase Inhibitor Diuretics

Carbonic anhydrase inhibitor diuretics inhibit carbonic anhydrase, which is an enzyme found in the proximal tubule. Inhibition of the enzyme causes an increase in excretion of hydrogen which in turn increases excretion of sodium, water, and potassium. Carbonic anhydrase inhibitor diuretics are used to treat open-angle glaucoma and preoperatively to decrease intraocular pressure associated with angle-closure glaucoma. Miotics or products containing epinephrine may be used in conjunction with carbonic anhydrase inhibitor diuretics to provide an enhanced effect. Acetazolamide (Diamox®) and methazolamide (Neptazane®) are examples of systemic carbonic anhydrase inhibitor diuretics. Dorzolamide (Trusopt®) is applied topically on the surface of the eye.

Loop Diuretics

Loop diuretics produce a rapid and effective diuretic response by inhibiting reabsorption of sodium and chloride directly in the loop of Henle especially when administered intravenously. Loop diuretics are effective in prompt reduction of pulmonary edema and decreasing intracranial pressure due to cerebral edema. Examples of loop diuretics include bumetanide (Bumex® and Burinex®), ethacrynic acid (Edecrin®), furosemide (Lasix®), and torsemide (Demadex® and Diuver®).

Osmotic Diuretics

Osmotic diuretics increase the amount of extracellular fluid and plasma volume by drawing fluid from the cells by osmosis. A surge in plasma volume causes an acceleration of blood flow to the kidney, which in turn allows a greater amount of filtrate to leave the kidney and reabsorption of water in the tubules is inhibited. Osmotic diuretics are available only for intravenous administration and are effective in rapid reduction of intracranial pressure, intraocular pressure, and promoting excretion of toxic substances from the body. Examples of osmotic diuretics include mannitol (Osmitrol®) and isosorbide (Isordil®).

Dyes/Stains

Differentiating between *dyes* and *stains* is difficult because the terms are often used interchangeably and both substances are used to color various body structures. Coloration may be added to indicate a planned incision site, identify internal structures, or to enhance visualization by creating color contrast; especially when working with fixed tissue specimens under a microscope to determine the presence of pathologic conditions. Typically, dyes are used when coloration of short duration is necessary; dyes are easily removed or absorb quickly and stains are longer lasting or permanent. Dyes and stains bind to tissue in the same ways that other molecules bind together (ionic bonds, hydrogen bonds, and covalent bonds) and binding is influenced by factors such as pH and salt concentrations.

Examples of dyes used in the surgical environment include gentian violet and methylene blue. Dyes may be incorporated into a sterile surgical marking pen or are available in liquid form for topical application, infiltration, or systemic administration. Stains are primarily used in the histology lab setting. Stains used to identify the cell wall include crystal violet, fuchsin, and safranin. Stains appropriate for identifying the nucleus of a cell include carminic acid, hemotoxylin with a salt added as a mordant (substance used to fix the stain to the tissue), methylene blue, methyl green, neutral red, and safranine. Stains appropriate for identifying the cytoplasm of a cell include aniline blue, eosin, fast green, light green, methyl blue, orange G, metanil yellow, and trinitrophenol. Stains appropriate for use on connective tissue include a wide range of acid dye combinations, Van Gieson's stain, and trichrome stains.

Emergency Drugs

Several types of critical patient situations can arise, especially in the surgical environment. Patients may experience malignant hyperthermia crises and allergic reactions as well as cardiac and respiratory emergencies. The drugs described in this section are drugs that would typically be found on emergency carts. An emergency cart contains highly specialized drugs, supplies, and equipment specific to the situation that is easily accessible and can be quickly moved into an operating room where a patient is experiencing a crisis situation. Contents of the emergency carts and established protocols will vary between facilities and it is vital that all surgical team members are familiar with the contents of each cart, the location of each item in or on the cart, why and how each item is to be used, and the policies and procedures established by each facility in order to provide fast and accurate patient care during an emergency situation. Examples of emergency carts include malignant hyperthermia cart, difficult airway/intubation, and cardiac arrest (sometimes called a crash cart or a code blue cart) carts. Additionally, specialized carts may be available specifically for use with pediatric patients.

Malignant Hyperthermia

Malignant hyperthermia (MH), also called malignant hyperpyrexia, is a rare life-threatening inherited genetic disorder. When an individual who is susceptible to malignant hyperthermia is exposed to a triggering agent, a malignant hyperthermia crisis may develop. In the surgical environment, agents considered to be triggers include inhalation anesthetic agents that are halogenated and the depolarizing neuromuscular blocking agent succinylcholine (Anectine®). A patient experiencing a malignant hyperthermia crisis will exhibit tachycardia, tachypnea, sweating, flushing of the skin, increased oxygen consumption and carbon dioxide production, acidosis, excretion of dark brown urine, muscle rigidity, a dramatic increase in body temperature, unstable blood pressure, eventual vascular collapse, and possibly death. Immediate treatment for malignant hyperthermia includes discontinuance of the triggering agent, oxygenation, administration of dantrolene (Dantrium®), initiation of cooling measures, management of acidosis, and provision of additional supportive measures as needed. Additional information concerning malignant hyperthermia may be obtained online from the Malignant Hyperthermia Association of the United States at **www.mhaus.org**.

Dantrolene is available in oral or parenteral forms and is used as a muscle relaxant to treat malignant hyperthermia. Additionally, muscle spasticity related to cerebral palsy, multiple sclerosis, spinal cord injuries, and stroke may be treated with dantrolene. Patients known to have malignant hyperthermia or those with a strong family history of malignant hyperthermia maybe given dantrolene prophylactically in advance of a planned surgical procedure to reduce the risk of a malignant hyperthermia crisis. If a malignant hyperthermia crisis develops during or immediately following a surgical procedure, dantrolene is the only current approved treatment option. Dantrolene inhibits movement of calcium into the muscle cell, thereby restricting the ability of the muscle to contract. Parenteral dantrolene is supplied in powder form and each 20 milligram vial of dantrolene must be reconstituted with 60 milliliters of sterile water for injection USP (without a bacteriostatic agent; D5W and normal saline may not be used) prior to use. Reconstituted dantrolene may be stored at room temperature for no longer than six hours.

Allergic Reaction

An allergic reaction is an exaggerated immune system (histamine) response to a foreign substance (antigen/allergen) such as venom from a snake or insect bite, food, pollen, dust, or a medication. Allergic reactions range from mild skin irritation to anaphylactic shock and can progress rapidly from mild to life-threatening. A patient experiencing an allergic reaction may exhibit the following signs and symptoms:

- Integumentary system—Flushing, urticaria (hives), and pruritus (itching)

- Mucous membrane—Swelling (eyelids, lips, tongue, soft palate, and throat)

- Respiratory system—Dyspnea (difficulty breathing), tightness of the chest, wheezing, and bronchospasm

- Central nervous system—Agitation, confusion, dizziness, headache, and vision disturbances

- Cardiovascular system—Chest pain, dizziness, syncope (fainting), hypotension (low blood pressure), tachycardia (rapid heart rate), and weak pulse

- Gastrointestinal system—Abdominal pain/cramping, diarrhea, nausea, and vomiting

An untreated allergic reaction can lead to complications including blockage of the airway, respiratory arrest, vascular collapse, cardiac arrest, and death. Treatment options for minor allergic reactions include basic first aid measures (e.g., cleaning the wound and applying ice). If the reaction is severe, antihistamines such as diphenhydramine (Benadryl®—available in topical, oral, rectal, and parenteral forms) and epinephrine (adrenaline—available in parenteral form—sometimes referred to as an anaphylaxis kit), may be prescribed along with a corticosteroid to produce an anti-inflammatory effect.

Note: Some of the drugs listed in this section, such as epinephrine, have additional uses, are identified in more than one classification, and are available in other forms.

Cardiac Arrest

In addition to drugs used during a cardiac arrest response, airway management, administration of oxygen, initiation of cardiopulmonary resuscitation (CPR), and defibrillation are crucial to patient survival. When a cardiac emergency occurs, the treatment and selection of appropriate drug therapy depends on the type of dysrhythmia that is diagnosed. With a few exceptions (such as aspirin, which is given orally if the patient is able to swallow and nitroglycerine, which is given sublingually), most drugs used during a cardiac emergency are given parenterally. During a cardiac arrest, the patient may experience collapse of the peripheral blood vessels making administration of emergency cardiac medications difficult or impossible. If a large diameter peripheral vein (such as the antecubital vein or external jugular vein) is not available, emergency medications may be administered through a central venous line (placed in the subclavian vein or internal jugular vein) or intraosseously via a special cannula that is inserted into the bone marrow. Drugs commonly used during a cardiac emergency include:

- Adenosine (Adenocard®)—Decreases blood pressure by causing peripheral vasodilation and decreases conduction time of an electrical impulse through the atrioventricular (AV) node stabilizing ventricular dysrhythmias.

- Adrenaline (epinephrine)—Increases blood pressure by causing peripheral vasoconstriction and, thereby, concentrating the available blood around the vital organs (brain and heart), stimulates the myocardium and strengthens the contraction of the heart, speeds conduction time of an electrical impulse through the AV node stabilizing ventricular dysrhythmias, and is a bronchodilator. May be injected directly into the heart using a special administration kit that includes an intracardiac needle.

- Amiodarone (Cordarone®)—Blocks the action of hormones that increase the heart rate, thereby slowing the heart rate and decreasing the metabolic needs of the cardiac tissue.

- Aspirin—Has an anti-inflammatory effect and prevents platelet aggregation (blood clot formation). Given orally (preferably chewed) at the first indication of an impending cardiac emergency or stroke, if the patient is conscious and able to swallow.

- Atropine—Blocks the effects of the Xth cranial (vagus) nerve (which is part of the sympathetic nervous system that is responsible for slowing the heart rate), thereby, increasing the heart rate and speeds the conduction time of an electrical impulse through the cardiac tissue.

- Calcium chloride—Used to treat electrolyte imbalances (hypocalcemia and hyperkalemia) that can lead to cardiac arrest, increases the force of the myocardial contraction, and minimizes hypotension associated with magnesium administration.

- Diltiazem (Cardizem®)—Dilates peripheral and coronary blood vessels lowering the blood pressure, decreases the force of the myocardial contraction and as a result lowers the metabolic needs of the cardiac tissue, and slows the heart rate by increasing the conduction time of an electrical impulse through the cardiac tissue.

- Digoxin—Decreases the conduction time of an electrical impulse from the AV node slowing the rate of ventricular contractions and improving the overall pumping action of the heart.

- Dopamine—Acts on the central nervous system to increase the heart rate, raise the blood pressure, and increase cardiac output to restore blood flow to the viscera.

- Ibutilide (Corvert®)—Slows the movement of the electrolyte sodium into the myocardial cells delaying repolarization of the muscle and slowing the heart rate.

- Lidocaine (Xylocaine®)—Reduces the electrical activity throughout the heart by blocking the sodium channels and slowing the heart rate.

- Magnesium sulfate—Mineral that decreases blood pressure, decreases heart rate, increases the amount of blood pumped from the left ventricle (stroke volume) with each beat, and conserves potassium.

- Morphine—Narcotic analgesic that is used during cardiac emergencies to relieve pain associated with angina, reduce inflammation of the heart, lower blood pressure, and dilate the coronary arteries.

- Nitroglycerine—Dilates coronary blood vessels improving blood flow to the heart, reduces metabolic needs of the heart, and reduces pain associated with angina.

- Procainamide (Pronestyl®)—Sodium-channel blocker that stabilizes both atrial and ventricular dysrhythmias by inhibiting movement of the electrical impulse through the heart; does not impact the sinoatrial node (SA) and, therefore, does not change the heart rate.

- Sodium bicarbonate—Buffer (base) used to treat acidosis that may occur when hyperventilation is not effective in raising the blood pH or resuscitation efforts are prolonged.

- Vasopressin (Pitressin®)—Causes peripheral vasoconstriction, which increases the blood pressure and shunts available blood to the heart and brain.

- Verapamil (Isoptin® and Calan®)—Calcium channel blocker that dilates the blood vessels lowering the blood pressure and reducing pain associated with angina, slows electrical activity through the cardiac tissues slowing the heart rate, decreases the force of the myocardial contraction, and increases blood flow to the heart.

Note: Some of the drugs listed in this section, such as lidocaine and epinephrine, have additional uses, are identified in more than one classification, and are available in other forms.

Respiratory Distress/Arrest

In cases of severe respiratory distress or respiratory arrest, the underlying cause will determine the type of treatment needed. The airway must be patent and the patient may require endotracheal intubation and mechanical ventilation with the administration of oxygen. If the respiratory problem is compounded by cardiac arrest, administration of chest compressions will be required. Drugs used during a respiratory emergency are available in inhalation, oral, and parenteral forms.

- **Neuromuscular blockers**—Cause complete relaxation (paralyzation) of the skeletal muscles to facilitate placement of an endotracheal tube and/or to maintain mechanical ventilation. Succinylcholine (Anectine®) is an example of a depolarizing ultrashort-acting-neuromuscular blocker. Examples of nondepolarizing neuromuscular blockers include atracurium (Tracrium®), mivacurium (Mivacron®), pancuronium (Pavulon®), rocuronium (Zemuron®), tubocurarine (Medtubine®), and vecuronium (Norcuron®).

- Respiratory stimulants—Stimulate the central nervous system to increase the urge to breathe, the rate of respirations, and the tidal volume (amount of air moved in and out of the lungs with each breath). Examples of respiratory stimulants include doxapram (Dopram®, Respiram®, and Stimulex®) and methylxanthines (caffeine citrate).

- Bronchodilators—Relax the muscles that surround the bronchial structures allowing the passageways to dilate which in turn allows movement of an increased volume of air with each breath. There are three main classifications of bronchodilators:
  - Beta-agonist bronchodilators—Group of oral and inhaled medications (sometimes called rescue inhalers) that provide a rapid relaxation response of the bronchial musculature and are typically short acting. Examples of beta-agonist bronchodilators include albuterol (Proventil® and Ventolin®), metaproterenol (Alupent® and Metaprel®), pirbuterol (Maxair®), terbutaline (Brethaire®), formoterol (Foradil®), and salmeterol (Serevent®).

  - Theophylline type bronchodilators—The effect theophylline type bronchodilators is similar to that of beta-agonist bronchodilators; however, the duration of action is longer; up to 12-24 hours in some patients. Theophylline type bronchodilators also act as coronary vessel dilators, myocardial stimulants and diuretics. Brand names for theophylline include Slophylline®, Theodur®, Unidur®, and Uniphyl®. The drug aminophylline is a combination of theophylline and ethylenediamine in a 2:1 ratio. The ethylenediamine increases the effectiveness of the theophylline by acting as a solvent and an emulsifier to improve solubility of the drug.
  - Anticholinergic bronchodilators—Slow onset of action and a weaker response time than beta-agonist bronchodilators. An example of an anticholinergic bronchodilator is ipratropium (Atrovent®).

- Narcotic antagonists—If the respiratory emergency is related to narcotic use, a narcotic antagonist such as flumazenil (Mazicon® and Romazicon®) or naloxone (Narcan®) may be indicated.

- Sodium bicarbonate—Used as a buffer (base) to treat acidosis.

- Corticosteroids—Reduce inflammation of the mucous membrane lining the inside of the bronchial structures. Examples of inhaled corticosteroid anti-inflammatories include budesonide (Pulmicort®), fluticasone (Flovent®), and mometasone (Asmanex®).

- Other—Diuretics may be used to remove excess fluids, nitrates and other vasodilators to increase blood flow, and analgesics to reduce pain and decrease anxiety.

Emetics

Emetics are drugs that induce vomiting (emesis). Vomiting is induced to empty the stomach especially if an overdose of a drug or a non-caustic poison has been ingested. Direct (gastric) emetics are administered orally and act directly on the stomach. Examples of gastric (direct) emetics include syrup of ipecac and alum. Indirect (systemic) emetics are administered parenterally and act on the central nervous system to stimulate vomiting. Apomorphine (Apokyn®) is an example of an indirect (central nervous system) emetic.

Note: Use of emetics is not recommended when the suspected poison is a strong acid or base, petroleum based, or a convulsant.

Gastric Agents

Gastric agents are used to produce an effect on the stomach such as reducing or eliminating nausea and vomiting (antiemetics), inducing vomiting (emetics), increasing gastric motility and relaxing the pyloric sphincter to allow partially digested food to move quickly from the stomach to the small intestine (metoclopramide/Reglan®), and to control gastric acidity (H_2 receptor blockers).

H_2 Receptor Blockers

H_2 receptor blockers, also called H_2 **antagonists**, are used to suppress secretion of hydrochloric acid in the stomach. A type of histamine, called histamine 2 (H_2) released in the stomach stimulates production of hydrochloric acid (HCl) which, in abundance, can cause inflammation and ulceration of the esophagus, stomach, and duodenum. H_2 receptor blockers limit the release of histamine, thereby, reducing the amount of HCl produced in the stomach. H_2 receptor blockers are available in oral and parenteral forms. Examples of H_2 receptor blockers include cimetidine (Tagamet®), famotidine (Axid®), and ranitidine (Zantac®).

Hormones

Hormones are naturally occurring chemical substances secreted by endocrine glands and various other cells throughout the body. Endocrine hormones are transported to the target tissue in the blood and other hormones act locally. In general, hormones help to regulate many body functions including behavior, growth and development, metabolism, mood, reproduction, and sexual maturity and function. Each hormone has a specific function and target tissue. Most hormone activity is controlled using negative feedback by the central nervous system. Please refer to a general anatomy and physiology book for additional information concerning hormones, hormone sources, and functions. Blood tests are used to determine hormone imbalances that may result from numerous causes such as aging, congenital conditions, disease processes, increased or decreased production, and surgical removal of all or part of an endocrine gland. When hormone imbalances are detected, hormone drugs may be prescribed. Hormones for pharmaceutical use are synthesized in a laboratory, made using biotechnology, or derived from an animal source. Hormone drugs are available for inhalation, ingestion, parenteral administration, or topical application. Several hormones have been described throughout this chapter and this segment continues with a brief discussion of corticosteroids, insulin and glucagon, prostaglandins, and sex hormones.

Corticosteroids

Corticosteroids are produced naturally in the cortex of the adrenal gland and are also available in pharmaceutical preparations. Corticosteroids are divided into three groups: glucocorticoids, mineralocorticoids, and the sex hormones.

- Glucocorticoids—Function to metabolize carbohydrates (especially glucose), fats, and proteins. Corticosteroids are also active in stress regulation and act as anti-inflammatory agents. Cortisol, also known as hydrocortisone, represents 95% of all glucocorticoids. Examples of glucocorticoids include betamethasone (Celestone® and Celestone Soluspan®), cortisone (Cortone®), dexamethasone (Decadron®), fluprednisolone (Rhinocort®), hydrocortisone (Cortef® and Solucortef®), methylprednisolone (Solu-Medrol®), paramethasone (Haldrone®), prednisolone (Orapred® and Prelone®), prednisone (Deltasone® and Sterapred®), triamcinolone (Azmacort, Aristocort, Kenalog-10®, and Kenalog-40®).

- Mineralocorticoids—Function in regulation of electrolytes and water balance. Aldosterone is the major mineralocorticoid hormone, which is available as fludrocortisone acetate (Florinef®).

- Sex hormones—Promote development of secondary sex characteristics.

Insulin/Glucagon

The islet cells of the pancreas produce both **insulin** and glucagon, which are antagonists that work in harmony to maintain homeostasis. Insulin is produced by the beta cells of the islets of Langerhans. The primary function of insulin is to lower the blood sugar level. Insulin is available in several strengths and preparations that have various onset and duration of action times. More than one preparation may be prescribed and different types of insulin can be mixed. Insulin may be administered subcutaneously by injection or infusion with the use of a pump or with the use of an inhaler. Types of rapid-acting insulin include lispro (Humalog®), aspart (Novolog®), and glulisine (Apidra®). Types of short-acting insulin include regular (Humulin® and Novolin®) and Velosulin® that is specifically for use in an infusion pump. Types of intermediate-acting insulin include NPH and lente. Types of long-acting insulin include ultralente, insulin glargine (Lantus®), and detemir (Levemir®). Humulin 70/30®, Novolin 70/30®, Novolog 70/30®, Humulin 50/50®, and Humalog 75/25® are examples of insulin that are premixed to contain more than one insulin preparation.

Glucagon is produced by the alpha cells of the islets of Langerhans. The primary function of glucagon is to raise the blood sugar level. Glucagon is available as

GlucaGen® and is administered orally and is available in a powdered form that must be reconstituted prior to parenteral administration.

Prostaglandins

Prostaglandins are hormone-like chemical messengers that are secreted by many types of cells in the body and act on nearby tissues. The effects of prostaglandins are too numerous to list; however, some limited examples are provided. In general, prostaglandins are responsible for initiation of the inflammatory response that results in fever and pain. Examples of prostaglandins used as medications include:

- PGE2 of PGF2 (dinoprostone/Dinoprost®)—Used to induce uterine contractions to stimulate childbirth or facilitate an abortion and to restrict gastric acid formation

- PGE1 (alprostadil)—Used in newborns with cyanotic heart defects to prevent closure of a patent ductus arteriosus and as a vasodilator for patients with Raynaud's phenomenon, ischemic limbs, and erectile dysfunction

- PGE—Decreases production of stomach acid to prevent and treat ulcers

- PGI2 (prostacyclin)—Causes bronchodilation

- Bimatoprost—Used to treat glaucoma

- Thromboxane—Stimulates blood vessel constriction and platelet aggregation following injury to a blood vessel

- PG12—Protects blood vessels from clot formation when no injury has occurred

Sex Hormones

The sex hormones are secreted from the ovaries in the female and from the testes in the male and are activated at the time of puberty under the control of other hormones that originate in the pituitary gland. Both the male and female sex hormones support growth and development of the secondary sex characteristics.

The female sex hormones are estrogens (the primary estrogen is estradiol) and progesterone. Estrogen contributes to pubic and underarm hair growth, breast development, menstruation, widening of the hips, and a greater fat to muscle ratio. Estrogen is available in topical, oral, and parenteral forms and by numerous brand names, including Divigel®, Estraderm MX®, Evalon®, Premarin®, and Progynova®, and is used to treat symptoms of menopause and increase bone density related to osteoporosis. Progesterone is useful in correcting amenorrhea and dysfunctional uterine bleeding as well as supporting pregnancy. Progesterone is available for oral and parenteral administration; brand names include Crinone®, Endometrin®, Progest®, and Prometrium®.

The male sex hormone is testosterone. Testosterone contributes to facial, pubic, and underarm air growth, enlargement of the external genitalia, and facilitates sperm development and maturity. Testosterone is administered parenterally to treat delayed onset of puberty and impotence. Brand names for testosterone include Andro LA 200®, Delatestryl®, Depandro 100®, Depo-Testosterone®, Testosterone Cypionate®, and Testosterone Enanthate®.

Inhalation Agents

Inhalation agents are gasses or vapors that are breathed or blown into the lungs. Oxygen and nitrous oxide are examples of inhalation agents that are gasses. Oxygen is not officially considered a drug, but because it is frequently administered in the surgical setting, it is mentioned here. Nitrous oxide, a general anesthetic, is the only true gas that is commonly administered to induce and maintain general anesthesia; although, many other gasses are used in the surgical environment for other reasons. The remainder of the inhalation agents used as anesthetics are volatile liquids. Use of a vaporizer may be necessary to speed evaporation of the liquid into a vapor that can be inhaled. Volatile liquids that are used as inhalation anesthesia agents include desflurane (Suprane®), enflurane (Ethrane®), halothane, isoflurane (Forane®), and sevoflurane (Ultane®).

Information concerning respiratory inhalers containing bronchodilators and anti-inflammatory agents is available in the Respiratory Distress/Arrest segment of this chapter.

Nasal Sprays

Nasal sprays are used to deliver medications to the mucous membrane lining of the nose with the use of an atomizer. Some nasal sprays are available for the consumer to purchase over-the-counter and others require a prescription. Medications intended to act locally such as cold and allergy treatments are commonly associated with nasal administration. Because the nasal mucosa is well vascularized, many types of medications can be administered via the capillaries of the nasal mucosa into the blood stream to be transported to the target tissue using a low-tech inexpensive method. Advantages to nasal administration include avoidance of parenteral administration for individuals who are fearful of needles and bypassing oral administration for those unable to swallow. An additional benefit to avoiding the gastrointestinal tract is that medication dosing is not dependent on hepatic first pass metabolism. Examples of type of drugs that can be administered nasally include analgesics, anticonvulsants, antiemetics, antipsychotics, glucagon, immunizations, insulin, narcotic antagonists, sedatives, topical anesthetics, and vasoconstrictors for treatment of epistaxis.

Irrigation Solutions

The term *irrigation* is used to describe the act of washing, flushing, or moistening with fluid. Sometimes the term *lavage* is used to represent irrigation, especially when referring to washing of the stomach (gastric lavage). In the surgical environment, solutions for irrigation are typically used to remove debris (blood, tissue fragments, bone fragments, and foreign bodies) from body surfaces, tissues, body cavities, body orifices, wounds (chronic, surgical, traumatic), hollow organs, improve visibility, and to flush medical devices (catheters, tubes, and drains). Occasionally, irrigation solutions are used prophylactically, to help establish a diagnosis, to dissect tissue, to distend a body cavity or joint, or to provide treatment. Irrigation solutions are not intended for injection or intravascular use. The surgeon will provide information concerning the type, strength, volume, method of delivery, and temperature of the irrigation solution. Irrigation solution is applied to the desired location via gravity (pouring, dripping), manual pressure (atomizer, syringe), or a mechanical device (pump that delivers a steady or pulsed flow of fluid). Gravity, suction, medical devices (such as a drain or catheter), and surgical sponges or dressings are used to remove or absorb the irrigation solution. Examples of irrigation solutions include:

- Nonelectrolytic solutions (aminoacetic acid/ Glycine®), sorbitol/Glucotrol®, mannitol/ Osmitrol®)—Used during endoscopic procedures, such as arthroscopy, laparoscopy, and transurethral procedures to decrease the potential for electrical injury

- Antiseptics—Examples include chlorhexidine, Dakin's solution, hydrogen peroxide, povidone iodine, and sodium hypochlorite

- Sterile water for irrigation—Hypotonic solution that is occasionally ordered by the surgeon to use as wound irrigation when lysis of cells is desired (e.g., following removal of a cancerous mass); often used on the sterile field to clean and soak the instruments because it does not contain salt, which can be corrosive to the finish on the surgical instruments

- Sterile saline for irrigation—Inexpensive, readily available, and most frequently used irrigating solution during surgical procedures; available in varying tonicities

- Lactated ringer's solution—Transparent isotonic solution that is useful during arthroscopic procedures because it provides a clear visual field and the electrolyte composition is similar to that of synovial fluid

- Cardioplegic solution (Physiolyte®, Plegisol®)— Used during open heart surgery to temporarily arrest the function of the heart

- Dextran (Hyskon®)—Used in the abdominopelvic cavity to reduce the risk of adhesion formation following an open or laparoscopic procedure.

Note: Medications, such as antibiotics, may be added to various irrigation solutions. Caution: Irrigation solutions that contain electrolytes (electrolytic) conduct electricity and are not usually used in conjunction with the electrosurgical unit especially during endoscopic procedures.

IV Fluids

Fluids for intravenous use consist of **crystalloids**, blood, blood products, colloids (information concerning blood, blood products, and colloid plasma expanders is included in the Blood Replacement Interventions segment of this chapter), and oxygen carrying solutions which are in development. Crystalloid solutions made from substances that form crystals, such as salts and sugars and are the primary fluid used for intravenous therapy. Intravenous therapy is initiated to replace fluid (as a result of trauma, surgery, or dehydration [due to excessive urination, sweating, vomiting, diarrhea], or the inability to take in fluids by mouth), replace electrolytes, deliver nutrients (including an energy source such as dextrose), and to permit administration of medication directly into the blood. Crystalloid solutions are available in three tonicities:

- **Isotonic**—Solution consists of the same number of particles as blood plasma and does not move fluid into or out of the cells

- Hypotonic—Solution consists of a lesser number of particles (a dilute solution) than blood plasma and pushes fluid out of circulation into the cells causing them to swell and possibly burst (called hemolysis)

- Hypertonic—Solution consists of a greater number of particles (a concentrated solution) than blood plasma and draws fluid out of the cells into circulation causing the cells to shrink (called crenation)

Isotonic crystalloid solutions are used to correct volume deficiencies and to provide electrolytes. Examples of isotonic crystalloid solutions include:

- Normal saline—Also referred to as NS or 0.9% sodium chloride; contains only water and salt

- Lactated Ringer's solution—Also referred to as LR or Ringer's lactate; contains the electrolytes calcium, chloride, potassium, and sodium as well as lactate, which acts as an alkalizing agent that is used to help correct acidosis

- Ringer's solution—Contains the same electrolytes as lactated Ringer's solution; excludes lactate

- 5% dextrose in water—Also referred to as D_5W; contains water and dextrose that is used to raise or maintain the blood sugar level

Hypotonic crystalloid solutions are used in patients with high sodium levels (hypernatremia) because they contain less salt and to treat dehydration. Examples of hypotonic crystalloid solutions include half-normal saline (0.45% sodium chloride) and quarter-normal saline (0.225% sodium chloride).

Hypertonic crystalloid solutions are used in patients with low sodium levels (hyponatremia) and to expand the volume of plasma and are often used in conjunction with colloid solutions. Examples of hypertonic crystalloid solutions include:

- 5% dextrose in normal saline—Also referred to as D_5NS; used to replace volume, salt, and provide an energy source (calories); also used to raise or maintain the blood sugar level

- 1.8% sodium chloride, 3.0% sodium chloride, 7.0% sodium chloride, 7.5% sodium chloride, and 10% sodium chloride

The list provided is not intended to be comprehensive. Intravenous solution options are numerous, several concentrations are variable, and many substances can be added that will alter the composition of the solution.

Lubricants

Lubricants are used in the surgical environment on skin and mucous membranes to decrease friction during rectal and vaginal examinations and to facilitate insertion or passage of catheters, endoscopes, and surgical instruments. Some lubricants are water-soluble (K-Y Jelly®) and some water-soluble lubricants also contain an antiseptic such as chlorhexidine gluconate (Surgilube®), or an anesthetic such as lidocaine (Xylocaine Viscous®). Caution is advised when using petroleum based lubricants such as Vaseline® and mineral oil (Muri-Lube®) because they may be flammable or support combustion. Castor oil and jojoba oil are lubricants derived from plants. Information concerning ophthalmic lubricants is contained within the Lubricants section of the Ophthalmic Agents portion of this chapter.

Narcotic Antagonists

A narcotic antagonist reverses the analgesic, hypotensive, respiratory depressant, and sedative effects of a narcotic (opiate/opioid) by competing for and occupying the same receptor sites as the narcotic. Examples of narcotic antagonists include naloxone (Narcan®) and flumazenil (Mazicon® and Romazicon®), which is also known as flumazepil. Other narcotic antagonists such as naltrexone (Trexan® and (Vivitrol®) are used in substance abuse programs to block the physiologic and psychologic effects of the drug. Narcotic antagonists may be administered orally or parenterally.

Narcotic Analgesics

Narcotic analgesics derived from the opium poppy plant are called opiates and those developed from synthetic or semisynthetic sources that resemble opiates are called opioids. Narcotic analgesics are used in enteral, parenteral, and topical forms to reduce the perception of and reaction to pain as well as increase pain tolerance for patients experiencing moderate to severe acute and chronic pain. Additional effects of opiates and opioids include suppression of the cough reflex, a perception of euphoria, decreased intestinal motility, respiratory depression, and sedation. Schedule II narcotics are used most frequently in the surgical environment. Examples of common narcotic analgesics include alfentanil (Alfenta®), butorphanol (Stadol®), fentanyl (Sublimaze®), hydromorphone (Dilaudid®), meperidine (Demerol®), morphine (Astramorph® and Duramorph®), remifentanil (Ultiva®), and sufentanil (Sufenta®). Narcotic antagonists (naloxone and flumazenil) reverse the effects of narcotic analgesics.

In addition to the documentation required for all medications, special documentation is required when a narcotic is administered because it is a controlled substance. If a dose of a narcotic is only partially used; state law, federal law, and/or facility policy will dictate the procedure that must be followed. Typically, two individuals must witness disposal of the remaining portion of the narcotic. Information concerning narcotic regulation is found in Chapter One, narcotic classifications are described in Chapter Three, and information about addiction and tolerance is found in Chapter Eight.

Neuroleptics/Tranquilizers

Neuroleptic drugs are also known as **tranquilizers**. Tranquilizers are available in oral and parenteral forms. Tranquilizers are further classified into two categories. Major tranquilizers, also known as antipsychotic drugs, are primarily used in the treatment of psychoses and neuroses (haloperidol/Haldol® and chlorpromazine/Thorazine®); however, some drugs in this classification are also used to relieve nausea and vomiting (prochlorperazine/Compazine® and droperidol/Inapsine®) and act as synergists of analgesics (promethazine/Phenergan® and hydroxyzine/Vistaril®). Minor tranquilizers, also known as anxiolytics, are used in the treatment of anxiety, stress, and irritability. An example of a minor tranquilizer is risperidone (Risperdal®). Some sedative/hypnotics are also considered to be minor tranquilizers.

Obstetrical Agents

Several types of drugs have uses specific to obstetrical patients. Pharmacologic agents are used to induce abortion, stimulate and suppress lactation, stimulate and relax uterine contractions, and prevent hemolytic disease of the newborn. Induction of an abortion involves intraamniotic injection of (20%) hypertonic saline followed by an oxytocic and/or prostaglandins. Drugs that induce lactation and stimulate increased milk production are called galactogogues. The antiemetic, metoclopramide (Reglan®) is sometimes used as a galactogogue. Drugs that suppress lactation include cabergoline (Dostinex®) and bromocriptine (Parlodel®).

Oxytocics

Oxytocic drugs are used to induce labor, strengthen uterine contractions during labor, and contract the uterus to control hemorrhage following an abortion or delivery (vaginal or abdominal) of a neonate. Oxytocin is a hormone that occurs naturally in the body but is also available as a pharmaceutical (Pitocin®). Oxytocin is available in parenteral form for intravenous and intramuscular use; it may be injected directly into the myometrium; especially during a Cesarean section. Methylergonovine maleate (Methergine®), which not only contracts the myometrium but is a vasoconstrictor as well, is available in oral or parenteral forms and is stored in the refrigerator. Tocolytic drugs such as terbutaline sulfate (Brethine®) are used to suppress uterine contractions and arrest premature labor.

Rho (D) Immune Globulin

Rho (D) immune globulin, known by the brand name RhoGAM®, is used to prevent hemolytic disease of the newborn (also called erythroblastosis fetalis). During a first pregnancy, blood from an Rh positive fetus may come in contact with the blood of the Rh negative mother, especially in the third trimester of pregnancy and during childbirth. The mother's body recognizes the Rh positive antigens as foreign and produces antibodies to protect the mother from the foreign antigens. In subsequent pregnancies, the maternal antibodies may enter the blood of the fetus and attack the Rh positive blood cells causing hemolytic disease of the newborn which is manifested by anemia, jaundice, and possibly heart failure. Rho (D) immune globulin is manufactured from human blood and contains Rh factor antibodies. Because the antibodies are present in the immune globulin, the mother's immune system does not need to produce the antibodies, thereby, protecting the fetus of a

future pregnancy from developing hemolytic disease of the newborn. The immune globulin is available for intramuscular injection and is typically administered following an abortion, any event that could produce placental hemorrhage (such as abdominal trauma or amniocentesis), and during a term pregnancy at 28 weeks of gestation and again within 72 hours after childbirth.

Ophthalmic Agents

Ophthalmic agents are specifically designed for use in the eye and the drug packaging will identify drugs that are approved for ophthalmic use. Many ophthalmic agents are the same drugs used elsewhere in the body; however, the ophthalmic version may be buffered so that the solution is more compatible with the fluids of the eye, manufactured in a special ophthalmic form (drops, ointment, etc.), and/or the concentration is adjusted specifically for use in the eye.

Antibiotics

Ophthalmic **antibiotics** are used to treat bacterial infections of the eyelids (blepharitis), the surface of the eye (exophthalmitis—conjunctivitis and keratitis), and of the inner tunics and cavities of the eye (endophthalmitis). Ophthalmic antibiotics may be administered topically (drops and ointments), injected subconjunctivally and intraocularly, and given systemically (oral and parenteral) and are available in drop, ointment, injectable, and ingestible forms (Table 10-7).

The eye may also be infected with fungi (includes molds and yeasts). Antifungal agents called fungicides (also called antimycotics) are used to treat surface (exophthalmic) and intraocular (endophthalmic) fungal infections. Treatment may be topical (examples include natamycin/Natacin® and amphotericin B/Ambisome®), intraocular (examples include amphotericin B/Ambisome® and fluconazole/Diflucan®), or systemic (examples include amphotericin/Ambisome® and voriconazole/Vfend®).

Dyes/Stains

Dyes and stains are substances used to color various structures of the eye to enhance visualization by creating contrast, especially when working under an operating microscope. Dyes and stains may be used on the surface of the eye to identify abnormalities such as dry eye syndrome, to visualize a puncture or an abrasion, and to identify the location of a foreign body. Examples of dyes used on the surface of the eye include fluorescein (Fluorescite®) and lissamine green, which are available on paper strips impregnated with the dye. Use of a Wood's lamp (black light/ultraviolet light) may be necessary when using fluorescein. Fluorescein is also available in parenteral form that is injected intravenously

TABLE 10-7 Examples of Ophthalmic Antibiotics

Route of Administration	Drug Name (generic/brand)	Concentration
Topical (drops)	• gentamicin/Garamycin®, Gentacidin® • neomycin/Neosporin® • polymyxin B+/Polytrim® • tobramycin/Tobrex®	0.3% 3.5 mg/ml 10,000 u/ml 0.3%
Topical (ointments)	• bacitracin +/Polysporin® • gentamicin/Genoptic® • oxytetracycline +/Terac® • sulfacetamide/Cetamide®	500 u/g 0.3% 5 mg/g 10%
Subconjunctival (injected)	• cefazolin • penicillin G • tobramycin • vancomycin	n/a n/a n/a n/a
Intraocular	• amikacin • ceftazidime • clindamycin • vancomycin	n/a n/a n/a n/a
Systemic (oral, parenteral)	• amikacin • ceftazidime • ciprofloxacin • tetracycline	n/a n/a n/a n/a

during ophthalmic angiography to examine blood flow to the retina and the choroid. Dyes and stains are also used intraocularly during cataract removal to identify the posterior capsule and in retinal surgery to visualize the membranes in the posterior capsule. Examples of capsular dyes include indocyanine green (IC-Green®) and trypan blue (VisionBlue®) and an example of a dye used on the posterior capsule membrane is trypan blue (MembraneBlue®).

Zonulysis

An enzyme called chymotrypsin (Alpha Chymar®, Zonulyn®, and Zolyse®) is sometimes used intraocularly to dissolve the zonule of Zinn (**zonulysis**) to facilitate removal of a cataract. The zonule of Zinn is a fibrous membrane that suspends the crystalline lens to the ciliary muscle.

Local Anesthesia Adjuncts (Agonists)

The same two agonistic anesthetic agents used as in conjunction with local anesthesia agents elsewhere in the body to enhance and/or prolong their effects are also used during ophthalmic procedures for the same reasons. The vasoconstrictor epinephrine (adrenaline) is used to reduce the risk of bleeding at the surgical site and to retain the anesthetic agent in the area. The enzyme hyaluronidase (Amphadase®) promotes penetration of the anesthetic agent into the connective tissue more readily; enhancing and prolonging the effect of the anesthetic

agent. Both adjunctive agents are manufactured in the liquid form and are mixed with the local anesthetic prior to infiltration.

Irrigating Solutions

Ophthalmic irrigating solution, sometimes referred to as balanced salt solution (BSS), is available for extraocular or intraocular use and is sterile, isotonic, and pH adjusted (to approximately 7.0). Glucose is sometimes added to provide an energy source. Irrigation of the conjunctiva and cornea may be necessary following exposure of the eye to a chemical or biohazardous material. Eyewash stations are located strategically throughout the healthcare facility and in industrial settings for use as needed. Examples of eyewash solutions include Buffered Eye-Lert®, Eye Relief®, and Mediwash®. Irrigating solutions are also used during eye exams and surgical procedures to keep the external tissues moist and to replace aqueous humor that may leak out of the eye through an incision. Examples of balanced salt solution intended for surgical use include AquaLase®, BSS®, and BSS Plus®.

Mydriatics/Cycloplegics

Mydriatics are sympathomimetic drugs, such as phenylephrine (Ak-Dilate®, Mydfrin®, and Spersaphrine®), that stimulate relaxation of the muscle that dilates the pupil (iris). **Cycloplegics** are antimuscarinics that paralyze the ciliary body interrupting the process of accommodation and paralyze the muscle that constricts the pupil, thereby, maintaining pupil dilation. Examples of cycloplegic drugs include atropine (Atropisol® and Isopto Atropine®), cyclopentolate (Ak-Pentolate®, Diopentolate®, and Cyclogyl®), homatropine (Isopto Atropine®), and tropicamide (Mydriacyl® and Tropicacyl®). Mydriatics and cycloplegics may be administered topically, orally, parenterally, or intraocularly and are used during ophthalmic examinations, during surgical procedures, and for ongoing treatment of closed-angle glaucoma.

Miotics

Miotics are drugs that cause the muscle of the iris to contract and constrict the pupil. Miotics may be administered topically or intraocularly and are used to treat glaucoma and to cause constriction of the pupil following mydriasis. Examples of miotics include the cholinergic drugs pilocarpine (Salagen®) and carbachol (Carbastat® and Miostat®) and the anticholinergic drug acetylcholine (Miochol-E®).

Viscoelastics

Sodium hyaluronate (Healon® and Staarvisc II®) and sodium chondroitin sulfate with sodium hyaluronate (Viscoat®) are clear viscous substances that are used intraocularly. Viscoelastics are provided in sterile syringes for use during ophthalmic procedures (e.g., cataract extraction, lens implantation/replacement, glaucoma and retinal procedures, and corneal transplantation) to maintain the size and shape of the anterior cavity and to protect the delicate intraocular structures. Viscoelastics are easily removed from the eye using an irrigation and aspiration technique or the substance may be allowed to remain in the eye. Viscoelastics are stored in the refrigerator but must be warmed to room temperature (for approximately 30 minutes) prior to use.

Lubricants

Ophthalmic lubricants are available in liquid (drop and spray) and semisolid (gel and ointment) forms (Table 10-8). Lubricants are used as artificial tears to treat dry eyes related to deficient tear production, to keep the eyes moist following surgery or an injury, and

to moisten and protect the eyes of a patient undergoing a surgical procedure under general anesthesia (because the blink reflex may be absent and/or the eyes may not close completely). Some lubricants are petroleum based and caution must be exercised if nearby use of the electrosurgical unit or a laser is planned to avoid combustion.

Sedatives/Hypnotics

Sedatives and **hypnotics** are central nervous system depressants that are typically classified as narcotics. Sedatives, also called anxiolytics, are used to produce a state of calm and reduce anxiety; and hypnotics, also called **soporifics**, are used to induce sleep. Sedatives and hypnotics act by increasing the action of the inhibitory neurotransmitter gamma-aminobutyric acid (GABA), thereby, slowing the effects of the central nervous system, reducing anxiety, and promoting sleep. A sedative and a hypnotic may be the same drug given in varying dosages to produce the desired effect and are available for systemic administration via oral and parenteral routes. Sedatives and hypnotics include barbiturates and benzodiazepines as well some other drugs such as antihistamines and psychotropic drugs.

Barbiturates, such as phenobarbital (Donnatal® and Solfoton®), are especially useful for control of seizures. Because of their rapid onset of action, some barbiturates including thiopental sodium (Sodium Pentothal®) and methohexital (Brevital®) are used as induction agents for general anesthesia. Barbiturates produce marked respiratory depression and surgical team members should be ready to provide immediate ventilatory support for the patient, as needed.

Benzodiazepines have anticonvulsant, amnesic, anxiolytic, and sedative effects and produce minimal cardiac and respiratory depression. Benzodiazepines are popular for use as a preoperative medication to reduce anxiety and intraoperatively when monitored anesthesia care (MAC) is provided during a procedure conducted under conscious sedation. Examples of benzodiazepines include diazepam (Valium®), droperidol (Inapsine®), lorazepam (Ativan®), and midazolam (Versed®). Flumazenil (Mazicon® and Romazicon®) is the preferred antagonist for benzodiazepines.

TABLE 10-8 Ophthalmic Lubricants

Type	Generic Name	Brand Name
Drops	Glycerin	Advanced Eye Relief Environmental® and Oasis Tears®
	hydroxypropyl methylcellulose	Genteal® and Visine Tears®
Sprays	liposome	Actimist®, ClaryMist®, and Tears Again®
Gels	carboxyl methylcellulose sodium	Refresh Liquigel® and TheraTears Liquigel®
Ointments	white petrolatum, mineral oil	Lacrilube® and Purilube®

Vagal Blockers

Vagal blockers, such as H₂ receptor blockers (H₂ antagonists) and cholinergic blockers (anticholinergics/parasympatholytics/antimuscarinics), are used to block the effects of the vagus nerve. Refer to the respective sections of this chapter for additional information.

Vasodilators

Vasodilators relax (dilate) the smooth muscle of the wall of a blood vessel, thereby, increasing the diameter of the lumen of the vessel, decreasing resistance to blood flow, and lowering the blood pressure. Vasodilators may be administered via enteral, parenteral, and topical routes. Some vasodilators, such as nitrates, are specific to coronary vessel dilation while others act systemically on the peripheral blood vessels. Examples of peripheral vasodilators include cyclandelate (Cyclospasmol®), isoxsuprine (Vasodilan®), and papaverine (Cerespan® and Pavabid®). Additionally, papaverine may be used topically to cause localized vasodilation.

Vasoconstrictors

Vasoconstrictors, also called vasopressors, tighten (constrict) the smooth muscle of the wall of a blood vessel thereby decreasing the diameter of the lumen of the vessel, increasing resistance to blood flow, and raising the blood pressure. Vasoconstrictors may be administered via enteral and parenteral routes. Ephedrine, metaraminol (Aramine®) and phenylephrine (Neo-Synephrine®), and vasopressin (Pitressin®) are examples of vasoconstrictors.

Summary

I. Amnesics—Drug that induces memory loss
II. Analgesics/Antipyretics—Drugs that reduce or eliminate pain (analgesic) and fever (antipyretic)
III. Anesthesia agents—Limited to local and topical anesthesia agents
    a. Amino amides—Biotransformed in the liver
    b. Amino esters—Biotransformed by pseudocholinesterase in the blood plasma
    c. Agonistic anesthetic agents
IV. Anticoagulants/Fibrinolytics—Anticoagulants prevent blood clot formation and fibrinolytics destroy clots that have already formed
V. Anticonvulsants—Prevent or reduce the effects of a seizure
VI. Antiemetics—Reduce or eliminate nausea and vomiting
VII. Antihistamines—Reduce or counteract the effects of histamines during an allergic reaction (also known as H₁ receptor antagonists)
VIII. Anti-infective agents—Chemicals capable of killing pathogens or hindering their growth
    a. Beta-lactams—Includes penicillins, cephalosporins, and carbapenems; inhibit enzymes necessary to manufacture the cell wall during mitosis
    b. Sulfonamides—Also known as sulfa drugs; synthetic agents that disrupt synthesis of folic acid, thereby, negatively impacting production of DNA and purine
    c. Polypeptides—Also known as polymyxins; bind to the bacterial cell membrane disrupting the cell's ability to release toxins
    d. Aminoglycosides—Disrupt protein synthesis of the ribosomes in the bacterial cell, thereby preventing growth of the cell
    e. Tetracyclines—Disrupt protein synthesis of the cell rendering the cell incapable of reproduction
    f. Antifungals—Inhibit the growth of or kill fungal infections (includes mold and yeast infections)
    g. Antimicrobials—Agents used to destroy microbes; includes antiseptics, disinfectants, and sterilants
        i. Antiseptics—Used on living tissue to prohibit growth of or destroy microorganisms
        ii. Disinfectants—Used on fomites to destroy pathogens; disinfection occurs on three levels
        iii. Sterilants—Chemical or physical agents that kill all microorganisms including bacterial spores
IX. Antineoplastics (chemotherapy agents)—Used in the treatment of various types of cancer; also called anticancer drugs
X. Autonomic agents—Affect the two divisions of the autonomic (involuntary) portion of the central nervous system
    a. Adrenergics—Mimic the effects of the sympathetic nervous system; also called sympathomimetics or adrenergic agonists
    b. Adrenergic blockers (alpha and beta)—Inhibit the effects of the sympathetic nervous system; also called sympatholytics and adrenergic antagonists
    c. Cholinergics—Mimic the effects of the parasympathetic nervous system; also called parasympathomimetics and muscarinics
    d. Cholinergic blockers—Block the effects of the parasympathetic nervous system; also called anticholinergics, antimuscarinics, and parasympatholytics

XI. Blood replacement interventions—Used to restore patient's normal blood volume and blood pressure
    a. Autologous blood—Taken from and reinfused to the same individual
    b. Donated blood products—Taken from one individual and infused into someone else
        i. Type and cross matching—Test performed on blood from both the donor and recipient to identify the blood type, Rh factor, and the presence of an antibodies in the donor blood that could be harmful to the recipient
        ii. Whole blood—Blood that has not had any portion removed
        iii. Component therapy—Portions of blood that are separated and used as needed; includes red blood cells and platelet rich plasma (which can be further separated into specific components)
    c. Colloid plasma expanders—Hypertonic solutions that draw fluid into the blood vessels to help maintain blood pressure and circulate remaining red blood cells

XII. Cardiovascular agents—Drugs that affect the heart and blood vessels
    a. Antidysrhythmics—Used to restore normal heart rhythm; four main classifications
    b. Coronary dilators—Cause vasodilation of the coronary arteries
    c. Inotropic agents—Change the force of a muscle contraction; especially contraction of the heart muscle
    d. Vasopressors and peripheral vasodilators—Vasopressors constrict the muscles of the blood vessel wall causing the lumen of the vessel to narrow; raising the patient's blood pressure. Vasodilators relax the muscles of the blood vessel wall causing the lumen of the vessel to widen; lowering the patient's blood pressure
    e. Antihypertensive agents—Prescribed to lower the blood pressure to within normal limits

XIII. Central nervous system stimulants—Speed physiological processes and increase mental alertness by mimicking the stimulatory effects of the sympathetic nervous system
    a. Amphetamines—Group of narcotics that includes methamphetamine, cocaine, anorexiants, and psychotropics
    b. Analeptics—Stimulate the respiratory center in the brain stem

XIV. Coagulants/hemostatics—Promote blood clot formation and maintenance

XV. Contrast media—Used during radiographic studies to enhance visualization by differentiating body structures; positive contrast media is radiopaque and negative contrast media is radiolucent

XVI. Diuretics—Increase the amount of urine that is excreted
    a. Carbonic anhydrase inhibitor diuretics—Inhibit the enzyme carbonic anhydrase causing an increase in excretion of hydrogen which in turn increases excretion of sodium, water, and potassium
    b. Loop diuretic—Produce rapid diuresis by inhibiting reabsorption of sodium and chloride in the loop of Henle
    c. Osmotic diuretic—Increase the amount of extracellular fluid and plasma volume by drawing fluid from the cells by osmosis

XVII. Dyes/Stains—Substances used to color various body structures; dyes are typically for short-term use and stains are longer lasting or permanent

XVIII. Emergency drugs—Used in response to critical patient situations; typically found on emergency carts
    a. Malignant hyperthermia—Dramatic increase in body temperature that develops when a susceptible individual is exposed to a triggering agent; dantrolene is administered and other supportive measures are initiated.
    b. Allergic reaction—Exaggerated immune system (histamine) response to a foreign substance; if the allergic reaction is severe, diphenhydramine, epinephrine and corticosteroids may be administered
    c. Cardiac arrest—Emergency measures include airway management, administration of oxygen, initiation of CPR, and defibrillation; pharmacologic treatment is determined according to the type of dysrhythmia diagnosed
    d. Respiratory distress/arrest—Treatment according to underlying cause; drug therapy may include the use of neuromuscular blockers, respiratory stimulants, bronchodilators, narcotic antagonists, sodium bicarbonate, and corticosteroids

XIX. Emetics—Drugs that induce vomiting

XX. Gastric Agents—Produce an effect on the stomach
    a. H_2 receptor blockers—Suppress secretion of hydrochloric acid in the stomach

XXI. Hormones—Chemical substances secreted by endocrine glands and various other cells throughout the body; endocrine hormones are transported to the target tissue in the blood and other hormones act locally
    a. Corticosteroids—Produced in the adrenal cortex and available as pharmaceutical preparations; includes glucocorticoids, mineralocorticoids, and sex hormones
    b. Insulin/Glucagon—Antagonists produced in the islet cells of the pancreas; insulin lowers the blood sugar level while glucagon raises the blood sugar level to achieve homeostasis

c. Prostaglandins—Secreted by many types of cells in the body and act on nearby tissues; produce numerous effects

d. Sex hormones—Support growth and development of secondary sex characteristics in both the male and the female; female sex hormones include estrogen and progesterone and the male sex hormone is testosterone

XXII. Inhalation agents—Gasses or vapors that are breathed or blown into the lungs

a. Nasal sprays—Applied to the mucous membrane lining of the nose with the use of an atomizer

XXIII. Irrigation solutions—Fluids used to wash, flush, or moisten body surfaces, tissues, body cavities, body orifices, wounds (chronic, surgical, traumatic), hollow organs, improve visibility, and to flush medical devices (catheters, tubes, and drains)

XXIV. IV fluids—Included crystalloids, blood, blood products, colloids (hypertonic, isotonic, and hypotonic), and oxygen carrying solutions

XXV. Lubricants—Used on skin and mucous membranes to decrease friction during rectal and vaginal examinations and to facilitate insertion or passage of catheters, endoscopes, and surgical instruments

XXVI. Narcotic antagonists—Reverse the analgesic, hypotensive, respiratory depressant and sedative effects of a narcotic

XXVII. Narcotic analgesics—Used to reduce the perception of and reaction to pain as well as increase pain tolerance for patients experiencing moderate to severe acute and chronic pain

XXVIII. Neuroleptics/Tranquilizers—Major tranquilizers are used in the treatment of psychoses and neuroses although some are used to relieve nausea and vomiting and act as a synergist of analgesics; minor tranquilizers are used in the treatment of anxiety, stress, and irritability (some sedative/hypnotics are considered to be minor tranquilizers)

XXIX. Obstetrical agents—Includes drugs used to induce abortion, stimulate and suppress lactation, stimulate and relax uterine contractions, and prevent hemolytic disease of the newborn

a. Oxytocics—Used to induce labor, strengthen uterine contractions during labor, and contract the uterus to control hemorrhage following an abortion or delivery of a neonate

b. Rho (D) immune globulin—Used to prevent hemolytic disease of the newborn

XXX. Ophthalmic agents—Specifically designed for use in the eye

a. Antibiotics—Used to treat bacterial infections of the eyelids, surface of the eye, and the inner tunics and cavities of the eye

b. Dyes/Stains—Used to color various structures of the eye to enhance visualization by creating contrast; especially when working under an operating microscope

c. Zonulysis—Used to dissolve the zonule of Zinn to facilitate removal of a cataract

d. Local anesthesia adjuncts (agonists)—Used to enhance and/or prolong the effects of a local anesthetic; included epinephrine (vasoconstrictor) and hyaluronidase (enzyme)

e. Irrigating solutions—Sterile, isotonic, and pH adjusted solution used to **irrigate** the eye; extraocular and intraocular use

f. Mydriatics/Cycloplegics—Mydriatics are sympathomimetic drugs that relax the muscle of the iris causing dilation of the pupil; cycloplegics are antimuscarinics that paralyze the ciliary body interrupting the process of accommodation and paralyze the muscle of the iris that constricts the pupil thereby maintaining pupil dilation

g. Miotics—Cause the muscle of the iris to contract and constrict the pupil

h. Viscoelastics—Viscous substances used intraocularly to maintain the size and shape of the anterior cavity and to protect the delicate intraocular structures

i. Lubricants—Used to moisten and protect the eyes if tear production is deficient, to keep the eyes moist following surgery or injury, and to protect the eyes of a patient undergoing a surgical procedure under general anesthesia

XXXI. Sedatives/Hypnotics—Central nervous system depressants (typically narcotics); sedatives are used to produce a state of calm and reduce anxiety and hypnotics are used to induce sleep

XXXII. Vagal blockers—Block the effects of the vagus nerve

XXXIII. Vasodilators—Relax (dilate) the smooth muscle of the wall of a blood vessel thereby increasing the diameter of the lumen of the vessel, decreasing resistance to blood flow, and lowering the blood pressure.

XXXIV. Vasoconstrictors—Tighten (constrict) the smooth muscle of the wall of a blood vessel thereby decreasing the diameter of the lumen of the vessel, increasing resistance to blood flow, and raising the blood pressure; also called vasopressors

Critical Thinking Review

1. Describe the differences between the ways that amino amides and amino esters are metabolized.
2. Explain why epinephrine and hyaluronidase are considered to be agonistic anesthetic agents.
3. Is an anticoagulant the same as a fibrinolytic? Why or why not?
4. Provide at least one example each of an alternative and a naturopathic antiemetic.
5. List the three types of beta-lactams and identify the main source of each.
6. List two synonyms for the term *adrenergic* and describe the action(s) of adrenergic drugs.
7. What is the function of an inotropic agent?
8. Differentiate between positive and negative contract media.
9. Describe malignant hyperthermia, list the symptoms, and identify the treatment(s) that a patient experiencing a malignant hyperthermia crisis may receive.
10. Identify at least one similarity and one difference between a vasoconstrictor and a vasodilator.

References

American Association of Blood Banks. (2012). *Standard setting activities*. Retrieved from http://www.aabb.org/sa/standards/Pages/default.aspx

American Heart Association. (2012). *Cardiac medications*. Retrieved from http://www.heart.org/idc/groups/heart-public/@wcm/@hcm/documents/downloadable/ucm_304568.pdf

Amnesic. (n.d.). *The American heritage® Stedman's medical dictionary*. Retrieved from http://dictionary.reference.com/browse/amnesic

Analeptic. (n.d.). *The American heritage® Stedman's medical dictionary*. Retrieved from http://dictionary.reference.com/browse/analeptic

Analgesic. (n.d.). *The American heritage® Stedman's medical dictionary*. Retrieved from http://dictionary.reference.com/browse/analgesic

Anantharaman, V. & Gunasegaran, K. (2011). *Advanced cardiac life support guidelines 2011*. Retrieved from http://www.nrcsingapore.org/sg/conference2011/articles/Advanced%20Cardiac%20Life%20Support%20Guidelines%202011.pdf

Anticoagulant. (n.d.). *The American heritage® Stedman's medical dictionary*. Retrieved from http://dictionary.reference.com/browse/anticoagulant

Anticonvulsant. (n.d.). *The American heritage® Stedman's medical dictionary*. Retrieved from http://dictionary.reference.com/browse/anticonvulsant

Antiemetic. (n.d.). *The American heritage® Stedman's medical dictionary*. Retrieved from http://dictionary.reference.com/browse/antiemetic

Antihistamine. (n.d.). *Merriam-Webster's medical dictionary*. Retrieved from http://dictionary.reference.com/browse/antihistamine

Antineoplastic. (n.d.). *The American heritage® Stedman's medical dictionary*. Retrieved from http://dictionary.reference.com/browse/antineoplastic

Antipyretic. (n.d.). *The American heritage® Stedman's medical dictionary*. Retrieved from http://dictionary.reference.com/browse/antipyretic

Balanced salt solution. (2009). Retrieved from http://www.drugs.com/pro/balanced-salt-solution.html

Baum, J. (n.d.). *Antibiotic use in ophthalmology*. Retrieved from http://www.oculist.net/downaton502/prof/ebook/duanes/pages/v4/v4c026.html

Benner, R. (2005). *IV therapy for EMS*. Upper Saddle River, NJ: Prentice Hall.

Berger, F. & Zieve, D. (2012). *Psychosis*. Retrieved from http://www.ncbi.nlm.nih.gov/pubmedhealth/PMH0002520

Brecher, M., Goodnough, L., & Monk, T. (2002). *The value of oxygen-carrying solutions in the operative setting, as determined by mathematical modeling*. Retrieved from http://onlinelibrary.wiley.com/doi/10.1046/j.1537-2995.1999.39499235673.x/full

Bowen, R. (2008). *Histamine and histamine receptors*. Retrieved from http://www.vivo.colostate.edu/hbooks/pathphys/endocrine/otherendo/histamine.html

Broyles, B., Reiss, B., & Evans, M. (2007). *Pharmacological aspects of nursing care* (7th ed.). Clifton Park, NY: Thomson Delmar Learning.

Centers for Disease Control and Prevention. (2009). *Guideline for disinfection and sterilization in healthcare facilities*. Retrieved from http://cdc.gov/hicpac/Disinfection_Sterilization/2_approach.html

Chabner, B. & Thompson, E. (2009). *Commonly used antineoplastic drugs*. Retrieved from http://www.merckmanuals.com/media/professional/pdf/Antineoplastic_drugs.pdf

Chabner, B. & Thompson, E. (2009). *Modalities of cancer therapy*. Retrieved from http://www.merckmanuals.com/professional/hematology_and_oncology/principles_of_cancer_therapy/modalities_of_cancer_therapy.html

Chabner, B. & Thompson, E. (2009). *Overview of cancer therapy*. Retrieved from http://www.oncolink.org/treatment/article.cfm?c=2&s=9&id=54

Cohen, B. (2005). *Memmler's the human body in health and disease* (10th ed.). Philadelphia, PA: Lippincott Williams & Wilkins.

Cook, J. (2006). *Cellular pathology: An introduction to techniques and applications*. Banbury, UK: Scion Publishing Limited.

Craig, R. & Stitzel, R. (2004). *Modern pharmacology with clinical applications.* Philadelphia, PA: Lippincott Williams & Wilkins.

Cunha, J. (2012). *Alpha blockers.* Retrieved from http://www.medicinenet.com/high_blood_pressure_treatment/page12.htm

Cunha, J. (2012). *Allergic reaction.* Retrieved from http://www.emedicinehealth.com/allergic_reaction/article_em.htm

Curren, A. M. (2010). *Dimensional analysis for meds* (4th ed.). Clifton Park, NY: Delmar Cengage Learning.

David, K. (2007). *IV fluids: Do you know what's hanging and why?* Retrieved from http://www.modernmedicine.com/modernmedicine/article/articleDetail.jsp?id=463604

Dennis, V. (2006). *Electrosurgery safety and your staff: Measures you can take to ensure that patients will have no adverse effects from the application of electrosurgical energy.* Retrieved from http://www.encision.com/encision%20media/articles%20media/outpatient2.html

Dickinson, R. (2006). *Life's blood: The crossmatch.* Retrieved from http://faculty.matcmadison.edu/mljensen/BloodBank/lectures/crossmatch.htm

diZerega, G. (n.d.). *Contemporary adhesion prevention.* Retrieved from http://centerforendo.com/articles/adhesions.htm

Dugdale, D., Chen, Y., & Zieve, D. (2011). *Transfusion reaction—hemolytic.* Retrieved from http://www.ncbi.nlm.nih.gov/pubmedhealth/PMH0002280

Dugdale, D., Henochowicz, S., & Zieve, D. (2012). *Anaphylaxis.* Retrieved from http://www.ncbi.nlm.nih.gov/pubmedhealth/PMH0001847

Ehrlich, S. (2011). *Magnesium.* Retrieved from http://www.umm.edu/altmed/articles/magnesium-000313.htm

Ehrlich, S. (2011). *Potassium.* Retrieved from http://www.umm.edu/altmed/articles/potassium-000320.htm

Emetic. (n.d.). *The American heritage® Stedman's medical dictionary.* Retrieved from http://dictionary.reference.com/browse/emetic

ESUR Contrast Media Safety Committee. (2007). *ESUR guidelines on contrast media* (Version 6.0). Retrieved from http://www.esur.org/fileadmin/Guidelines/ESUR_2007_Guideline_6_Kern_Ubersicht.pdf

Fibrinolytic. (n.d.). *The American heritage® Stedman's medical dictionary.* Retrieved from http://dictionary.reference.com/browse/fibrinolytic

Fickling, J., Parsons, J., & Loeffler, C. (2002). *Irrigation solution: Will your choice affect the electrosurgical outcome or patient safety?* Retrieved from http://www.valleylab.com/education/hotline/pdfs/hotline_0207.pdf

Fitzakerley, J. (2012). *Principles of anti-hormone chemotherapy.* Retrieved from http://www.d.umn.edu/~jfitzake/Lectures/DMED/Antineoplastics/Antihormones/Principles.html

Frey, K., et al. (2008). *Surgical technology for the surgical technologist: A positive care approach* (3rd ed.). Clifton Park, NY: Delmar Cengage Learning.

Friedman, N. (2010). *Ophthalmic surgical dyes: VisionBlue and MembraneBlue.* Retrieved from http://www.ophthalmologyweb.com/Tech-Spotlights/26540-Ophthalmic-Surgical-Dyes-Vision-Blue-and-MembraneBlue

Gabriel, A. (2011). *Wound irrigation.* Retrieved from http://emedicine.medscape.com/article/1895071-overview

Gallimore, D. (2006). *Understanding the drugs used during cardiac arrest response.* Retrieved from http://www.nursingtimes.net/nursing-practice/clinical-zones/cardiology/understanding-the-drugs-used-during-cardiac-arrest-response/203172.article#

Gifford-Ellis, P. (2004). *Suppression of lactation.* Retrieved from http://www.rch.org.au/picu_intranet/guidelines.cfm?doc_id=7933

Gillson, S. (2011). *H2 blockers: Class of drugs that block stomach acid.* Retrieved from http://heartburn.about.com/od/medsremedies/a/h2blockers.htm

Goldwein, J. & Somer, B. (2001). *Biological response modifiers.* Retrieved from http://www.oncolink.org/treatment/article.cfm?c=2&s=9&id=54

Hancock, R. & Chapple, D. (2012). *Peptide antibiotics.* Retrieved from http://aac.asm.org/content/43/6/1317.full

Heart Rhythm Society. (n.d.). *Antiarrhythmics.* Retrieved from http://www.hrsonline.org/patientinfo/treatments/medications/aa/#One

Heiserman, D. (2004). *Coagulants (promoting clot formation).* Retrieved from http://www.waybuilder.net/sweethaven/MedTech/Pharmacol/coursemain.asp?whichMod=module030504

Heller, J. & Zieve, D. (2011). *Breathing—slowed or stopped.* Retrieved from http://www.nlm.nih.gov/medlineplus/ency/article/003069.htm

Heller, J. & Zieve, D. (2011). *Malignant hyperthermia.* Retrieved from http://www.ncbi.nlm.nih.gov/pubmedhealth/PMH0002292

Higashide, T. & Sugiyama, K. (2008). *Use of viscoelastic substance in ophthalmic surgery—focus on sodium hyaluronate.* Retrieved from http://www.ncbi.nlm.nih.gov/pmc/articles/PMC2698691

Histamine. (n.d.). *Merriam-Webster's medical dictionary.* Retrieved from http://dictionary.reference.com/browse/histamine

Hoad-Robson, R. (2010). *Radionuclide (isotope) scan.* Retrieved from http://www.patient.co.uk/health/Radionuclide-(Isotope)-Scan.htm

Hopper, T. (2007). *Mosby's pharmacy technician principles & practice* (2nd ed.). St. Louis, MO: Saunders Elsevier.

Hypnotic. (n.d.). *The American heritage® Stedman's medical dictionary.* Retrieved from http://dictionary .reference.com/browse/hypnotic

Inotropic. (n.d.). *MedLine plus medical dictionary.* Retrieved from http://www2.merriam-webster.com/ cgi-bin/mwmednlm?book=Medical&va=inotropic

Inotropic. (n.d.). *The American heritage® Stedman's medical dictionary.* Retrieved from http://dictionary .reference.com/browse/inotropic

Irrigation. (2003). *Miller-Keane encyclopedia and dictionary of medicine, nursing, and allied health* (7th Edition). Saint Louis, MO: Saunders Elsevier.

Jhang, J. (2006). *Blood component therapy.* Retrieved from http://www.columbia.edu/itc/hs/medical/selective/AdvClinicalPathology/2006/lecture/jhang10-17 BloodComponentTherapyMedicalStudentNotes.pdf

Johns Hopkins Sjogren's Center. (2011). *Ocular surface staining.* Retrieved from http://www .hopkinssjogrens.org/disease-information/ diagnosis-sjogrens-syndrome/ocular-surface-staining

Kaynar, A. (2012). *Respiratory failure.* Retrieved from http://emedicine.medscape.com/ article/167981-overview

Kimball, J. (2010). *Antibiotics: Antibacterial agents.* Retrieved from http://users.rcn.com/jkimball. ma.ultranet/BiologyPages/A/Antibiotics.html

Klabunde, R. (2010). *Beta-adrenoceptor antagonists (beta-blockers).* Retrieved from http://www .cvpharmacology.com/cardioinhibitory/beta-blockers.htm

Klabunde, R. (2010). *Calcium-channel blockers (CCBs).* Retrieved from http://www.cvpharmacology.com/ vasodilator/CCB.htm

Klabunde, R. (2010). *Diuretics.* Retrieved from http:// cvpharmacology.com/diuretic/diuretics.htm

Klabunde, R. (2010). *Potassium-channel blockers (class III antiarrhythmics).* Retrieved from http://www .cvpharmacology.com/antiarrhy/potassium-blockers.htm

Klabunde, R. (2010). *Vaughan-Williams classification of antiarrhythmic drugs.* Retrieved from http://www .cvpharmacology.com/antiarrhy/Vaughan-Williams .htm

Klabunde, R. (2011). *Sodium-channel blockers (class I antiarrhythmics).* Retrieved from http://www .cvpharmacology.com/antiarrhy/sodium-blockers .htm

Klabunde, R. (2012). *Nitrodilators.* Retrieved from http://cvpharmacology.com/vasodilator/nitro.htm

Klajn, R. (n.d.). *Chemistry and chemical biology of tetracyclines.* Retrieved from http://www.chm.bris .ac.uk/motm/tetracycline/tetracycline.htm

Levison, M. (2009). *Aminoglycosides.* Retrieved from http://www.merckmanuals.com/professional/ infectious_diseases/bacteria_and_antibacterial_ drugs/aminoglycosides.html

Levison, M. (2009). *Beta-lactams.* Retrieved from http://www.merckmanuals.com/professional/ infectious_diseases/bacteria_and_antibacterial_ drugs/%CE%B2-lactams.html

Levison, M. (2009). *Overview of antibacterial drugs.* Retrieved from http://www.merckmanuals.com/ professional/infectious_diseases/bacteria_and_ antibacterial_drugs/overview_of_antibacterial_ drugs.html

Levison, M. (2009). *Overview of bacteria.* Retrieved from http://www.merckmanuals.com/professional/ infectious_diseases/bacteria_and_antibacterial_ drugs/overview_of_bacteria.html

Levison, M. (2009). *Polypeptides.* Retrieved from http:// www.merckmanuals.com/professional/infectious_ diseases/bacteria_and_antibacterial_drugs /polypeptides.html

Levison, M. (2009). *Sulfonamides.* Retrieved from http://www.merckmanuals.com/professional /infectious_diseases/bacteria_and_antibacterial_ drugs/sulfonamides.html

Levison, M. (2009). *Tetracyclines.* Retrieved from http://www.merckmanuals.com/professional /infectious_diseases/bacteria_and_antibacterial_ drugs/tetracyclines.html

Lew, W. & Weaver, F. (2008). *Clinical use of topical thrombin as a surgical hemostat.* Retrieved from http://www.ncbi.nlm.nih.gov/pmc/articles/ PMC2727895

Malignant Hyperthermia Association of the United States. (2011). *What is MH?* Retrieved from http://www.mhaus.org/ mhaus-faqs-healthcare-professionals/ what-is-malignant-hyperthermia

Martin, G. (2005). *An update on intravenous fluids.* Retrieved from http://www.medscape.org/ viewarticle/503138

Mather, R. (2012). *Empiric antiinfective therapy in ophthalmology.* Retrieved from http://eyemicrobiology .upmc.com/Antimicrobial.htm

McAuley, D. (2012). *Dantrolene—Dantrium®.* Retrieved from http://www.globalrph.com/dantrolene_ dilution.htm

McDonnell, G. & Russell, D. (1999). *Antiseptics and disinfectants: Activity, action, and resistance.* Retrieved from http://www.ncbi.nlm.nih.gov/pmc/ articles/PMC88911/

McDonough, J. (n.d.). *Midazolam: An improved anticonvulsant treatment for nerve agent-induced seizures.* Retrieved from http://www.dtic.mil/cgi-bin/ GetTRDoc?AD=ADA436040

McLeod, I. (2011). *Local anesthetics*. Retrieved from http://emedicine.medscape.com/article/873879-overview

Moini, J. (2009). *Fundamental pharmacology for pharmacy technicians*. Clifton Park, NY: Delmar Cengage Learning.

Morrison, G. (n.d.). *Radiographic contrast media*. Retrieved from http://faculty.mwsu.edu/radsci/gary.morrison/Contrast_Media.pdf

Nabili, S. (2009). *Pulmonary edema*. Retrieved from http://www.medicinenet.com/pulmonary_edema/article.htm

National Center for Chronic Disease Prevention and Health Promotion. (2011). *Targeting epilepsy: Improving the lives of people with one of the nation's most common neurological conditions*. Retrieved from http://www.cdc.gov/chronicdisease/resources/publications/AAG/epilepsy.htm

National Heart Lung and Blood Institute. (2011). *What is high blood pressure?* Retrieved from http://www.nhlbi.nih.gov/health/health-topics/topics/hbp

National Institutes of Health Office of Dietary Supplements. (n.d.). *Dietary supplement fact sheet: Magnesium*. Retrieved from http://ods.od.nih.gov/factsheets/Magnesium-HealthProfessional

National Library of Medicine. (2011). *Protamines*. Retrieved from http://www.nlm.nih.gov/cgi/mesh/2011/MB_cgi?mode=&term=Protamine+Sulfate

Nazario, B. (2011). *Types of insulin for diabetes treatment*. Retrieved from http://diabetes.webmd.com/guide/diabetes-types-insulin

Niekraszewicz, A. (2005). *Chitosan medical dressings*. Retrieved from http://www.fibtex.lodz.pl/54_08_16.pdf

Ogbru, O. (2005). *Beta blockers*. Retrieved from http://www.medicinenet.com/beta_blockers/article.htm

Olson, J. (2006). *Clinical pharmacology made ridiculously simple*. Miami: MedMaster, Inc.

Ophardt, C. (2003). *Antibiotic—penicillin*. Retrieved from http://www.elmhurst.edu/~chm/vchembook/652penicillin.html

Ophardt, C. (2003). *Central nervous system introduction—drugs acting upon the central nervous system*. Retrieved from http://www.elmhurst.edu/~chm/vchembook/670drugcns.html

Ophardt, C. (2003). *Narcotic analgesic drugs*. Retrieved from http://www.elmhurst.edu/~chm/vchembook/674narcotic.html

Ophardt, C. (2003). *Other antibiotics*. Retrieved from http://www.elmhurst.edu/~chm/vchembook/654antibiotic.html

Ophardt, C. (2003). *Prostaglandins*. Retrieved from http://www.elmhurst.edu/~chm/vchembook/555prostagland.html

Ortho-Clinical Diagnostics. (2011). *About RhoGAM® brand*. Retrieved from http://www.rhogam.com/Professional/AboutRhogamBrand/Pages/default.aspx

Patterson, T. (2006). *Treatment of invasive aspergillosis: Polyenes, echinocandins, or azoles?* Retrieved from http://www.aspergillus.org.uk/secure/articles/pdfs/MM44supplement1/17050463.pdf

Raji, A. (2008). *The endocrine system & types of hormones: An overview*. Retrieved from http://www.hormone.org/endocrine_system.cfm

Ranasinghe, J., Lacerenza, L., Garcia, L., & Soens, M. (n.d.). *Obstetric haemorrhage*. Retrieved from http://update.anaesthesiologists.org/wp-content/uploads/2009/09/Obstetric-Haemorrhage.pdf

Riback, W. (n.d.). *Plasma expanders: "Expanding the options."* Retrieved from http://www.traumasa.co.za/files%5CPlasma%20Expanders%20Botswana.pdf

Rice, J. (2006). *Principles of pharmacology for medical assisting* (4th ed.). Clifton Park, NY: Thomson Delmar Leaning.

Rowlett, R. (2004). *How many? A dictionary of units of measurement*. Retrieved from http://unc.edu/~rowlett/units/dictU.html

Sedative. (n.d.). *The American heritage® Stedman's medical dictionary*. Retrieved from http://dictionary.reference.com/browse/sedative

Seyednejad, H., Imani, M., Jamieson, T., & Seifalian, A. (2008). *Topical haemostatic agents*. Retrieved from http://www.drozek.us/documents%20on%20Web%20site/Teaching/articles%20and%20topics/anticoagulation/topical%20hemostatics.pdf

Simon, H. & Zieve, D. (2009). *Glaucoma—medications*. Retrieved from http://www.umm.edu/patiented/articles/what_drug_treatments_glaucoma_000025_8.htm

Stevens, D. (2005). *Benzodiazepines: Preoperative medication*. Retrieved from https://docs.google.com/viewer?a=v&q=cache:j5wjwqUhOMEJ:chua2.fiu.edu/Nursing/anesthesiology/COURSES/Semester%25201/NGR%25206173%2520ANE%2520Pharm%25201/ANE%2520Pharm%25201%2520Slides/FIU_10-05_BENZODIAZEPINES.ppt+chua2.fiu.edu/Nursing/.../FIU_10-05_BENZODIAZEPINES.ppt&hl=en&gl=us&pid=bl&srcid=ADGEESia76gzL-k8jHKbe1hXWp5DO_JWrAIGKwRmX0LREfH_8Oq_2cYywJLsvT3_5j4-X2Ct-BU7KhGIjsJEexLEAgEZzCJdyVWFat9HbEg6kBf-BvrjozkkVeoMW4Z_pRCFWGcQgxO&sig=AHIEtbQetccDvaEn9-aZBRg7QN-0hy5ym0Q

Tehrani, N. & Levin, A. (2008). *Commonly used dilating drops (mydriatic medications)*. Retrieved from http://www.pgcfa.org/kb/entry/166

Tetzlaff, J. (n.d.). *Amino amide local anesthetics*. Retrieved from http://faculty.weber.edu/ewalker/ Medicinal_Chemistry/topics/Psycho/local_a_ amide.htm

Tetzlaff, J. (n.d.). *Amino ester local anesthetics*. Retrieved from http://faculty.weber.edu/ewalker/ Medicinal_Chemistry/topics/Psycho/local_a_ ester.htm

Texas Heart Institute. (n.d.). *Beta blockers*. Retrieved from http://www.texasheartinstitute.org/hic/topics/ meds/betameds.cfm

Texas Heart Institute. (n.d.). *Calcium channel blockers*. Retrieved from http://www.texasheartinstitute.org/ HIC/Topics/Meds/calcmeds.cfm

Thomas, P. (2003). *Current perspectives on ophthalmic mycoses*. Retrieved from http://www.ncbi.nlm.nih .gov/pmc/articles/PMC207127

Thomson, H. & Webb, J. (2009). *Contrast media: Safety issues and ESUR guidelines* (2nd revised ed.). New York, NY: Springer.

Todar, K. (2012). *Todar's online textbook of bacteriology*. Retrieved from http://textbookofbacteriology .net/kt_toc.html

Toxicology Data Network. (2009). *Apomorphine*. Retrieved from http://toxnet.nlm.nih.gov/cgi-bin/sis/ search/a?dbs+hsdb:@term+@DOCNO+3289

University of Illinois at Chicago Department of Ophthalmology and Visual Sciences. (2011). *Eye medications*. Retrieved from http://www.uic.edu/com/ eye/LearningAboutVision/EyeFacts/MedicineFor- Eyes.shtml

University of Maryland Medical Center. (2011). *Potassium nitrate/silver nitrate*. Retrieved from http:// www.umm.edu/drug/notes/Potassium-nitrate-silver- nitrate-On-the-skin.htm#ord3

University of the West of England. (n.d.). *X-ray contrast media made clear*. Retrieved from http://hsc.uwe .ac.uk/idis2/contrast_agents/cm%20zip/contrastmedia_ schering.pdf

Veritti, D. & Toneatto, G. (2012). *Dyes play vital role in vitreoretinal surgery*. Retrieved from http://www .healio.com/ophthalmology/retina-vitreous/news/ print/ocular-surgery-news-europe-edition/%7b3C 507E9D-A56E-47CB-993F-CE8F501BA513%7d/ Dyes-play-vital-role-in-vitreoretinal-surgery

Volders, E., Shaw, S., McLelland, J., & Connolly, K. (n.d.). *Breastfeeding support and promotion*. Retrieved from http://www.rch.org.au/rchcpg/index .cfm?doc_id=9790

Wolfe, T. (n.d.). *Therapeutic intranasal drug delivery*. Retrieved from http://intranasal.net/Home/default .htm

Woodrow, R. (2007). *Essentials of pharmacology for health occupations* (5th ed.). Clifton Park, NY: Thomson Delmar Learning.

World Health Organization. (2002). *The clinical use of blood handbook*. Retrieved from http://www.who .int/bloodsafety/clinical_use/en/Handbook_EN.pdf

Wu, L. (2012). *Fungal endophthalmitis treatment & management*. Retrieved from http://emedicine. medscape.com/article/1204298-treatment#a1128

Yavuz, S., Celkan, A., Göncü, T., Türk, T., & Ozdemir, I. (2001). *Effect of papaverine applications on blood flow of the internal mammary artery*. Retrieved from http://www.atcs.jp/pdf/2001_7_2/84.pdf

Zieve, D. & Dugdal III, D. (2009). *Seizures*. Retrieved from http://www.nlm.nih.gov/medlineplus/ency /article/003200.htm

Zonule of Zinn. (2009). *Mosby's medical dictionary* (8th ed.). Saint Louis, MO: Mosby Elsevier.

ANSWERS TO CRITICAL THINKING REVIEW QUESTIONS

CHAPTER 1

1. Break down the term *pharmacology* and provide definitions for the word root and the suffix.
   The word pharmacology *is derived from the Greek root word* farmakon, *meaning drug, and the suffix "-logy," meaning to study. The term* pharmacology *is defined as the study of drugs.*

2. The drug propofol (Diprivan®) was discovered in 1986. Identify the drug classification and provide a brief description of how the drug is used.
   Propofol (Diprivan®) is classified as a sedative/hypnotic, and it is used in the surgical environment to induce and maintain general anesthesia and to achieve conscious sedation.

3. What is the role of the WHO in international drug safety?
   The WHO collaborates with agency representatives from several national governments to provide support to those agencies to allow each nation to create standards for drug safety, effectiveness, and quality, thereby promoting patient safety, especially in developing nations. The goal is development and standardization of a set of international guidelines concerning drug manufacture, storage, distribution, and dispensation. The WHO is also involved in detecting and penalizing manufacturers and distributors of illegal drugs.

4. List three of the WHO *Guidelines for Safe Surgery* that relate directly to medication use in the surgical environment and explain the importance of each.
   Three of the WHO Guidelines for Safe Surgery that relate directly to medication use in the surgical environment are rapid recognition and response to adverse drug reactions, recommended practices to avoid drug delivery errors (such as labeling techniques), and administration of prophylactic antibiotics. Answers related to the importance of each of the guidelines will vary, but should directly relate to a use example in the surgical environment.

5. Which federal agency was created as a result of the Controlled Substances Act of 1970?
   The United States Drug Enforcement Administration (DEA) was founded in 1973 to enforce the Controlled Substances Act of 1970.

6. Briefly describe the role of the United States Food and Drug Administration (FDA).
   The United States Food and Drug Administration (FDA) was formed in 1930 and is responsible for overseeing the effectiveness, safety, and security of all drugs (human and veterinary), biological agents (including blood and vaccines), medical devices, cosmetics, and radiation-emitting devices. The jurisdiction of the FDA extends to safety and security of the nation's food supply as well.

7. Why is it important for a surgical technologist to be familiar with the content of the state practice acts in the state where he or she is employed?
   Roles of various medical practitioners are spelled out in the individual state's practice acts. The purpose of a practice act is to protect the public by identifying the scope of practice, setting practice limits, and defining the responsibilities of the practitioner. Penalties for noncompliance with the practice act are also described. Information pertaining to tasks that can be delegated to the surgical technologist is usually found in the medical practice act and the nurse practice act and although the title of surgical technologists may not be used, applicable terms include unlicensed assistive personnel and allied health professional. Laws contained within the practice acts vary from state to state, and it is the individual surgical technologist's personal duty to read, understand, and abide by the related practice acts.

8. Differentiate between a policy and a procedure.
   A policy is a written institutional rule or plan of action that addresses a specific need and requires compliance within that institution. A procedure outlines the steps necessary to implement the policy.

9. If there is a conflict between federal law, state law, and facility policy and procedure, to which regulation must the surgical technologist adhere?
   Facility policies and procedures must comply with both federal and state laws and may be even stricter. The stricter regulation always prevails.

10. List three or more possible consequences of a medication or solution violation.

    There are several patient and practitioner consequences for violating federal law, state law, or facility policy when dealing with medications and solutions. Patient consequences include causing temporary harm to the patient, causing permanent harm to the patient, and causing patient death. Practitioner consequences include negative job performance review, loss of employment, loss of national certification, involvement in legal action, payment of a fine, and imprisonment.

CHAPTER 2

1. Define the term *dimensional analysis* and describe the situations that dimensional analysis is applied in the surgical setting.

    Dimensional analysis is the process of understanding and applying the relationships between the qualities of various items (such as drugs and systems for identifying and measuring drug dosages) based on the physical characteristics (dimensions) of each item. Dimensional analysis is applied in the surgical setting when comparing weight, size (length/width/height/volume), distance, temperature, and time between various systems.

2. Differentiate between a proper and an improper fraction.

    A proper fraction consists of a numerator that is smaller than the denominator, and an improper fraction consists of a numerator that is larger than the denominator, indicating that when reduced to lowest terms, the final number will include a whole number and fraction.

3. The Institute for Safe Medication Practices (ISMP) recommends use of a zero before a decimal point if the decimal number is a fraction only. Why? Use information found elsewhere in this textbook to answer this question.

    The ISMP recommends use of a zero before a decimal point if the decimal number is a fraction only to reduce the risk of error because a decimal point is easy to overlook and the fraction could be mistaken as a whole number (.5 could be mistaken for 5 if a leading zero [0.5] is not used).

4. What number does the Roman numeral II represent? Provide two examples of the use of Roman numerals in pharmacology.

    The Roman numeral II represents the number 2 (two). Roman numerals are used in pharmacology to identify narcotic classifications and on some written prescriptions.

5. Why is the military time-keeping system preferred in the healthcare setting? Write the equivalent of 0300 using civilian time.

    The military time-keeping system is preferred in the healthcare setting to eliminate any potential confusion between AM and PM that may occur within the civilian time-keeping system. 0300 is written in civilian time as 3:00 AM.

6. Explain how to convert international units to milligrams.

    There is no standard conversion of drugs that are measured in units to another type of measure such as milligrams or milliliters.

7. What does the term *milliequivalent* mean? Provide two examples of the use of milliequivalent measures in the medical setting.

    A milliequivalent is a unit of measure that represents one thousandth of a measure. Milliequivalents are used when referring to electrolytes and when reporting lab test results.

8. Explain why one milliliter is equal to one cubic centimeter. When referring to volume, use of which term (*ml* or *cc*) is recommended by the ISMP?

    The space occupied by one milliliter is equal to one cubic centimeter; therefore, the terms are interchangeable. The ISMP recommends use of the term milliliter when referring to volume.

9. State the normal body temperature (measured orally) using both the Celsius and Fahrenheit scales.

    Normal body temperature when measured orally is 37° C or 98.6° F.

10. List and describe the visual changes that can take place when mixing medications that would indicate incompatibility of the drugs. Should a drug mixture be used if an incompatibility occurs?

    Visual changes that may take place when mixing medications that could indicate incompatibility may be seen as an unexpected color change, presence of precipitates (appearance of particles in the solution), formation of gas (appearance of bubbles), or turbidity (loss of clarity, cloudiness). A medication mixture should never be used if there is any sign of incompatibility.

CHAPTER 3

1. List the three types of drug nomenclature and provide a brief description of each.

    The term drug nomenclature *represents a system for naming. The three types of names given to drugs are as follows:*

    - *Chemical name, which provides the exact formula and molecular structure of the drug.*
    - *Generic name, which is the nonproprietary name of the drug.*
    - *Proprietary (brand/trade) name, which the manufacturer assigns to the drug for marketing purposes.*

2. Which type of drug nomenclature is preferred in the healthcare setting? Why?

    The generic name is the preferred name in the healthcare setting because several manufacturers may market the same drug under different proprietary names. Healthcare facilities often change vendors to secure the best contracted price for pharmaceuticals.

3. List the generic and the chemical name for the brand name drug Demerol®.

    The generic name for the drug Demerol® is meperidine hydrochloride and the chemical name is ethyl 1-methyl-4-phenylisonipecotate hydrochloride.

4. Is a prescription necessary to purchase an OTC drug? Why or why not?

    No, the term over the counter *is used to describe drugs that can be purchased directly by the consumer without a prescription from a physician.*

5. List the information that must be present on a written prescription.

    Written prescriptions should contain the following information:

    - *Name, address, and telephone number of the prescriber (may include the prescriber's license number and/or Drug Enforcement Administration number, especially if the prescription is for a controlled substance)*
    - *Name, address, and age/date of birth of the patient*
    - *Current date*
    - *Name, strength, and amount of the drug*
    - *Instructions for the patient concerning the route of administration, frequency of administration, and any precautions or restrictions*
    - *Number of refills allowed, if any*
    - *Signature of the prescriber*
    - *Brand/generic substitutions, if allowed*

6. The surgeon preference card is a form of standing orders. If there is a change in the order because of the patient's special circumstances, how will the change most likely be communicated to the surgical team members?

    If any changes to the standing orders are required, they are most often issued verbally.

7. On his preference card (Figure 3-4), Dr. XYZ is requesting bupivacaine 0.5% to be available for postoperative pain control. What are the brand and chemical names for this product?

    The brand names for the drug bupivacaine are Marcaine® and Sensorcaine® and the chemical name is 1-butyl-N-(2,6-dimethylphenyl) piperidine-2-carboxamide.

8. What is the classification of the drug bupivacaine 0.5%? Use information found elsewhere in this textbook to answer this question.

    Bupivacaine 0.5% (brand names Marcaine® and Sensorcaine®) is a nerve conduction blocking agent in the amino amide group.

9. The drug morphine is a controlled substance. According to the Controlled Substances Act, what is the schedule? Why?

    Morphine is classified as a Schedule II drug because it has a currently accepted medical use and a high potential for abuse. The risk of physical or psychological dependence is serious.

10. Think about drugs that are classified according to the body system affected. Limited information is presented in this chapter. Use information contained elsewhere in this textbook or from outside resources to identify at least three more drugs that affect three additional body systems.

    Answers will vary but could include:

    - *The drug aminophylline is a bronchodilator; therefore, it could be classified as a respiratory system drug.*
    - *The drug nitroglycerin is a vasodilator; therefore, it could be classified as a cardiovascular system drug.*
    - *The drug furosemide is a loop diuretic; therefore, it could be classified as a urinary system drug.*

CHAPTER 4

1. The term *zoologic* is used in this chapter to identify drugs from animal sources. Does this description include drugs from human sources?

    The term zoologic *includes drugs from all animal sources, including human sources.*

2. Differentiate between vitamins and minerals. Use information from an outside source to answer this question.

    The following table provides a brief comparison of vitamins and minerals:

Minerals	Vitamins
Inorganic (not derived from living organisms)	*Organic (derived from living organisms)*
From the earth and water (including plants and animals that acquire minerals from soil and water)	*From plants and animals*
Necessary for regulation of the heart rate, production of hormones, and maintenance of bone strength among other functions	*Necessary for homeostasis*

3. What are some of the benefits of rDNA technology?
Some of the benefits of rDNA technology include minimizing or eliminating the risk of transmission of pathogens and reducing the risk of allergic reaction because the rDNA product contains minimal (or is free of) human and animal antigens.

4. Briefly describe the antigen/antibody response. Use information from an outside source to answer this question.
An antigen is a foreign substance, usually a protein, which causes activation of antibodies. Antibodies are produced by the immune system in response to an antigen. The antigen/antibody response is usually initiated to prevent infection. An allergy is an overreaction of the immune system to an antigen (allergen) that is not normally harmful (such as pollen or dust) to most individuals. Symptoms of an allergic response can range from mild (itchy eyes, runny nose, sneezing) to severe (anaphylaxis).

5. What is anaphylaxis? Use information from an outside source to answer this question.
Anaphylaxis is a severe allergic response that occurs rapidly following exposure to an allergen (such as food, medication, or a bee sting) and may be fatal if not treated immediately. Symptoms of anaphylaxis include itching (pruritus), redness of the skin (erythema), hives (urticaria), airway constriction, wheezing, and a significant drop in blood pressure (hypotension) that can lead to fainting (syncope), shock, and death.

6. Which organization is responsible for development of the Daily Reference Intake (DRI)?
The United States Department of Agriculture (USDA) Food and Nutrition Information Center (FNIC) is responsible for development of the Daily Reference Intake (DRI).

7. List four body functions that are regulated by minerals.
Many body functions are regulated by minerals. The list includes:
- *Blood clotting*
- *Bone formation*
- *Component of certain enzymes and proteins*
- *Component of hemoglobin*
- *Digestion*
- *Energy production*
- *Energy storage and transfer*
- *Fluid and electrolyte balance*
- *Function of amino acids*
- *Function of certain enzymes*
- *Gene expression*
- *Glucose use*
- *Immunity*
- *Iron metabolism*
- *Maintenance of fluid and electrolyte balance*
- *Metabolism of amino acids, carbohydrates, and cholesterol*
- *Muscle contraction*
- *Necessary component of vitamin B complex function*
- *pH maintenance*
- *Prevention of dental carries (cavities)*
- *Production of energy*
- *Stress management*
- *Synthesis of nucleotides*
- *Synthesis of proteins and nucleic acids*
- *Thyroid function*
- *Thyroid hormone regulation*
- *Tooth and bone formation/strength*
- *Transmission of nerve impulses*

8. What is the importance of an adequate intake of potassium in the diet?
Adequate potassium intake in the diet is important in energy production, muscle contraction, synthesis of proteins and nucleic acids, and transmission of nerve impulses. Fruits and vegetables are good sources of dietary potassium.

9. What are the dietary sources of calcium?
The dietary sources of calcium are dairy products and green vegetables.

10. List four parts of a plant that may be used as sources for drugs.
All parts of the plant (flowers, fruits, berries, leaves, bark, sap, roots, resin, etc.) may be used as sources for drugs.

CHAPTER 5

1. List the three main drug forms and provide a brief description of each.
Drugs are found in the three basic forms of matter: gas, liquid, and solid. Gases are liquids in their vapor form. A liquid is described as the fluid form of matter. A solid is described as the particulate form of matter.

2. Briefly explain the process of diffusion. You may need to utilize an outside source, such as your anatomy and physiology book, to fully understand and convey this concept.
Diffusion is movement of molecules from an area of higher concentration to an area of lower concentration through a medium such as air. Diffusion does not require the use of energy (passive transport).

3. If oxygen is not technically considered a pharmaceutical, why is it discussed in this textbook?
Oxygen is listed as a medical gas because it is a gas that is necessary for life, and is frequently administered in patient care settings.

4. Provide three examples of a volatile liquid. Give the generic and brand names of each. Use information found elsewhere in this textbook to answer this question.
   The following inhalation agents are potent volatile liquids whose vapors produce general anesthesia when inhaled:
   - *Fluothane®—halothane*
   - *Ethrane®—enflurane*
   - *Ultane®—sevoflurane*
   - *Suprane®—desflurane*
   - *Forane®—isoflurane*

5. Prior to using an emulsion or a suspension, why may it be necessary to redistribute the droplets or particles? How will redistribution be accomplished?
   Because settling of one of the liquids or the particles may occur, redistribution of the liquids may be necessary prior to use. Redistribution may be accomplished by gently shaking or rolling the drug container.

6. Describe the differences and similarities between heterogenous and homogenous mixtures.
   In a mixture, each substance retains its own characteristics (properties). Mixtures can be classified as heterogenous (meaning that the substances are not equally distributed) or homogenous (meaning that the substances are equally distributed).

7. Explain the meaning of the term *viscosity*. Describe the appearance of a semisolid that is slightly viscous.
   The term viscosity *refers to the thickness of the semisolid. A semisolid that is slightly viscous would appear to be runny rather than thick.*

8. Provide an example of a drug that is reconstituted prior to use. What does the term *reconstitution* mean?
   Answers will vary but could include:
   - *Bacitracin injection (Baci-IM®)*
   - *Topical thrombin (Thrombostat®)*
   The term reconstitution *means to add a liquid to a dried substance to return it to its former condition and strength.*

9. What is the fourth state of matter and how is it used in the medical setting? Use information from an outside source, such as your surgical technology textbook, to answer this question completely.
   Plasma is the fourth state of matter and is used in the medical setting as a sterilant.

10. Will all of the drug forms described in this chapter be utilized in the surgical setting? Why or why not? Use information found elsewhere in this textbook to answer this question.
    No, all of the drug forms described in this chapter will not be utilized in the surgical setting because surgical patients are required to be NPO (have nothing by mouth) for several hours prior to and during surgery and some of the drug forms described are administered orally.

CHAPTER 6

1. Which term is used to describe the action of a drug upon the target cells?
   The term that is used to describe the action of a drug upon the target cells (receptor, membrane, cell, tissue, organ, or whole body) is pharmacodynamics.

2. Which term is used to describe the four step process of movement of a drug throughout the body?
   The term that is used to describe the four step process of movement of a drug throughout the body is pharmacokinetics. The four steps in pharmacokinetics are absorption, distribution, biotransformation, and excretion.

3. What piece of equipment may be needed to transform a volatile liquid into vapor? Which process is used to allow the transformation from the liquid to the vapor state?
   A vaporizer that typically uses heat to stimulate the transformation from the normal (liquid) state of matter to the gaseous form is needed to transform a volatile liquid into a vapor. The process is called vaporization or evaporation.

4. List the two main routes of enteral administration.
   The two main routes of enteral administration are oral and rectal.

5. Explain the difference between instillation and infusion.
   Instillation involves medications that are dripped into the body, while infusion means that the medication is inserted into the vein to produce the desired therapeutic effect. Sometimes intravenous fluids are said to be instilled because they do enter the body drop by drop, but intravenous administration is a better example of infusion.

6. Do the terms *spinal* and *epidural* mean the same thing? Why or why not?
   No, the terms spinal *and* epidural *do not mean the same thing. The term* spinal *(intrathecal) means that the medication is injected through the dura mater directly into the cerebrospinal fluid (CSF), while the term* epidural *means that the medication is injected in the space outside of the dura mater and then crosses the dural membrane and enters the CSF.*

7. What is the definition of the term *gas*? Use information contained elsewhere in this textbook to answer this question.
   The term gas *is defined as a liquid in its vapor form.*

8. When a drug is administered intravenously, does absorption related to pharmacodynamics occur? Why or why not?

Intravenous medications are administered directly into the circulatory system; therefore, absorption that is related to the process of pharmacokinetics does not occur. The medication is ready for transport as soon as it is infused.

9. Provide three examples of parenteral routes of administration and provide a description of each.

There are several examples of parenteral routes of administration that include:
Intradermal—into the skin
Subcutaneous—into the adipose tissue
Intramuscular—within a muscle
Intravenous—within a vein
Intraarterial—within an artery
Intraosseous—within a bone
Epidural—above or outside of the dura mater
Intrathecal (spinal)—within the dura mater
Intraarticular—within a joint
Intracardiac—within the heart

10. What is a loop diuretic? Use information contained elsewhere in this textbook to answer this question.

A loop diuretic produces a rapid and effective diuretic response by inhibiting reabsorption of sodium and chloride directly in the loop of Henle especially when administered intravenously. Loop diuretics are effective in prompt reduction of pulmonary edema and decreasing intracranial pressure due to cerebral edema. Examples of loop diuretics include bumetanide (Bumex® and Burinex®), ethacrynic acid (Edecrin®), furosemide (Lasix®), and torsemide (Demadex® and Diuver®).

CHAPTER 7

1. Explain how the term *pharmacokinetics* differs from the term *pharmacodynamics*.

The term pharmacokinetics *has to do with movement of the drug within the body. The four main processes involved in pharmacokinetics are absorption, distribution, biotransformation, and excretion. The term* pharmacodynamics *refers to the interaction of the drug molecules with the target receptor, membrane, cell, tissue, organ, or whole body.*

2. Describe the difference between absolute and relative bioavailability.

The term absolute bioavailability *has to do with the availability of the drug given by different routes, while the term* relative bioavailability *has to do with the availability of the drug that is produced differently (such as the difference between a brand name drug and the generic version of the same drug).*

3. Which route of administration eliminates the need for the drug to be absorbed?

A drug that is given intravenously is already in the circulatory system and absorption is not necessary.

4. Which route of administration allows for 100% bioavailability?

A drug given intravenously is said to have 100% bioavailability because the entire dose of the drug is immediately in the circulatory system.

5. The hepatic first pass effect affects drugs given only by one route of administration. Which route is affected? Explain your answer.

The hepatic first pass effect affects drugs that are ingested. Because of the hepatic portal system, a portion of the drug is sent to the liver via the hepatic vein, where it is biotransformed before it gets into general circulation. As a result, bioavailability is reduced.

6. Give two examples of comorbid conditions that may affect the process of pharmacokinetics.

Examples of comorbid conditions include problems with cardiac function, general circulation, circulation to the target cells, liver function, kidney function, respiratory function, endocrine function (such as thyroid disorders and diabetes), and gastrointestinal tract function (including gastric emptying rate).

7. How is facilitated passive diffusion (transport) similar and dissimilar to passive transport?

Facilitated passive transport and passive transport are similar because the drug molecules move from an area of high concentration across a semipermeable membrane to an area of low concentration and no energy is expended. The difference is that during facilitated passive transport, proteins are used to help transport the drug molecule across the membrane.

8. Are metabolism and biotransformation the same thing? Explain your answer.

Yes, in pharmacology, metabolism and biotransformation are synonyms. Additionally, the term biodegradation *may also be used to describe the chemical changes that a drug substance undergoes as it is being broken down (catabolism) within the body in preparation for excretion.*

9. By which process do most drugs enter the circulatory system?

Most drugs enter the circulatory system at the site of absorption by a process called passive transport.

10. What is a metabolite?

A metabolite is a smaller version of the original drug molecule that consists of a less-active or inactive substance that is easily excreted.

CHAPTER 8

1. Describe the link between pharmacokinetics and pharmacodynamics.

   Numerous factors can enhance or impede pharmacokinetics of a particular drug. These same factors may also affect the interaction of the drug with the target receptor, membrane, cell, tissue, organ, or whole body (pharmacodynamics). Factors affecting both pharmacokinetics and pharmacodynamics include the drug form, route of administration, dose, interaction with other drugs, NPO status, patient's age, comorbid conditions, circadian differences, plasma protein binding, tissue binding, pregnancy, barriers, physical properties of the drug, and availability of transporters.

2. What are the three aspects of pharmacodynamics and how are they interrelated?

   The three aspects of pharmacodynamics are onset of action (time that elapses from administration of the drug until the therapeutic effect of the drug is noted), peak effect (time that elapses when the drug is most effective), and duration of action (time that elapses from onset of action to termination of action), and they are interrelated by their time frames and the therapeutic effect of the drug.

3. Briefly describe the mechanism by which each of the four drug theories are thought to elicit their responses.

   The four methods by which drugs are thought to elicit their responses are as follows:

   - *Drug receptor interactions—Occur when a drug molecule attaches to a receptor that is usually a protein or glycoprotein located on the plasmalemma, on an organelle, or within the cytoplasm of the target cell. Most drugs have an affinity (attraction) to the target cells.*
   - *Drug enzyme interactions—Occur when a drug speeds or inhibits the action of an enzyme or changes the response of the cells affected by the enzyme.*
   - *Nonspecific responses—Type of drug interaction that occurs when a drug does not seem to act as a result of a drug receptor interaction or a drug enzyme interaction. The drug is thought to congregate and act on the plasmalemma or infiltrate the plasmalemma and act on the contents of the cell.*
   - *Chemical interactions—Effects of some drugs that are evident without any alteration of cellular function such as neutralization of stomach acid.*

4. What is the main benefit of using a synergist?

   The main benefit of using a synergist is that the effect of the two (or more) combined drugs is greater than the effect of each drug individually.

5. What is an agonist? Briefly describe the three categories of agonists.

   An agonist is a drug that simulates or prolongs the action of another drug or naturally occurring body substance but may not have an action of its own. The word agonist *is the opposite of the word* antagonist. *Agonists are identified in three categories:*

   - *Strong agonists produce the greatest effect even though only a small percentage of the available receptors on the plasmalemma may be occupied by the drug.*
   - *Weak agonists produce approximately the same effect as a strong agonist, but must occupy a greater percentage of the cell's receptors.*
   - *Partial agonists produce a weak effect even though all of the available receptors are occupied by the drug.*

6. What is an antagonist? Briefly describe the five categories of antagonists.

   An antagonist is a drug that prevents or reverses the effect of another drug or naturally occurring body substance. Antagonists are identified in five categories:

   - *Competitive antagonism occurs when the antagonist competes for and binds to the receptor that would normally be occupied by the initial drug (agonist) preventing that drug from acting. Because high doses of the initial drug may overcome the power of the antagonist, this type of antagonism is said to be surmountable.*
   - *Noncompetitive antagonism occurs when the antagonist binds to a receptor site that would not normally be occupied by the initial drug causing a change in the initial drug's receptor site rendering it unrecognizable and unusable by the initial drug. Because high doses of the initial drug cannot overcome the power of the antagonist, this type of antagonism is said to be insurmountable.*
   - *Irreversible antagonism, also called nonequilibrium competitive antagonism, is similar to competitive antagonism; however, the effect is permanent. This type of antagonism is also said to be insurmountable.*
   - *Physiological antagonism occurs when two drugs are given that cancel the effects of one another.*
   - *Antagonism by neutralization occurs when two drugs bind together inactivating one another.*

7. List eight reasons why an additive may be used.

   Additives may be used to produce synergistic or agonistic effects. Additives may also be used to dilute, reconstitute, activate, act as a preservative, give flavor to, or alter the pH of the initial drug.

8. Define the term *prophylaxis* and give an indication of why a prophylactic drug may be used.

   The term prophylaxis *is used to describe preventive measures. Examples of prophylactic drugs include giving immunizations or preoperative antibiotics to patients who do not show signs of infection. Answers will vary because there are several indications for using prophylactic drugs.*

9. Differentiate between a side effect and an adverse effect.

   Side effects are expected but undesirable, generally mild, and often tolerable or manageable effects of a drug that are not therapeutic. Examples of side effects include, but are not limited to, skin irritation, nausea, vomiting, constipation, diarrhea, dry mouth, dizziness, and drowsiness. Adverse effects are more serious (than side effects) undesirable effects that may cause harm to the patient. Some adverse effects are predictable and others are unexpected. Treatments are available for some adverse effects, but not all. Examples of adverse effects include, but are not limited to, mild-to-severe allergic reactions (including anaphylaxis), hair loss (alopecia), bone marrow depression, and damage to or failure of vital organs such as the heart, liver, lungs, kidneys, and brain.

10. Explain the difference between physiological and psychological addiction.

    Addiction may be physiological (also called chemical addiction) that affects the function of an organism or psychological that pertains to or influences the mind or the emotions and is usually seen with narcotic analgesics, alcohol, and benzodiazepine as well as other psychotropic drugs.

CHAPTER 9

1. List the six rights of medication administration and explain the importance of each. Be sure to describe how the six rights apply to care of the surgical patient.

   The six rights of medication administration is a memory tool to help ensure that a drug is handled and administered correctly. The six rights, importance of each right, and the application to the surgical patient are as follows:

Right	Importance	Application to the surgical patient
Right Patient	• Patient identity is determined • Drug and food allergies (if any) are noted	• Occurs during the "time out"
Right Drug	• Use the three verification process	• Standing orders (preference card) • Written orders • Verbal orders
Right Dose	• Use the three verification process • Be sure that the dose is consistent with age/size, diagnosis, and gender of patient	• Understand and calculate accurately • Reconstitute correctly (follow manufacturer's instructions)
Right Route of Administration	• Route of administration must be consistent for the surgical patient	• Not all routes of administration are appropriate for use in the surgical environment
Right Time and Frequency	• In the surgical environment, drugs are general given when ordered	• Frequency is not usually a concern unless the procedure is lengthy
Right Documentation/ Labeling	• Documentation includes: name of drug, dose, route of administration, time of administration, unusual responses • Never document prior to administering the drug	• Within the sterile field, all locations of the drug are labeled

2. Give an overview of the three verification process and provide a description of when each verification occurs in the surgical setting.

   The three verification process is a safe medication practice that involves checking each medication (name, strength, expiration date, and any other pertinent facts) three times. If two individuals (such as the circulator and the surgical technologist) are involved in the transfer of a drug onto the sterile field, both individuals must be actively involved in the verification, which usually takes place visually and verbally. Information that is verified includes (at minimum) the name of the drug, the strength of the drug, the expiration date, and any other pertinent facts. If the drug is passed to another surgical team member, the drug information is verbalized again as the drug is transferred (and each time thereafter). The process is implemented in the following manner:

Verification	Occurrence
First Verification	Takes place when the medication is removed from the storage location or when the items on the procedure cart are checked for accuracy according to the surgeon's preference card.
Second Verification	Occurs just prior to removal of the drug from the container (e.g., just prior to drawing up in a syringe or transferring onto the sterile field). The syringe and/or other storage location (such as a medicine cup) are labeled as soon as it is prepared for use.
Third Verification	Occurs immediately following removal of the drug from the container.

3. Differentiate between a vial and an ampule.
   Differences between a vial and an ampule include:

Vial	Ampule
Small glass tube	Small glass or plastic bottle.
Contains a solution	Contains a solution or a powder.
Hermetic seal	Sealed with a rubber stopper that is held in place with an aluminum collar. May also have a protective cap to protect sterility and allow access to the stopper.
Neck is scored to allow glass to be broken easily to allow removal of the solution	Rubber stopper must be penetrated or removed to allow removal of the solution or powder (may require reconstitution).

4. Why are some ampules manufactured from tinted glass?
   Some ampules are clear and others are made of tinted (often amber or brown) glass to protect the contents from degradation due to photochemical reactions that may occur if the drug is exposed to light.

5. List the color outlet or tank color that matches the gasses named.
   The appropriate outlet or cylinder colors have been added to the following table:

Name of Gas	Outlet or Cylinder Color
Carbon Dioxide (CO_2)	Gray
Helium (He)	Brown
Medical Air (a mixture of oxygen, nitrogen, carbon dioxide, and argon)	Yellow
Nitrogen (N_2)	Black
Nitrous Oxide (N_2O)	Blue
Oxygen (O_2)	Green (international, white)
Suction (not a medical gas; however, the vacuum outlet/connector system is similar in configuration to the medical gas outlet/connectors; therefore, they are often grouped together for logistical reasons)	White

6. What types of medications are packaged in tubes?
   Semisolids, such as creams, gels (includes lubricants), and ointments, are often supplied in a tube.

7. What does the term *contraindication* mean? Provide two examples of situations in which a drug may be contraindicated.
   Contraindications are the reasons why a drug should not be given because the hazards of the drug outweigh the benefits in a given situation. Examples of situations in which a drug may be contraindicated include pregnancy, lactation status, age (pediatric/geriatric), gender, and the presence of comorbid conditions such as diabetes, kidney disease, and liver disease.

8. Identify five situations in which use of a syringe may be indicated.
   Syringes may be used to:
   - *Transfer medications from their storage container to the patient*
   - *Transfer medications to another location such as the sterile fiddle*
   - *Irrigate*
   - *Withdraw fluid or air from the body*
   - *insert fluid or air into the body or a medical device*

9. In which situation is a Toomey syringe most commonly used? Why?
   Toomey syringes are most commonly used during urologic surgical procedures because the tip of the syringe is designed to fit standard urology instruments such as a cystoscope. Additionally, the removable tip may be exchanged for a catheter tip.

10. Which has a larger diameter, a 10 gauge needle or a 33 gauge needle? Defend your answer.
    The 10 gauge needle has a larger diameter. Needle diameter is measured using the gauge (g) scale. Low gauge numbers represent large diameter needles and high gauge numbers represent small diameter needles.

CHAPTER 10

1. Describe the differences between the ways that amino amides and amino esters are metabolized.

Amino amides differ from amino esters in that drugs in the amide group are biotransformed in the liver and drugs in the ester group are biotransformed by pseudocholinesterase in the blood plasma.

2. Explain why epinephrine and hyaluronidase are considered to be agonistic anesthetic agents.

   Epinephrine and hyaluronidase are considered to be agonistic anesthetic agents because they are used to enhance and prolong the effects of the anesthetic agent. Because epinephrine is a vasoconstrictor, the anesthetic remains in the area in which it was infiltrated for an extended period. Hyaluronidase is an enzyme that allows the anesthetic agent to penetrate the tissue more readily, which in turn enhances and prolongs the effect of the anesthetic agent.

3. Is an anticoagulant the same as a fibrinolytic? Why or why not?

   No, an anticoagulant is not the same as a fibrinolytic. Anticoagulants prevent blood clots from forming and fibrinolytics destroy existing clots.

4. Provide at least one example each of an alternative and a naturopathic antiemetic.

   Examples of alternative treatments for nausea and vomiting include acupuncture and hypnosis, and examples of treatments considered naturopathic include ingestion of peppermint and ginger.

5. List the three types of beta-lactams and identify the main source of each.

   The three types of beta-lactams are drugs in the penicillin, cephalosporin, and carbapenem groups. Drugs in the penicillin group are obtained from Penicillium molds commonly found on the skin of citrus fruits, cephalosporins are derived from the Acremonium fungus commonly found in soil, and carbapenems originate from thienamycin, which is a product of Streptomyces cattleya found in soil.

6. List two synonyms for the term *adrenergic* and describe the action(s) of adrenergic drugs.

   The terms sympathomimetic *and* adrenergic *are synonymous with the term* adrenergic. *The term* adrenergic *means activated by adrenaline, and adrenergic drugs are used to mimic the effects of the sympathetic nervous system. Adrenergics are capable of causing bronchodilation, stimulation of the heart, increase in blood flow to the voluntary (skeletal) muscles, pupil dilation (mydriasis), and constriction of the peripheral blood vessels.*

7. What is the function of an inotropic agent?

   Inotropic agents are used to change the force of a muscle contraction, especially contraction of the heart muscle. Inotropic agents may have a positive

(increase) or negative (decrease) impact on the contractile force.

8. Differentiate between positive and negative contrast media.

   Contrast media is used during radiographic (x-ray) studies to enhance visualization by differentiating body structures. Positive contrast media (compounds that contain iodine or barium) is radiopaque (absorb x-rays well) and shows as white or light gray on the x-ray image. Negative contrast media (gasses such as air, carbon dioxide, metrizamide, and oxygen) is radiolucent (allows x-rays to pass through) and shows as dark gray on the x-ray image. Radioactive isotopes (also called radionuclides) are also used as contrast media.

9. Describe malignant hyperthermia, list the symptoms, and identify the treatment(s) that a patient experiencing a malignant hyperthermia crisis may receive.

   Malignant hyperthermia (MH), also called malignant hyperpyrexia, is a rare life-threatening inherited genetic disorder that manifests when a susceptible individual is exposed to a triggering agent. Agents considered triggers in the surgical environment include halogenated inhalation agents and the depolarizing neuromuscular blocking agent succinylcholine (Anectine®). A patient experiencing a malignant hyperthermia crisis will exhibit tachycardia, tachypnea, sweating, flushing of the skin, increased oxygen consumption and carbon dioxide production, acidosis, excretion of dark brown urine, muscle rigidity, a dramatic increase in body temperature, unstable blood pressure, eventual vascular collapse, and possibly death. Immediate treatment for malignant hyperthermia includes discontinuance of the triggering agent, oxygenation, administration of dantrolene (Dantrium®), initiation of cooling measures, management of acidosis, and provision of additional supportive measures as needed.

10. Identify at least one similarity and one difference between a vasoconstrictor and a vasodilator.

    Vasodilators are similar to vasoconstrictors in that both have an effect on the muscle of the blood vessel; however, the effects on the muscle are opposite. Vasodilators relax (dilate) the smooth muscle of the wall of a blood vessel, increasing the diameter of the lumen of the vessel, decreasing resistance to blood flow, and lowering the blood pressure. Vasoconstrictors tighten (constrict) the smooth muscle of the wall of a blood vessel, decreasing the diameter of the lumen of the vessel, increasing resistance to blood flow, and raising the blood pressure.

GLOSSARY

Note: The definitions provided in this glossary pertain to pharmacology and the terms defined may have other applications.

Symbols

−	Represents the term *subtraction*.
%	Represents the term *percent*.
.	Represents a decimal point.
⟌	Represents long division; long division bracket.
:	Represents a ratio (colon).
@	Represents the term *at*.
′	Represents the household system term *foot/feet*.
″	Represents the household system term *inch/inches*.
+	Represents the term *addition*.
<	Represents the term *less than*.
=	Represents the term *equals*.
>	Represents the term *greater than*.
×	Represents the term *multiplication*.
÷	Represents the term *division*.
√	Represents the term *square root*.
°	Represents the term *degrees*.
μ	Represents the term *micro*.
μg	Represents the term *microgram*.
ℳ	Represents the apothecary system term *minim*.
0	Represents the Arabic number zero.
1	Represents the Arabic number one.
2	Represents the Arabic number two.
3	Represents the Arabic number three.
4	Represents the Arabic number four.
5	Represents the Arabic number five.
6	Represents the Arabic number six.
7	Represents the Arabic number seven.
8	Represents the Arabic number eight.
9	Represents the Arabic number nine.
f℈	Represents the apothecary system term *fluid scruple*.
f℥	Represents the apothecary system term *fluid ounce*.
f℈	Represents the apothecary system term *fluid dram*.
R_x	Represents the Latin term *take thou*; represents a prescription or a pharmacy.
℈	Represents the apothecary system term *scruple*.
℥	Represents the apothecary system term *ounce*.
ℨ	Represents the apothecary system term *dram/drachm*.
/	Separates the numerator and denominator of a fraction; indicates division.

Important Numeric Values

0° C	Freezing point of water.
100° C	Boiling point of water.
32° F	Freezing point of water.
212° F	Boiling point of water.
37° C	Normal body temperature (measured orally).
98.6° F	Normal body temperature (measured orally).

A

Absolute bioavailability Used to compare the availability of the same drug when administered intravenously or by another route such as ingestion.

Absolute zero Theoretical temperature at which no additional heat can be removed and all molecular movement ceases (−273° C, or −459° F).

Absorption Occurs when the drug is taken into the circulatory system by the capillaries.

Abuse Improper use of a drug that can lead to addiction/dependence.

ac Abbreviation of the Latin term *ante cibum*, meaning before meals.

Acid Substance with a pH of less than 7 that is capable of turning litmus paper red. Acids have a high concentration of hydrogen ions, which have the potential to be donated. Acids typically have a sour taste.

Acidemia Occurs when the blood pH is less than 7.35.

Acidosis Condition of high acidity in the blood (academia) and body fluids; may be respiratory or metabolic in origin.

Active transport Drug molecules (in solution) move from an area of low concentration across a semipermeable membrane to an area of high concentration. Energy, usually in the form of adenosine triphosphate (ATP), is expended during active transport.

Acupuncture Ancient Chinese method of relieving pain and promoting healing that involves insertion of small needles into the body at specified locations; considered alternative therapy.

Acute Disease or medical condition that is severe, but of short duration.

ad Abbreviation of the Latin term *auris dexter*, meaning right ear.

Addend Number that is added to another (augend) to obtain one sum.

Addiction Occurs when a drug is needed for an individual to function in a seemingly normal fashion. Dependence may be physiological (chemical) or psychological and is often a result of abuse of narcotic analgesics, alcohol, and benzodiazepines as well as other psychotropic drugs. However, one may also become addicted to caffeine, laxatives, nasal sprays, etc. Addiction is also called dependence.

Addition Unification of two or more numbers to obtain one sum.

Additive Substance that is combined with the initial drug for a variety of reasons such as to produce synergistic or agonistic effects. Additives may also be used to dilute, reconstitute, activate, act as a preservative, give flavor to, or alter the pH of the initial drug.

Adenosine Triphosphate (ATP) Major source of energy within the body that is manufactured in the mitochondria of a cell.

ad lib Abbreviation of the Latin term *ad libitum*, meaning at liberty/as much as desired.

ad libitum Latin term meaning at liberty/as much as desired.

Administration set Tubing that allows a sterile pathway for fluid from an IV bag; available in numerous configurations; also known as IV tubing or an infusion set.

Adrenergic Drug that mimics the effects of the sympathetic nervous system; also called sympathomimetic or adrenergic agonist.

Adrenergic agonist Drug that mimics the effects of the sympathetic nervous system; also called adrenergic or sympathomimetic.

Adrenergic antagonist Drug that inhibits the effects of the sympathetic nervous system; also called adrenergic blocker or sympatholytic.

Adrenergic blocker (alpha and beta) Drug that inhibits the effects of the sympathetic nervous system; also called adrenergic antagonist and sympatholytic (refer to alpha-adrenergic blocker and beta-adrenergic blocker for additional information)

Adverse effects Effects that are undesirable and may cause harm to the patient. Some adverse effects are predictable, while others are unexpected. Treatments are available for some adverse effects, but not all.

Aerobic Organism or tissue that depends on oxygen to sustain life.

Aerosol Contains small liquid or solid particles that are suspended in a gas. The particles are dispensed from a pressurized container or with the use of an atomizer.

Affinity Attraction.

Agonist 1. A drug that simulates or prolongs the action of another drug or naturally occurring body substance but may not have an action of its own. 2. The term *agonist* is also used in pharmacology when describing a drug receptor interaction to indicate the presence and potential action of the initial drug. To avoid confusion, the term *initial drug* will be used in this textbook in place of the term *agonist* when used in this context.

Alkylating agent Type of antineoplastic drug that modifies the DNA base of a cancer cell by adding an alkyl group, thereby disrupting transcription and replication of the cell.

Allergen A foreign substance, usually a protein (but can be a carbohydrate), that causes activation of an antibody and the subsequent immune response (allergic reaction); examples of allergens include venom from a snake or insect bite, food, pollen, dust, or a medication; also called an antigen.

allergic reaction An exaggerated immune system (histamine) response to a foreign substance (antigen/allergen); allergic reactions range from mild skin irritation to anaphylactic shock and can progress rapidly from mild to life threatening.

Alopecia Medical term for hair loss or baldness.

Alpha-adrenergic blocker Type of adrenergic blocker that is capable of relaxation of the smooth muscle found at the bladder neck and in the prostate, and reducing hypertension; may also be called alpha blocker.

Alpha blocker Type of adrenergic blocker that is capable of relaxation of the smooth muscle found at the bladder neck and in the prostate, and reducing hypertension; may also be called alpha-adrenergic blocker.

Alternative therapy Nontraditional treatments that include acupuncture and hypnosis.

Alveoli Small air sacs found in the lungs that are surrounded by a capillary network where gas exchange (oxygen/carbon dioxide) occurs.

AM Acronym that represents the Latin term *ante meridiem*.

Amino acid Organic compound composed of an amino group and a carboxylic acid group. Amino acids are considered the building blocks of proteins and also function in metabolism and act as chemical messengers within the body.

Amino amide Group of drugs used as local anesthetics; slightly differ chemically from amino esters; metabolized in the liver; stable in solution; less likely than amino esters to cause an allergic reaction.

Amino ester Group of drugs used as local anesthetics; differ chemically from amino amides; metabolized by pseudocholinesterase in the blood plasma; unstable in solution; more likely than amino amides to cause an allergic reaction.

Aminoglycoside Antiinfective agents that contain amino sugars in glycoside linkage; originally derived from bacteria in two groups—drugs ending with the suffix -mycin originate from the Streptomyces family, while drugs ending with the suffix -micin originate from the Micromonospora family (now, many of the aminoglycosides are synthetic); proven to interrupt protein synthesis of the ribosomes in the bacterial cell, thereby preventing growth of the cell; also capable of degrading the bacterial cell wall causing destruction of the cell; effective against most Gram-negative aerobic bacilli and facultative anaerobic bacilli.

Amnesia Complete or partial memory deficit.

Amphetamine Central nervous system stimulants used to speed physiological processes and increase mental alertness by mimicking the stimulatory effects of the sympathetic nervous system; classified as narcotics; used as an anorexiant a vasoconstrictor, and for their paradoxical effect in individuals diagnosed with attention-deficit hyperactivity disorder (ADHD).

Ampule Small glass tube that contains a solution, usually a sterile pharmaceutical. The ampule is heat sealed to make it hermetic (air tight). The neck of the ampule is scored so that it can be broken open easily to allow the solution to be removed for use.

Anabolism Process of metabolism in which simple substances are built up into more complex substances.

Anaerobic Organism or tissue capable of sustaining life in the absence of oxygen.

Analeptic Drug that stimulates the respiratory center within the brain stem.

Analgesic Drug that reduces the perception of and reaction to pain; also called analgetic; some analgesics are also classified as antipyretic.

Analgetic Drug that reduces the perception of and reaction to pain; also called analgesic; some analgetics are also classified as antipyretic.

Anaphylactic shock Sudden, severe, potentially deadly allergic reaction in which the patient suffers hives (urticaria), hypotension, swelling (eyelids, lips, tongue, and throat), and difficulty breathing (dyspnea) or cessation of breathing (apnea); also known as anaphylaxis.

Anaphylaxis Sudden, severe, potentially deadly allergic reaction in which the patient suffers hives (urticaria), hypotension, swelling (eyelids, lips, tongue, and throat), and difficulty breathing (dyspnea) or cessation of breathing (apnea); also known as anaphylactic shock.

Anatomy Structure of the body.

Anesthesia Lack of sensation.

Angina pectoris Chest discomfort that occurs when the coronary arteries do not deliver enough oxygenated blood to the myocardium.

Anorexiant Drug that suppresses the appetite.

Antagonism by neutralization Occurs when two drugs bind together and inactivate one another.

Antagonist A drug that prevents or reverses the effect of another drug or naturally occurring body substance.

Ante cibum Latin term meaning before meals.

Ante meridiem (AM) Latin term meaning before midday/noon.

Antiandrogen Drug that blocks the production of testosterone or the ability of testosterone to bind with cells that depend on testosterone for growth.

Antibiotic Drug that inhibits the growth of or kills bacteria.

Antibody A protein produced in the blood or tissues in response to an antigen that initiates a response from the immune system.

Anticancer drug Capable of destroying or inhibiting spread or growth of a malignant neoplasm; also referred to as antineoplastic or chemotherapeutic drug.

Anticholinergic Drug used to block the effects of the parasympathetic nervous system; capable of decreasing production of secretions, decreasing peristalsis of the gastrointestinal tract, dilating the pupils, and decreasing contractibility of the urinary bladder; also called antimuscarinic, cholinergic blocker, and parasympatholytic.

Anticoagulant Agent that prevents blood clot formation.

Anticonvulsant Drug that prevents or reduces the effects of a seizure; also called antiepileptic.

Antiemetic Drug that reduces or eliminates nausea and vomiting (emesis).

Antiepileptic Drug that prevents or reduces the effects of a seizure; also called anticonvulsant.

Antiestrogen Drug that blocks the production of estrogen or the ability of estrogen to bind with cells that depend on estrogen for growth.

Antifebrile Drug that reduces or eliminates fever; also called antipyretic, antithermic, and febrifuge; some antifebriles have analgesic/analgetic effects.

Antifungal Drug used to inhibit the growth of or kill fungal infections; also known as antimycotic.

Antigen A foreign substance, usually a protein (but can be a carbohydrate), that causes activation of an antibody and the subsequent immune response (allergic reaction); examples of allergens include venom from a snake or insect bite, food, pollen, dust, or a medication; also called an allergen.

Antihistamine Drug used to reduce or counteract the effects of histamines during an allergic reaction; also known as H$_1$ receptor antagonists.

Antihypertensive Prescribed to lower the blood pressure to within-normal limits (120/80 mm Hg or below).

Antiinfective agent Chemical capable of killing or hindering the growth of pathogens.

Antimetabolite Antineoplastic drug that interferes with cell metabolism by interrupting production of enzymes that affect DNA structure.

Antimicrobial Chemical capable of killing or hindering the growth of microbes; includes antiseptics, disinfectants, and sterilants.

Antimuscarinic Drug used to block the effects of the parasympathetic nervous system; capable of decreasing production of secretions, decreasing peristalsis of the gastrointestinal tract, dilating the pupils, and decreasing contractibility of the urinary bladder; also called anticholinergic, cholinergic blocker, and parasympatholytic.

Antimycotic Drug used to inhibit the growth of or kill fungal infections; also known as antifungal.

Antineoplastic Drug capable of destroying or inhibiting spread or growth of a malignant neoplasm; also referred to as anticancer or chemotherapeutic drug.

Antipyretic Drug that reduces or eliminates fever; also called antifebrile, antithermic, and febrifuge; some antipyretics have analgesic/analgetic effects.

Antiseptic Used on living tissue (during the surgical scrub or the skin prep) to prohibit growth of or destroy microorganisms.

Antiserum A component of blood that contains antibodies to specific antigens; also known as immune serum.

Antithermic Drug that reduces or eliminates fever; also called antifebrile, antipyretic, and febrifuge; some antithermics have analgesic/analgetic effects.

Anxiolytic Minor tranquilizer used to produce a state of calm and reduce anxiety; also called an sedative.

Apnea Cessation of breathing.

Apothecary An outdated term that refers to a chemist who prepared and sold drug preparations and medicinal compounds.

Apothecary system Measurement system that originated in ancient Greece and was used by physicians to prescribe medicine and by pharmacists to formulate the prescribed compound. A few medications (such as aspirin, codeine, digitalis, and phenobarbital) are still prescribed and labeled in apothecary terms.

Aqueous solution Solution in which the solvent is water.

Arabic numerals System for numbering that uses a series of symbols to represent the numbers zero through nine (0–9), which is compatible with the decimal system. All other numbers are created by placing the symbols in an assigned place value column.

Arrhythmia Heart rhythm abnormality; sometimes referred to as dysrhythmia.

Arthroscopy Minimally invasive surgical procedure that allows viewing of the inside of a joint through a small incision with the use of an endoscope.

as Abbreviation of the Latin term *auris sinister*, meaning left ear.

Asepto syringe Syringe for irrigation and aspiration of large surgical or traumatic wounds and natural body openings. The large asepto syringe employs a catheter tip and has two components: the barrel, which is usually transparent, and the bulb. The end of the barrel near the bulb is flanged to provide finger rests for the user when compressing the bulb and markings on the barrel indicate the capacity of the syringe. The bulb fits snugly into the barrel, creating a seal, and the bulb is pliable to allow the user to compress and release it easily; also known as a large bulb syringe.

Aspirate Withdraw by suction; can also refer to pulmonary aspiration.

Atom Smallest unit of matter; consists of a nucleus composed of protons and neutrons and electrons that orbit the nucleus.

Atomizer Device used to create a fine mist from a liquid.

ATP (adenosine triphosphate) Major source of energy within the body that is manufactured in the mitochondria of a cell.

Atto- Metric system prefix meaning quintillionth; abbreviated as a.

au Abbreviation of the Latin term *auris utraque*, meaning each ear (both ears).

Augend Number to which another is added (addend) to obtain one sum.

Auricular Pertaining to the outer ear.

Auris dexter Latin term meaning right ear.

Auris sinister Latin term meaning left ear.

Auris utraque Latin term meaning each ear (both ears).

Autologous Derived from and transplanted to the same individual's body; donor and recipient are the same.

Autonomic nervous system Controls involuntary body functions; consists of the sympathetic and parasympathetic divisions.

avian Pertaining to a bird.

B

B/P (blood pressure) Force of blood against the lumen of a blood vessel.

Bacilli Bacteria that are shape like a rod.

Bacteria Large group of single-celled pathogenic microorganisms that can be spiral, spherical, or rod shaped and can occur singly, in clusters, or in chains.

Bactericidal Agent that kills bacteria.

Bacteriostatic Agent that inhibits bacterial growth.

Balanced salt solution (BSS) Ophthalmic irrigating solution that is sterile, isotonic, and pH adjusted (to approximately 7.0) for intraocular and extraocular use; glucose may be added to provide an energy source.

Barbiturate Central nervous system depressants that are narcotics; used in low doses for control of seizures and in larger doses for induction of general anesthesia.

Baricity Molecular weight.

Base Substance with a pH of greater than 7 that is capable of turning litmus paper blue. Bases have a high concentration of hydroxide ions and have the potential to accept hydrogen ions. Bases typically have a bitter taste. Another word for base is alkaline.

Behavioral tolerance Drug tolerance that occurs as an individual learns to conceal the effects of the drug.

Benzodiazepine Central nervous system depressants that are narcotics; have anticonvulsant, amnesic, anxiolytic, and sedative effects and produce minimal cardiac and respiratory depression; popular for use as a preoperative medication to reduce anxiety and intra-operatively when monitored anesthesia care (MAC) is provided during a procedure conducted under conscious sedation.

Beta-adrenergic blocker Type of adrenergic blocker that is capable of reducing hypertension, resolving cardiac dysrhythmias, lowering intraocular pressure, and relieving angina pectoris as well as migraine headaches; also called beta blocker.

Beta blocker Type of adrenergic blocker that is capable of reducing hypertension, resolving cardiac dysrhythmias, lowering intraocular pressure, and relieving angina pectoris as well as migraine headaches; also called beta-adrenergic blocker.

Beta-lactam Group of antibacterial agents that includes penicillins, cephalosporins, and carbapenems (among others); not effective against resting bacteria but work by inhibiting the enzymes necessary to manufacture the cell wall as the bacteria reproduces.

bid Abbreviation of the Latin term *bis in die*, meaning twice a day.

Bioavailability Describes the amount of a drug that enters the circulatory system and is available to the target tissue cells.

Biodegradation Chemical changes that a drug substance undergoes as it is being broken down (catabolism) within the body in preparation for excretion; also known as biotransformation and metabolism.

Biohazardous material Solid or liquid agent (microorganism, toxin, etc.) from a living organism capable of causing harm to humans.

Biological 1. Pertaining to living matter. 2. Pharmaceutical agents such as blood products and vaccines that originate from living matter.

Biological potency Activity, action, or effect of a drug within the body.

Biological response modifier Immune system substance (e.g., antibodies and cytokines) that increase the patient's biological response to a malignant tumor.

Biotechnology Use of living matter to manufacture pharmaceuticals (and other industrial substances) by using recombinant DNA technology.

Biotransformation Chemical changes that a drug substance undergoes as it is being broken down (catabolism) within the body in preparation for excretion; also known as biodegradation and metabolism.

Bis in die Latin term meaning twice a day.

Bladder A bag or sac; urinary bladder stores urine until it is released through the urethra.

Blood pressure (B/P) Force of blood against the lumen of a blood vessel.

Blood type Based on the presence or absence of antigens on the surface of a red blood cell. There are four blood types (A, B, AB, and O) in addition to the Rh factor (positive or negative).

Boiling point of water 100° C or 212° F.

Bolus 1. Large dose of a drug usually given parenterally to rapidly achieve a therapeutic level. 2. Soft mass of chewed or partially digested food.

Botanic Pertaining to plants.

Bovine Pertaining to cattle.

Brand name Name that the manufacturer assigns to a drug for marketing purposes; also known as the trade name and the proprietary name.

Broad-spectrum 1. Antibiotic that is effective against a wide range of bacteria. 2. Extensive array of uses.

Bronchodilator Relax the muscles that surround the bronchial structures allowing the passageways to dilate, which in turn allows movement of an increased volume of air with each breath.

Buccal Pertaining to the cheek or in the direction of the cheek. Medication that is administered buccally is typically in the tablet form. The tablet is placed between the cheek and the upper or lower gum.

Buffer Substance that is capable of neutralizing an acid or a base.

Bulb syringe Used to insert or withdraw fluids from surgical or traumatic wounds and natural body openings; see large and small bulb syringe.

C

C 1. Abbreviation that represents the Celsius/centigrade temperature scale. 2. Roman numeral symbol that represents the number one hundred. 3. Abbreviation that represents the household system term *cup/cups*.

Calcium-channel blocker Drug that reduces the force of each heartbeat; limits the amount of calcium in the muscle, which reduces the contractile force of the muscle and decreases the heart's need for oxygen and nutrients.

Calibrations Markings or divisions used to determine degree or measure quantity according to predetermined standards to maintain accuracy. Calibrations are found on thermometers to identify temperature, on syringes to measure volume, etc.

Cap(s) Abbreviation for the term *capsule(s)*.

Caprine Pertaining to goats.

Capsule Soluble gelatinous casing that encloses a dose of medication.

Carbapenem Drug in the beta-lactam group of anti-infective agents; originates from thienamycin which is a product of the *Streptomyces cattleya* bacteria that is found in soil; primarily effective against Haemophilus influenza, anaerobes, most enterobacteriaceae, and methicillin-resistant staphylococci and streptococci.

Carbonic anhydrase inhibitor diuretic Type of diuretic that inhibits carbonic anhydrase, which is an enzyme found in the proximal tubule. Inhibition of the enzyme causes an increase in excretion of hydrogen, which in turn increases excretion of sodium, water, and potassium; used to treat open-angle glaucoma and preoperatively to decrease intraocular pressure associated with angle-closure glaucoma.

Cardiovascular Pertaining to the heart and blood vessels.

Carpule Sterile cartridge filled with medication that is essentially the barrel portion of a syringe that is later inserted into a reusable holder/plunger mechanism at the time of use. Also called a cartridge.

Cartridge Sterile device filled with medication that is essentially the barrel portion of a syringe that is later inserted into a reusable holder/plunger mechanism at the time of use. Also called a carpule.

Catabolism Process of metabolism in which complex substances are broken down into more simple substances.

Catalyst Substance that initiates or increases the speed of a chemical reaction.

Catheter Hollow cylindrical device inserted into a body cavity, duct, or vessel to allow insertion or withdrawal of fluids and gasses.

Catheter tip Blunt tapered syringe tip that can be inserted into a medical device (such as a Foley catheter) to allow air or fluid to be inserted or withdrawn.

cc Abbreviation of the Latin term *cum cibo*, meaning with food; also cubic centimeter.

Cell membrane Double phospholipid membrane that surrounds the plasma (cytoplasm/protoplasm) of a cell; also known as the plasma membrane and plasmalemma.

Cellular tolerance Drug tolerance that occurs when the number of receptors that bind to the drug are decreased; also known as reduced responsiveness or downregulation.

Celsius (C) Temperature scale that is part of the metric system; also known as centigrade.

Centi- Metric system prefix meaning hundredth; abbreviated as c.

Centigram Metric system term that represents one hundredth of a gram.

Centiliter Metric system term that represents one hundredth of a liter.

Centimeter Metric system term that represents one hundredth of a meter.

Central nervous system Division of the nervous system that includes the brain and spinal cord.

Central nervous system stimulant Drug used to speed physiological processes and increase mental alertness by mimicking the stimulatory effects of the sympathetic nervous system; includes amphetamines, analeptics, and emetics.

Central vein Large vein that is located closer to the heart than a peripheral vein. Examples of central veins include the jugular, femoral, and subclavian veins.

Cephalosporin Drug in the beta-lactam group of anti-infective agents; derived from the Acremonium fungus (formerly called Cephalosporium) commonly found in soil; further classified by generation (first through fifth).

cg Abbreviation that represents the metric system term *centigram*.

Chemical interactions Effects of some drugs that are evident without any alteration of cellular function such as neutralization of stomach acid.

Chemical name Provides the exact formula and molecular structure of the drug.

Chemotherapeutic 1. Pertaining to chemical therapy. 2. Drug capable of destroying or inhibiting spread or growth of a malignant neoplasm; also referred to as anticancer or antineoplastic drug.

Cholinergic Drug used to mimic the effects of the parasympathetic nervous system; capable of slowing of the heart, pupil constriction, increased gastrointestinal peristalsis, increased production of secretions (such as gastric juices, mucous, saliva, and sweat), increased contractibility of the urinary bladder, increased strength of the skeletal muscles, pupil constriction (miosis), and decreased intraocular pressure; also called muscarinic and parasympathomimetic.

Cholinergic blocker Drug used to block the effects of the parasympathetic nervous system; capable of decreasing production of secretions, decreasing peristalsis of the gastrointestinal tract, dilating the pupils, and decreasing contractibility of the urinary bladder; also called anticholinergic, antimuscarinic, and parasympatholytic.

Chromosome Colored strand of DNA.

Chronic Disease or medical condition that is ongoing or recurrent.

Chronotropic effect Agents that increase or decrease the speed of a rhythmic physiological process such as the heart rate.

Ciliary body Muscle that controls accommodation of the crystalline lens of the eye.

Circa Around; about; often pertains to approximate date.

Circadian rhythm Circadian rhythm is the sleep, wake, and activity pattern that occurs within a 24-hour period. Circadian rhythm is sometimes referred to as the internal or biological clock. Circadian patterns vary between individuals (everyone's clock is different) and within an individual from day to day according to their stress, activity, and wellness levels.

Circumferential Around; surrounding.

Civilian time Time-keeping system that uses a 12-hour clock in which the 12 numbers repeat; designations of AM and PM are used to represent morning and afternoon. Synonymous with standard time.

cl Abbreviation that represents the metric system term *centiliter*.

Clearance Removal of a drug from a specified volume of blood plasma.

Clotting factors Twelve proteins contained within the blood plasma that are necessary for normal blood clotting; deficiency of any one of the factors can result in a bleeding disorder.

cm Abbreviation that represents the metric system term *centimeter.*

Coagulant Drug or other substance used to promote blood clotting, maintain a blood clot, or otherwise act to slow or stop bleeding; also called hemostatic agent or procoagulant.

Cocci Bacteria that are round in shape and form characteristic arrangements such as diplococci, staphylococci, and streptococci.

Collar Fastener that fits circumferentially around a device to secure the components.

Colloid 1. Large-molecular-weight insoluble particle such as gelatin or a starch placed in a solution that can be administered as a plasma expander to patients experiencing low blood volume. 2. Solution that contains a high-molecular-weight substance as the main osmotic particle. Colloid solutions such as albumin, dextran, and hydroxyethyl starch are used as plasma expanders when crystalloids are ineffective.

Colloid plasma expander Hypertonic solution that draws fluid into the blood vessels to help maintain blood pressure and circulate red blood cells.

Comorbid condition A disease or condition that exists in addition to the patient's primary problem. The comorbid disease may exacerbate the primary problem or make treatment of the primary problem difficult.

Compatibility Ability of two or more drugs to be prescribed simultaneously or mixed together without causing a negative reaction.

Competitive antagonism Form of antagonism that occurs when the antagonist competes for and binds to the receptor that would normally be occupied by the initial drug (agonist) preventing that drug from acting. Because high doses of the initial drug may overcome the power of the antagonist, this type of antagonism is said to be surmountable.

Complexation Situation in which two or more compounds in a mixture form a chemical that inactivates one or more of the drugs.

Complex fraction Contains a simple fraction in the numerator, denominator, or both.

Component therapy Use of portions of blood that are separated and used as needed; includes red blood cells and platelet-rich plasma (which can be further separated into specific components).

Compound Consists of two or more different atoms.

Compound fraction Requires a mathematical calculation in either the numerator or the denominator.

Compounding Act of combining two or more elements, ingredients, or parts.

Concave Curving inward; opposite of convex.

Concentrate To make a solution stronger or denser by removing solvent (liquid) or adding solute (solid usually the drug).

Concentration Strength or amount of the active ingredient of a medication (usually the solute) in relation to the volume (usually the solvent).

Congenital defect Developmental defect that is present at birth.

Conjunctiva Mucous membrane that covers the exposed surface of the eyeball and lines the inner surfaces of the eyelids.

Conscious sedation Patient experiences a depressed state of consciousness with the use of a sedative, but is able to maintain the airway and breathe independently; can be aroused to respond to physical and verbal stimulation (if necessary); used during medical or dental procedures; often used in conjunction with a local anesthetic.

Constant Fixed; unchanging.

Contraindications Reasons why a drug or treatment should be avoided.

Contrast media Radiopaque solution introduced into structures with lumens during radiographic exams to differentiate various tissues.

Control syringe Syringe that employs three finger rings instead of flanges. Two of the rings are attached to the barrel and one is attached to the plunger. The rings provide increased stability (control) of the syringe in the hand of the user and allow additional pressure to be applied to eject the contents if resistance occurs. Also called a three-ring syringe.

Controlled release A form of sustained release that is designed to maintain a steady concentration of the drug within the body.

Controlled substance Drug that has a potential to cause physical or psychological dependency; narcotic.

Convex Curving outward; opposite of concave.

Coronary dilator Causes relaxation of the blood vessels of the heart.

Corticosteroid Produced naturally in the cortex of the adrenal gland; also available in pharmaceutical preparations; divided into three groups: glucocorticoids, mineralocorticoids, and the sex hormones.

Covalent bond Type of chemical bond in which one or more pairs of electrons are shared by two atoms.

Critical item Medical device, such as a surgical instrument, that will come in contact with sterile tissue; must be sterilized or disinfected with a high-level agent.

Cryoprecipitate Fraction of blood plasma that contains Factor VIII, fibrinogen, von Willebrand factor, Factor XIII, plasma proteins, albumin, immunoglobulin, and other clotting factor derivatives.

Crystalloid Solution that contains sodium as the main osmotic particle. Crystalloid solutions such as 0.9% saline and lactated Ringer's solution are commonly used intravenous fluids.

Cubic centimeter On thousandth of a liter.

Cum cibo With food.

Cup Household system term that represents the equivalent of 8 ounces.

Cycloplegic Antimuscarinic drug that paralyzes the ciliary body interrupting the process of accommodation and paralyzes the muscle that constricts the pupil, thereby maintaining pupil dilation.

Cylinder Tubular (cylindrical) pressurized metal container that is typically used to store a gas. Medical gases, such as oxygen and nitrous oxide, often stored in a large tank in a cylinder may be employed; also known as a tank.

Cylindrical Resembling a cylinder (tube-like structure).

Cystoscopy Minimally invasive surgical procedure that allows viewing of the inside of the urinary bladder with the use of an endoscope that is inserted through the urethra.

Cytoplasm Liquid component of a cell that contains the organelles.

D

D Roman numeral symbol that represents the number five hundred.

da/daw abbreviation for the terms *dispense/dispense as written*.

dag Abbreviation that represents the metric system term *dekagram*.

dal Abbreviation that represents the metric system term dekaliter.

dam Abbreviation that represents the metric system term *dekameter*.

dc Abbreviation for the term *discontinue/discharge*.

DEA (Drug Enforcement Administration) Responsible for enforcement of the laws pertaining to controlled substances.

Deca- Metric system prefix meaning ten; abbreviated as da.

Deci- Metric system prefix meaning tenth; abbreviated as d.

Decigram Metric system term that represents one tenth of a gram.

Deciliter Metric system term that represents one tenth of a liter.

Decimal point (.) Symbol used to separate whole number from the fraction when using the decimal system; stated as point when reading a decimal system number.

Decimal system Numbering system that is part of the metric system and relies on a place value system that is based on multiples of ten and uses a decimal point to separate the whole numbers from the fractions.

Decimeter Metric system term that represents one tenth of a meter.

Degradation Reduction of quality (amount, intensity, strength).

Dehydrated Product for which the moisture has been removed.

Deionized All ions (electrically charged particles) have been removed.

Dekagram Metric system term that represents 10 grams.

Dekaliter Metric system term that represents 10 liters.

Dekameter Metric system term that represents 10 meters.

Delayed release Drug is liberated at a time other than when administered.

Denominator Lower number of a fraction.

Deoxyribonucleic acid (DNA) Main component of a chromosome that carries the genetic information of a cell.

Dependence Occurs when a drug is needed for an individual to function in a seemingly normal fashion. Dependence may be physiological (chemical) or psychological and is often a result of abuse of narcotic analgesics, alcohol, and benzodiazepine as well as other psychotropic drugs. However, one may also become addicted to caffeine, laxatives, nasal sprays, etc. Dependence is also called addiction.

Depolarizing neuromuscular blocker Type of neuromuscular blocker that mimics the release of acetylcholine across the neuromuscular junction causing muscle contraction (fasciculation), which is followed by a period of muscle fatigue; metabolized by plasma pseudocholinesterase; pharmacologic antagonist is not available.

Depot storage Administered drug has an affinity for a certain type of tissue such as muscle or fat where it is bound, making a portion of the drug unavailable to the target cells. However, when the drug is released from the tissue, a lingering effect of the drug may be noted; also known as tissue binding.

Dermal Pertaining to the skin.

Detoxification Occurs when an individual who is addicted to a drug discontinues use of the drug. Withdrawal may occur suddenly or gradually. Physical and psychological manifestations of withdrawal can vary in intensity and severity from very mild to extremely serious, and in some situations may be deadly. Symptoms of withdrawal can last from as little as a few hours to as long as several weeks. Examples of withdrawal symptoms include nausea, vomiting, diarrhea, constipation, sweating, and tremors. Some individuals experience a rebound effect in which the problem for which the drug was initially administered returns in a seemingly more severe fashion until homeostasis is reestablished; also known as withdrawal.

dg Abbreviation that represents the metric system term *decigram*.

Difference Result of subtraction.

Diffusion Movement of molecules from an area of higher concentration to an area of lower concentration through a medium such as air. Diffusion does not require the use of energy and is a form of passive transport. Diffusion is similar to osmosis; however, diffusion may or may not require a cell membrane to occur.

Diluent Substance used to dilute a solution.

Dilute To make a solution weaker or less dense by adding solvent (liquid) or removing solute (solid—usually the drug).

Dilution A decrease in the strength or concentration of a medication usually by increasing the amount of the solvent.

Dimensional analysis Process of understanding and applying the relationships between the qualities of various items (such as drugs and systems for identifying and measuring drug dosages) based on the physical characteristics (dimensions) of each item.

Diplococci Characteristic arrangement of round bacterial cells that form in pairs.

Disinfectant Agent used on fomites to destroy pathogens; occurs on three levels (low, intermediate, and high).

Dispense To disperse.

Dispositional tolerance Type of tolerance in which metabolism of the drug occurs more rapidly; also known as metabolic tolerance.

Distribution Delivery of the drug to the target cells, the site of metabolism, and the site of excretion by the circulatory system.

Diuretic Type of drug that increases urine production.

Dividend Number that is to be portioned or divided; numerator of a fraction; contained within the long division bracket.

Division Splitting or dividing a number into equal groups.

Divisor Number of desired portions of the dividend; denominator of a fraction; number to the left of the long division bracket; may be a factor of another number.

dl Abbreviation that represents the metric system term *deciliter*.

dm Abbreviation that represents the metric system term *decimeter*.

DNA (deoxyribonucleic acid) Main component of a chromosome that carries the genetic information of a cell.

Documentation Record of an activity (such as medication administration in the patient's chart) usually a written statement to provide/serve as evidence.

Dose Prescribed amount (quantity) of a medication.

Downregulation Drug tolerance that occurs when the number of receptors that bind to the drug are decreased; also known as reduced responsiveness or cellular tolerance.

Drachm Apothecary system term that represents the equivalent of 3 scruples; synonymous with the term *dram*.

Dram Apothecary system term that represents the equivalent of 3 scruples; the term *drachm* may also be used.

Dromotropic effect Changes the speed at which electrical impulses are conducted through the heart muscle.

Drop Household system term that represents the equivalent of a small quantity of liquid that forms a spherical mass.

Dropper Plastic or glass barrel that is tapered at one end with a rubber bulb/stopper attached to the opposite end. The barrel may have calibrations to indicate the volume. A dropper may be incorporated in the cap of a medication bottle or may be available separately. A dropper is used to instill liquid medication into the nose, eyes, or ears. Droppers may also be used to measure a small amount of medication that is to be added to another liquid or to insert medication into the mouth of an infant.

Drug A substance that is used to diagnose, treat, cure, mitigate (to make less severe), or prevent a disease or condition.

Drug Enforcement Administration (DEA) Responsible for enforcement of the laws pertaining to controlled substances.

Drug enzyme interactions Occur when a drug speeds or inhibits the action of an enzyme or changes the response of the cells affected by the enzyme.

Drug interactions Two or more drugs are combined to intentionally produce a desired effect or unintentionally to produce an undesirable effect.

Drug label Printed information affixed to a drug package or included within the drug packaging that contains information about the drug. Label information may include the trade name, generic name, concentration, amount, expiration date, directions for reconstitution/dilution, storage information, handling precautions, warnings, route of administration, etc.

Drug receptor interactions Occur when a drug molecule attaches to a receptor that is usually a protein or glycoprotein located on the plasmalemma, on an organelle, or within the cytoplasm of the target cell. Most drugs have an affinity (attraction) to the target cells.

Drug theories The four methods by which drugs are thought to elicit their responses. The four methods are drug receptor interactions, drug enzyme interactions, nonspecific responses, and chemical interactions.

Drug tolerance May be cellular (when the number of receptors that bind to the drug are decreased) or behavioral (when the individual learns to conceal the effects of the drug) in nature.

Dura mater Outermost layer of the meninges.

Duration of action Time that elapses from onset of action to termination of action.

Dye Pigment used to color tissue; used when coloration is needed for short duration; may be easily removed or absorbed.

Dyspnea Difficulty breathing.

Dysrhythmia Heart rhythm abnormality; sometimes referred to as arrhythmia.

E

Ear syringe Syringe for irrigation and aspiration of small wounds or body orifices that is constructed as a single unit of soft plastic that has a bulb on one end and a tapered opening on the other end; also known as small bulb syringe, nasal syringe, and ulcer syringe.

Eccentric tip Off-center syringe tip that is used when the syringe must remain parallel to the injection site (such as during an intradermal injection).

Effector Body structure that carries out a response to a nerve impulse.

Effects Characteristics or actions of a drug.

Efficacy Ability to produce the desired effect; effectiveness.

Electrolytes Ions in solution. Common electrolytes found within the body include calcium (+), chloride (–), hydrogen phosphate (–), hydrogen carbonate (–), magnesium (+), potassium (+), and sodium (+). Electrolytes are important in many body functions including muscle contraction, fluid balance, and blood pressure control. If not resolved, electrolyte imbalance can escalate to a medical emergency.

Electrolytic Irrigation solutions that contain electrolytes; conduct electricity; not usually used in conjunction with the electrosurgical unit (especially during endoscopic procedures) because of the risk of electrical injury.

Electron Negatively charged portion of an atom.

Electronic medication administration record (eMAR) Record-keeping system that employs barcode technology on the drug packages and labels; may be used for inventory control and generating patient charges.

Electuary Sweetened paste that is taken orally.

Element Consists of one or more like atoms.

Elixir Sweetened solution in which the solvent is ethyl alcohol.

eMAR (electronic medication administration record) Record-keeping system that employs barcode technology on the drug packages and labels; may be used for inventory control and generating patient charges.

Emesis Regurgitation; ejection of the stomach contents through the mouth; reverse peristalsis; also called vomiting.

Emetic Drug that induces vomiting (emesis).

Emulsion Consists of two liquids that cannot combine (heterogenous mixture), typically oil in water.

Endophthalmitis Inflammation of the inner tunics and cavities of the eye; possibly due to a bacterial infection.

Endoscope Rigid or flexible instrument used for viewing the interior of the body through a natural opening or a small incision. An endoscope consists of a lens system, eyepiece, fiber optic light delivery system, and possibly an additional channel to allow for insertion or withdrawal of gasses or fluids, introduction of other medical devices, or removal of foreign bodies.

Enema Insertion of a liquid through the anus into the rectum.

Enteral Involving the intestinal tract.

Enzyme A protein that initiates or increases the speed (in other words, acts as a catalyst) of a chemical reaction. The enzyme itself is not expended nor does it undergo any lasting change during the reaction.

Epicutaneous Pertaining to the surface of the skin.

Epidural Above or outside of the dura mater.

Equal Two numbers or other items that are alike in degree, quantity, or volume.

Equation Mathematical statement that shows that two expressions are alike.

Equine Pertaining to horses.

Equivalency Expression of relationships between two mathematical statements that are alike.

Equivalent fraction Has the same value as another fraction.

Equivocal Uncertain; questionable.

Exa- Metric system prefix meaning quintillion; abbreviated as E.

Excipient An additive that does not affect the performance of a drug.

Excretion Elimination of a drug from the body.

Exophthalmitis Inflammation of the surface of the eye (conjunctiva and cornea); possibly due to a bacterial infection.

Express 1. Squeeze out. 2. To put a thought into words (written or stated). 3. To represent using a character, figure, formula, or symbol.

Extended release Drug is liberated over a prolonged period for the purpose of maintaining the peak effect, thereby reducing the number of doses needed.

Extremes Two outer terms of a proportion that are cross-multiplied when solving for an unknown.

F

F Abbreviation that represents the Fahrenheit temperature scale.

Facilitated passive diffusion (transport) Movement of the drug molecules from an area of high concentration to an area of low concentration without using any energy. However, proteins are used to develop a pathway (called a protein channel) to help transport the drug molecule across the semipermeable membrane.

Factor An integer that can be divided into another integer without producing a remainder.

Facultative Able to survive in more than one environment.

Fahrenheit (F) Temperature scale that is part of the household system.

Fasciculation Uncoordinated twitching of one or more muscles; may be caused by administration of a depolarizing neuromuscular blocker.

Fat soluble Capable of being dissolved or liquefied in lipids.

Fat soluble vitamins Vitamins capable of being dissolved or liquefied in lipids. The fat soluble vitamins are A, E, D, and K.

FDA (Food and Drug Administration) Responsible for overseeing the effectiveness, safety, and security of all drugs (human and veterinary), biological agents (including blood and vaccines), medical devices, cosmetics, and radiation-emitting devices. The jurisdiction of the FDA also extends to safety and security of the nation's food supply.

Febrifuge Drug that reduces or eliminates fever; also called antifebrile, antipyretic, and antithermic; some febrifuges have analgesic/analgetic effects.

Feeding tube Tube inserted directly into the stomach to administer nutrition.

Femto- Metric system prefix meaning quadrillionth; abbreviated as f.

Fibrinolysis Breakdown of fibrin contained within a blood clot, usually by the action of an enzyme.

Fibrinolytic Drug that destroys fibrin, which is a major component of a blood clot (thrombus); also called thrombolytic.

Fight-or-flight response Sympathetic nervous system response to stress, anger, or an emergency situation; manifested by a surge of adrenaline that increases the heart rate and force of heart contractions, increases blood pressure, promotes blood flow to skeletal muscles, dilates the bronchial tree, and promotes visual acuity.

Flange Rim, such as on the barrel and plunger of a syringe that provides support for the user's fingers when drawing in or ejecting the contents of the syringe.

Flow rate Speed at which a gas or solution progresses during a specified amount of time (such as the flow of oxygen expressed in liters per minute or IV fluid expressed in drops per minute or ml per hour).

fl oz Abbreviation that represents the household system term *fluid ounce/fluid ounces*.

Fluid dram Apothecary system term that represents the equivalent of 3 fluid scruples.

Fluid ounce 1. Apothecary system term that represents the equivalent of 8 fluid drams. 2. Household system term that represents the equivalent of 2 tablespoons.

Fluid scruple Apothecary system term that represents the equivalent of 20 minims.

Foley catheter Indwelling catheter that is passed through the urethra into the bladder to allow for drainage of urine into a collection bag. A balloon on the part of the catheter that is retained in the bladder is inflated (usually with sterile water) to hold the catheter in place. Foley catheters may be manufactured from latex or silicone.

Fomite Inanimate object capable of harboring and transmitting pathogens from one individual to another.

Food and Drug Administration (FDA) Responsible for overseeing the effectiveness, safety, and security of all drugs (human and veterinary), biological agents (including blood and vaccines), medical devices, cosmetics, and radiation-emitting devices. The jurisdiction of the FDA also extends to safety and security of the nation's food supply.

Foot Household system term that represents the equivalent of 12 inches (possibly length of a human foot).

Formulary List of approved drugs.

Fraction Equal divisions of an item or a portion that is less than the whole item or number.

Fractionated Separated or divided into components.

Freezing point of water 0° C or 32° F.

ft Abbreviation that represents the household system term *foot/feet*.

Fungi Group of organisms (pathogenic and beneficial) that consists of yeasts and molds.

G

g Abbreviation that represents the metric system term *gram*; the terms *gm* and *GM* may also be used.

gal 1. Abbreviation that represents the apothecary system term *gallon*. 2. Abbreviation that represents the household system term *gallon*.

Galactagogue Drug that induces lactation and stimulates increased milk production.

Gallon 1. Apothecary system term that represents the equivalent of 4 quarts. 2. Household system term that represents the equivalent of 4 quarts/16 cups/128 ounces.

Gamma camera Device similar to a Geiger counter that is capable of detecting gamma radiation emitted from radioisotopes; also called a scintillation camera.

Ganglia Mass of nerve tissue that is outside of the central nervous system.

Gas A liquid in its vapor form.

Gastric agent Drug that produces an effect on the stomach such as reducing or eliminating nausea and vomiting, inducing vomiting, increasing gastric motility and relaxing the pyloric sphincter to allow partially digested food to move quickly from the stomach to the small intestine, and controlling gastric acidity.

Gastrointestinal tract Pertains to the digestive system, particularly the stomach, small bowel, and colon.

Gastrostomy tube (G-tube) Tube inserted into the stomach percutaneously (through the skin).

Gauge Standard unit of measure typically applied when measuring the diameter. When referring to a hypodermic needle or stainless steel suture, low gauge numbers represent a large diameter and high gauge numbers represent a small diameter.

Geiger counter Instrument used to detect and measure the intensity of a radioactive material.

General anesthesia Drug-induced state of unconsciousness (complete lack of sensation) to allow a patient to undergo a medical, dental, or surgical procedure.

Generic name Nonproprietary name of a drug. The generic name is often a shortened version of the chemical name or may be a reference to the intended use of the drug that is selected by original developer. The generic name is the preferred name for use in the health care setting.

Genetic engineering Term used interchangeably with biotechnology and recombinant DNA technology.

Giga- Metric system prefix meaning billion; abbreviated as G.

Glucagon Hormone produced by the alpha cells of the islets of Langerhans in the pancreas to raise the blood sugar level; also available as a pharmaceutical.

Glucocorticoid Corticosteroid produced in the cortex of the adrenal gland and also available as a pharmaceutical; function to metabolize carbohydrates (especially glucose), fats, and proteins; also active in stress regulation and acts as antiinflammatory agent; cortisol (also known as hydrocortisone) represents 95% of all glucocorticoids.

gly Abbreviation that represents the term *glycine*.

Glycine A nonessential amino acid that naturally occurs in connective tissue, muscle, and skin and functions to break down glucose into energy, regulates bile synthesis to metabolize fat, and acts as an inhibitory neurotransmitter in the spinal cord and brain stem. Glycine is also produced commercially and is used as a dietary supplement (sweetener), as an antacid, to treat muscle diseases, as an adjunctive therapy in the treatment of schizophrenia, and for bladder irrigation during transurethral prostatectomy.

gm Abbreviation that represents the metric system term *gram*; the terms *g* and *GM* may also be used.

GM Abbreviation that represents the metric system term *gram*; the terms *g* and *gm* may also be used.

gr Abbreviation that represents the apothecary system term *grain*.

Graduated pitcher Container constructed with a handle and a spout that is marked with calibrations to indicate the volume. Graduated pitchers allow the user to pour irrigation fluid into a surgical wound and typically hold one liter of solution.

Grain Apothecary system term that represents the weight of a single grain of wheat.

Gram Metric system term that represents weight; one thousandth of a kilogram.

Gram-negative Classification of bacteria that stain blue/purple when the Gram stain technique is applied; examples of Gram-negative bacteria include cyanobacteria, spirochetes, green sulfur bacteria, and most proteobacteria.

Gram-positive Classification of bacteria that stain pink/red when the Gram stain technique is applied; examples of Gram-positive bacteria include bacilli, clostridium, enterococci, listeria, staphylococci, and streptococci.

Gram stain Laboratory method for rapidly identifying bacterial cells based on the ability of the cell membrane to retain or shed the stain; Gram-positive bacteria stain blue/purple; Gram-negative bacteria stain pink/red; not all bacteria fit into the Gram-positive/Gram-negative classifications.

gt/gtt/gtts Abbreviation of the Latin terms *gutta/guttae*, meaning drop/drops/drops.

G-tube (gastrostomy tube) Tube inserted into the stomach percutaneously (through the skin).

Gutta/guttae Latin term meaning drop/drops.

H

h Abbreviation of the Latin term *hora*, meaning hour.

H_1 receptor antagonist Drug used to reduce or counteract the effects of histamines during an allergic reaction; also known as antihistamine.

H_2 antagonist Drug used to suppress secretion of hydrochloric acid in the stomach; also called H_2 receptor blocker.

H_2 receptor blocker Drug used to suppress secretion of hydrochloric acid in the stomach; also called H_2 antagonist.

Half-life Amount of time necessary for the concentration of the drug in the plasma to be reduced by 50%.

Halogenated Some volatile liquids used as inhalation general anesthesia agents contain halogen and are referred to as halogenated; halogenated agents are known triggers for malignant hyperthermia; examples of halogenated agents include desflurane, halothane, isoflurane, and sevoflurane.

Heart rate Speed at which the heart is beating. Normal heart rate for an adult is approximately 72 beats per minute.

Hecto- Metric system prefix meaning hundred; abbreviated as h.

Hectogram Metric system term that represents 100 grams.

Hectoliter Metric system term that represents 100 liters.

Hectometer Metric system term that represents 100 meters.

Helminth Parasitic worm.

Hemodynamic changes Changes within the body that affect the mechanism of blood circulation such as blood volume, blood pressure, and heart rate.

Hemolytic Pertains to destruction of the membrane of a red blood cell that results in the release of hemoglobin; caused by some types of anemia, exposure to a toxin, or the presence of antibodies.

Hemolytic disease of the newborn Occurs when an incompatibility exists between maternal blood (Rh−) and fetal blood (Rh+) because the mother has developed antibodies against the fetal Rh+ blood (usually is not a problem during a first pregnancy but can occur in subsequent pregnancies); causes destruction of the red blood cells of the newborn that results in anemia; can be prevented with the use of Rho (D) immune globulin.

Hemolytic transfusion reaction Allergic reaction that can occur during blood transfusion in which the transfused donor blood cells are destroyed by the recipient's immune system.

Hemophilia Blood clotting disorder related to a deficiency of clotting factor VII or IX, which are proteins required for platelet aggregation.

Hemostasis Stoppage or control of bleeding during a surgical procedure.

Hemostatic agent Drug or other substance used to promote blood clotting, maintain a blood clot, or otherwise act to slow or stop bleeding; also called coagulant or procoagulant.

Hepatic first pass effect A portion of the drug is first sent to the liver in the blood via the hepatic vein, where it is biotransformed before it gets into general circulation and can be distributed to the target tissue cells. As a result, the patient does not receive the benefit of the full dose of the drug and the dosages must be calculated (usually increased) to compensate because the bioavailability is reduced.

Hepatic portal system Venous return system that sends blood from various abdominal organs (such as the stomach, spleen, pancreas, and intestine) directly to the liver.

Hermetic air tight.

Heterogenous A mixture in which the substances are not equally distributed.

hg Abbreviation that represents the metric system term *hectogram*.

High-level disinfection Kills all microorganisms with the exception of bacterial spores and prions; used on critical items.

Hilt Portion of a hypodermic needle where the shaft meets the flanged hub.

Histamine Amine compounds (organic compounds containing ammonia) released by the mast cells (type of cell found in connective tissue) during an allergic reaction.

Histology Study of tissues.

hl Abbreviation that represents the metric system term *hectoliter*.

hm Abbreviation that represents the metric system term *hectometer*.

Homeostasis Maintenance or balance of the body's physiologic systems.

Homogenous A mixture in which the substances are equally distributed.

Hora Latin term meaning hour.

Hora somni Latin term meaning hour of sleep (at bedtime).

Hormone Substance produced by a gland that is transported in the blood to have an effect on a body function elsewhere in the body.

Household system Measurement system primarily used in the United States to determine length, weight, and volume; also referred to as United States customary units.

hs Abbreviation of the Latin term *hora somni*, meaning hour of sleep (at bedtime).

Hub Portion of a hypodermic needle that allows the needle to be attached to a syringe.

Hydrogen bond Type of chemical bond that involves an interaction between a hydrogen atom and an electronegative atom, such as nitrogen, oxygen, or fluorine from another molecule or chemical group.

Hydrophilicity Ability of a drug to be attracted to and dissolved in water.

Hypercalcemia High concentration of calcium in the blood.

Hyperkalemia High concentration of potassium in the blood.

Hypernatremia High concentration of sodium in the blood.

Hyperpyrexia Excessive fever.

Hypertension High blood pressure.

Hyperthermia Increase in body temperature.

Hypertonic Solution that consists of a greater number of particles (a concentrated solution) than blood plasma and draws fluid out of the cells into circulation, causing the cells to shrink (called crenation).

Hypnosis Alternative therapy that involves a state of concentration and relaxation that is induced by suggestion and resembles sleep; sometimes used to reduce the perception of pain.

Hypnotic Central nervous system depressant classified as a narcotic; used to induce sleep; also called soporific.

Hypocalcemia Low concentration of calcium in the blood.

Hypodermic Pertaining to the structures beneath the skin.

Hypokalemia Low concentration of potassium in the blood.

Hyponatremia Low concentration of sodium in the blood.

Hypotension Low blood pressure.

Hypothermia Decrease in body temperature.

Hypotonic Solution that consists of a lesser number of particles (a dilute solution) than blood plasma and pushes fluid out of circulation into the cells, causing them to swell and possibly burst (called hemolysis).

I

I Roman numeral symbol that represents the number one.

Iatrogenic response A complication that is inadvertently induced in the patient by a health care provider or as a result of medical treatment (including diagnostic procedures). Side effects, adverse effects, toxic effects, and teratogenic effects are all examples of iatrogenic responses that relate to pharmacology.

Ichthyoid Pertaining to fish.

IM Abbreviation for the term *intramuscularly*.

Immediate-release system Used to describe drug forms that are easily broken down, allowing the active ingredient to be available for absorption without delay.

Immune serum A component of blood that contains antibodies to specific antigens; also known as antiserum.

Implantation Inserted below the skin or into a body structure.

Impregnated 1. Infused, permeated, or saturated with a substance. 2. To fertilize; such as ova with sperm.

Improper fraction Numerator is larger than the denominator.

in Abbreviation that represents the household system term *inch/inches*.

inch Household system term that represents the equivalent of one twelfth of a part (possibly the length of a human foot), length of the distal portion of a human thumb, three grains of barley (taken from the center of the ear, dried, and laid end to end), or one hundred points (.) lined up side by side.

Incident report Form used in health care facilities and other business settings to recount any type of adverse or unusual event such as a medication error, a property damage, or an injury to a patient, an employee, or a visitor.

Incompatibility A negative reaction that occurs when two or more drugs or other products are prescribed simultaneously or mixed together.

Indications Reasons why a drug or treatment is prescribed.

Indigenous Naturally occurring or originating in a particular location.

Induce To prompt, influence, or initiate.

Indwelling catheter Catheter that will be temporarily or permanently retained (fully or partially) within the body.

Infusion Medication or solution inserted into the vein or other body structure to produce the desired therapeutic effect.

Infusion pump Programmable device used to deliver solutions at an established flow rate from a solution bag or from a syringe.

Infusion set Tubing that allows a sterile pathway for fluid from an IV bag; available in numerous configurations; also known as an administration set or IV tubing.

Ingestion To take in by swallowing.

Inhalation Forced or drawn into the lungs.

Initial drug Term used in this text to describe an agonist as a drug receptor interaction that indicates the presence and potential action of the initial drug.

Inorganic Not derived from living organisms.

Inotropic effect Causing a change in the force of a muscle contraction, especially of the heart muscle; may have a positive (increase) or negative (decrease) impact on the contractile force.

Instability Tendency to be unpredictable.

Instillation Dripped into the body.

Insulin Hormone produced by the beta cells of the islets of Langerhans in the pancreas to lower the blood sugar level; also available as a pharmaceutical.

Integer A positive or negative whole number including zero.

Intermediate-level disinfection Kills most microorganisms (bacteria, fungi, and viruses) including the tuberculosis bacilli and the hepatitis B virus but not bacterial spores; used on semi-critical items.

International System of Units Official name of the metric system; English version.

International unit An arbitrary type of measure that represents the biological potency of a drug within the body regardless of the mass of the substance that is accepted globally. Because a unit is standardized according to the action of the drug, standardization of the unit pertains only to that drug. There is no standard conversion of drugs that are measured in units to another type of measure such as milligrams or milliliters.

Intraarterial Within an artery.

Intraarticular Within a joint.

Intracardiac Within the heart.

Intradermal Within the deep layer of the skin (dermis).

Intralaryngeal Within the larynx.

Intramuscular Within a muscle.

Intranasal Within the nose.

Intraocular Within the eye.

Intraoperative phase of surgical case management All activities from the initiation to the completion of the surgical procedure.

Intraosseous Within a bone.

Intraperitoneal Within the abdominal (peritoneal) cavity.

Intrathecal Within a sheath. In the case of an intrathecal block, the sheath is the dura mater.

Intratracheal Within the trachea.

Intravenous Within a vein.

Intravesicular Within the bladder.

Intravitreal Within the vitreous humor.

Ion Positively (+) or negatively (−) charged atom or molecule in which the number of electrons does not equal the number of protons.

Ionic Pertaining to an ion.

Ionic bond Type of chemical bond in which one or more electrons from one atom separate and attach to another atom, resulting in positive and negative ions that are attracted to each other.

Ionization state Determination of the drug molecule's charge—may be positive or negative.

Irreversible antagonism Type of antagonism that is similar to competitive antagonism; however, the effect is permanent. This type of antagonism is also said to be insurmountable and is also called nonequilibrium competitive antagonism.

Irrigate To moisten or wash a wound or an orifice.

Irrigating syringe Used to irrigate wounds and to aspirate fluid from the body or to insert fluid or air into a body cavity through a medical device.

Islets of Langerhans (alpha and beta cells) Cells in the pancreas responsible for producing the antagonistic hormones glucagon (produced by the alpha cells) and insulin (produced by the beta cells).

Isotonic Solution that consists of the same number of particles as blood plasma and does not move fluid into or out of the cells.

IV Abbreviation for the term *intravenously*.

IV bag Glass or polyvinyl chloride container that can range in size from 50 milliliters to 5 liters. More than 200 commercially prepared solutions are available. An IV bag is used in conjunction with an administration set or a transfer device to deliver the solution to the patient or to the sterile field. Also called a solution bag.

IV tubing Tubing that allows a sterile pathway for fluid from an IV bag; available in numerous configurations; also known as an administration set or infusion set.

K

Kelvin temperature scale Temperature scale commonly used in scientific settings that is based on absolute zero; no number on the scale can be below zero.

kg Abbreviation that represents the metric system term *kilogram*.

Kidney Organ responsible for production of urine and regulation of other body functions including regulation of fluid balance and blood pressure.

Kilo- Metric system prefix meaning thousand; abbreviated as K.

Kilogram Metric system term that represents one thousand grams.

Kiloliter Metric system term that represents 1,000 liters.

Kilometer Metric system term that represents 1,000 meters.

kl Abbreviation that represents the metric system term *kiloliter*.

km Abbreviation that represents the metric system term *kilometer*.

L

L Roman numeral symbol that represents the number fifty.

l/L Abbreviation for the term *liter*.

Lactation Secretion or production of milk by the mammary glands following childbirth.

Large bulb syringe Syringe for irrigation and aspiration of large surgical or traumatic wounds and body orifices. The large bulb syringe employs a catheter tip and has two components: the barrel, which is usually transparent, and the bulb. The end of the barrel near the bulb is flanged to provide finger rests for the user when compressing the bulb and markings on the barrel indicate

the capacity of the syringe. The bulb fits snugly into the barrel, creating a seal, and the bulb is pliable to allow the user to compress and release it easily; also known as an asepto syringe.

lb 1. Abbreviation that represents the apothecary system term *pound*. 2. Abbreviation that represents the household system term *pound*.

Leach To penetrate or pass through a porous substance.

Liberation Freeing of a drug from its administration form.

Lipophilicity Ability of a drug to be attracted to and dissolved in fat.

Liquid Fluid form of matter.

Liter Metric system term representing volume; one thousand milliliters.

Litmus paper Paper impregnated with litmus powder, which when exposed to various substances is capable of changing color to indicate the pH of the substance.

Local anesthesia Loss of sensation in a small area of the body following infiltration of a nerve conduction blocking agent; used to manage intraoperative and postoperative pain.

Long division bracket Symbol ($\overline{)}$) that separates the dividend from the divisor when performing long division.

Loop diuretic Type of drug that increases urine excretion by inhibiting reabsorption of salts from the loop of Henle in the kidney.

Low-level disinfection Kills most bacteria but not bacterial spores and is ineffective against the organism that causes tuberculosis; also kills some viruses and fungi; used on noncritical items.

Lubricant Used in the surgical environment on skin and mucous membranes to decrease friction during rectal and vaginal examinations and to facilitate insertion or passage of catheters, endoscopes, and surgical instruments.

Luer-lok® tip Threaded syringe tip options that allows a needle to be twisted (screwed) securely in place.

M

M Roman numeral symbol that represents the number one thousand.

MAC (monitored anesthesia care) Patient is monitored by an anesthesia provider, sedated, and provided with an analgesic and/or amnesic (as needed) while a dental, medical, or surgical procedure is performed under local anesthesia.

Malignant 1. Has a tendency to produce death. 2. Tumor characterized by uncontrolled growth; metastatic, invasive, cancerous.

Malignant hyperthermia Dramatic increase in body temperature that develops when a susceptible individual is exposed to a triggering agent.

Mass A substance that takes up space and has weight.

Matter A substance that has mass (occupies space and has weight).

mcg Abbreviation that represents the term *microgram*.

Means Two inner terms of a proportion that are cross-multiplied when solving for an unknown.

Medicine cup Container used to store small amounts of fluid. Calibrations found on the medicine cup can be in drams, ounces, tablespoons, or milliliters. The type of measurement most commonly used in the surgical environment is milliliters; however, because medicine cups are used in settings other than surgery, other types of measurements may also be present.

Mega- Metric system prefix meaning million; abbreviated as M.

Meninges Covering of the central nervous system (brain and spinal cord) that consists of three layers. From outermost to innermost, the layers are the dura mater, arachnoid mater, and pia mater.

Meniscus Curved or a crescent-shaped body (convex or concave) found on the upper surface of a column of liquid. The curvature is caused by surface tension of the liquid.

mEq Abbreviation that represents the term *milliequivalent*.

Metabolic acidosis High level of acid in the blood (academia) and body fluids due to an increase in production of hydrogen or a reduction in the ability of the body to form bicarbonate.

Metabolic rate Speed at which the body expends energy to function.

Metabolic tolerance Type of tolerance in which metabolism of the drug occurs more rapidly; also known as dispositional tolerance.

Metabolism In pharmacology, refers to chemical changes that a drug substance undergoes as it is being broken down (catabolism) within the body in preparation for excretion; also known as biotransformation and biodegradation.

Metabolite Breakdown product of biotransformation (metabolism). Metabolites are smaller than the original drug molecule and less active or inactive substances that are more easily excreted.

Metastasize To spread; often used to describe cancer cells spreading to parts of the body not associated with the original cancer site.

Meter Metric system term that represents length; size of a meter is related to the size of the earth and represents one ten-millionth of the distance from the North Pole to the Equator along the meridian nearest to Dunkirk, France.

Methicillin-resistant *Staphylococcus aureus* **(MRSA)** *Staphylococcus aureus* infection that is difficult to treat because the bacteria has undergone mutation, causing it to become resistant to commonly used antibiotics.

Metric system Scientific system for measuring length (meters), weight (grams), and volume (liters) that uses Arabic numerals and is decimal based.

mg Abbreviation that represents the term *milligram*.

mi Abbreviation that represents the household system term *mile/miles*.

Micro- Metric system prefix meaning millionth; abbreviated as μ or mc.

Microbe Microorganism, especially one that is capable of causing disease.

Microgram Metric system term that represents one millionth of a gram.

Microorganism Living matter that is too small to be viewed without the assistance of a microscope. Bacteria are examples of microorganisms.

Microscope Instrument for viewing objects too small to be seen by the unaided eye; consists of a lens for magnification and a source of illumination.

Mydriasis Pupil dilation.

Mile Household system term that represents the equivalent of 5,280 feet.

Military time Time-keeping system that uses a 24-hour clock to eliminate any potential confusion between AM and PM that may occur within the civilian time-keeping system.

Milli- Metric system prefix meaning thousandth; abbreviated as m.

Milliequivalent (mEq) Unit of measure that represents one thousandth of a measure. For example, if drug (usually an electrolyte) is measured by weight in grams, then a milliequivalent is one thousandth (0.001) of a gram.

Milligram Metric system term that represents one thousandth of a gram.

Milliliter Metric system term that represents one thousandth of a liter.

Millimeter Metric system term that represents one thousandth of a meter.

Mineral Inorganic elements that are naturally found in the earth and in water as well as plants and animals that acquire the minerals from soil and water. Certain minerals are needed by the body to regulate the heart rate, produce hormones, and maintain bone strength among other functions.

Mineralocorticoid Corticosteroid produced in the cortex of the adrenal gland and also available as a pharmaceutical; functions to regulate electrolyte and water balance; aldosterone is the major mineralocorticoid hormone.

Minim Apothecary system term that represents the equivalent of the quantity of water in a drop that weighs 1 grain.

Minuend Number from which another number (subtrahend) is subtracted.

Miotic Drug that causes the muscle of the iris to contract and constricts the pupil.

Mitigate To make less severe.

Mitosis Method of cell division that results in two cells that are identical to the parent cell. Mitosis consists of four active phases (prophase, metaphase, anaphase, and telophase) and a resting phase (interphase).

Mitotic inhibitor Drug that interrupts various stages of cell division (mitosis) according to the type of drug; also called plant alkaloid.

Mixed number Contains a whole number and a fraction.

Mixture Physical combination of two or more substances.

ml/mL Abbreviation that represents the metric system term *milliliter*.

mm Abbreviation that represents the metric system term *millimeter*.

Modified-release system Designed to delay or extend liberation of the drug.

Mold Type of fungus that often forms a fuzzy growth on the surface of organic matter; may be harmful or beneficial such as those used to make antibiotics; also called mycelium.

Molecular weight Combined weight of all atoms in the molecule.

Molecule Smallest unit of a compound or an element.

Monitored anesthesia care (MAC) Patient is monitored by an anesthesia provider, sedated, and provided with an analgesic and/or amnesic (as needed) while a dental, medical, or surgical procedure is performed under local anesthesia.

Monograph Complete and detailed description.

Multiplicand Number that will be multiplied by another number (multiplier).

Multiplication Mathematical calculation performed with two numbers to obtain a product; consists of addition of a number (multiplicand) to itself the number of times specified.

Multiplier Number by which another number (multiplicand) is multiplied.

Muscarinic Drug used to mimic the effects of the parasympathetic nervous system; capable of slowing of the heart, pupil constriction, increased gastrointestinal peristalsis, increased production of secretions (such as gastric juices, mucous, saliva, and sweat), increased contractibility of the urinary bladder, increased strength of the skeletal muscles, pupil constriction (miosis), and decreased intraocular pressure; also called cholinergic and parasympathomimetic.

Mycelium Fungal growth that often forms a fuzzy growth on the surface of organic matter; may be harmful or beneficial such as those used to make antibiotics; also called mold.

Mycoses Fungal infections.

Mydriatic Sympathomimetic drug that stimulates relaxation of the muscle of the iris, causing dilation of the pupil.

Myocardial infarction Destruction of an area of the heart muscle caused by disruption of the blood supply to the heart.

Myocardium Muscle of the heart.

Myometrium Muscle of the uterus.

N

Nano- Metric system prefix meaning billionth; abbreviated as n.

Narcotic analgesic Controlled substance used to reduce the perception of and reaction to pain as well as increase pain tolerance for patients experiencing moderate-to-severe acute and chronic pain.

Narcotic antagonist Agent used to reverse the effect of a narcotic.

Narcotics Drugs that have a potential to cause physical or psychological dependency; controlled substances.

Nasal syringe Syringe for irrigation and aspiration of small wounds or natural body openings that is constructed as a single unit of soft plastic that has a bulb on one end and a tapered opening on the other end; also known as small bulb syringe, ear syringe, and ulcer syringe.

Nasogastric (NG) tube Tube inserted into the stomach via the nasal portal.

Naturopathic Treatments that involve healthy lifestyle choices and dietary supplements.

Nausea Sensation that precedes vomiting.

Nausea/emesis gravidarum Morning sickness.

Needle Slender, hollow, pointed instrument that typically fits onto the end of a syringe that is used to pierce body tissue to allow for injection or withdrawal of fluids.

Negative contrast media Radiolucent material used during radiographic studies to enhance visualization by differentiating body structures; examples include gasses (such as air), carbon dioxide, metrizamide, and oxygen; shows as dark gray on the x-ray image.

Neonate Newborn; within the first 28 days of life.

Neoplasm New growth; often refers to abnormal tissue.

Nerve Bundle of specialized fibers that conduct information to and from the central nervous system; major component of the peripheral nervous system.

Nerve conduction blocking agent Prevent conduction of pain sensation impulses initiated in the nerves at the surgical site from reaching the brain.

Nerve impulse Electrical signal that transmits information from a receptor to the central nervous system and from the central nervous system to the effector along the pathway of a nerve.

Nervous system Body system that is responsible for regulation of all body functions based on responses to internal and external stimuli; consists of two major divisions (central nervous system comprised of the brain and spinal cord; peripheral nervous system comprised of all nerves, ganglia, receptors, and effectors).

Neuroleptic Drug used in the treatment of psychoses, neuroses, to relieve nausea and vomiting, as a synergist of an analgesic, and to treat anxiety, stress, and irritability; also known as a tranquilizer.

Neuromuscular blocker Skeletal muscle relaxant that interferes with passage of impulses from motor nerves to skeletal muscles; used to cause weakness/paralysis to relax the jaw to facilitate endotracheal intubation, when mechanical ventilation is required, and/or to allow for tissue retraction.

Neuron Specialized cell in the nervous system responsible for conduction of nerve impulses.

Neurotransmitter Chemical substance (such as acetylcholine or epinephrine) that transmits an impulse from a nerve across a synapse to an effector (such as a gland, muscle, or another nerve).

Neutron Portion of the nucleus of an atom that has no charge.

NG (nasogastric) tube Tube inserted into the stomach via the nasal portal.

Nil per os Nothing by mouth.

Nomenclature Refers to a system for naming or the rules for naming.

Noncompetitive antagonism Type of antagonism that occurs when the antagonist binds to a receptor site that would not normally be occupied by the initial drug, causing a change in the initial drug's receptor site, rendering it unrecognizable and unusable by the initial drug. Because high doses of the initial drug cannot overcome the power of the antagonist, this type of antagonism is said to be insurmountable.

Noncritical item Medical device, such as a blood pressure cuff, that will come in contact only with intact skin; must be disinfected with at least a low-level agent.

Nondepolarizing neuromuscular blocker Type of neuromuscular blocker that competes for the postsynaptic receptors, thereby preventing stimulation of the muscle contraction; metabolized in the liver; pharmacologic antagonist is available.

Nonelectrolytic Irrigation solutions that do not contain electrolytes; do not conduct electricity; usually used in conjunction with the electrosurgical unit (especially during endoscopic procedures) to reduce the risk of electrical injury.

Non-ionic Does not contain ions.

Nonspecific responses Type of drug interaction that occurs when a drug does not seem to act as a result of a drug receptor interaction or a drug enzyme interaction. The drug is thought to congregate and act on the plasmalemma or infiltrate the plasmalemma and act on the contents of the cell.

Normal body temperature (measured orally) 37° C or 98.6° F.

Nosocomial infection Infection acquired while hospitalized or otherwise receiving health care.

NPO Abbreviation of the Latin term *nil per os*, meaning nothing by mouth.

Nucleic acids Linked nucleotides.

Nucleotides Three molecules (sugar, phosphate group, and a base) that provide the structural components (giving the double helical shape) of DNA.

Nucleus Center portion of an atom that is composed of protons and neutrons.

Numerator Upper number of a fraction.

O

Obstetrical Pertaining to the care of pregnant women before, during, and after delivery of the neonate.

Ocular Pertaining to the eye.

Oculus dexter Latin term meaning right eye.

Oculus sinister Latin term meaning left eye.

Oculus utraque Latin term meaning each eye (both eyes).

od Abbreviation of the Latin term *oculus dexter*, meaning right eye.

Official "Do Not Use" List Provided by the Joint Commission that identifies specific abbreviations must appear on each accredited institution's do-not-use list.

Off-label use Drug is used for a purpose other than intended or used in a different form, in varying dosage, or for a different age group.

Oncotic pressure Force exerted by the flow of water through a semipermeable membrane separating two solutions with different concentrations of solute; also called osmotic pressure.

Onset of action Time that elapses from administration of the drug until the therapeutic effect of the drug is noted.

Operating microscope Microscope used during surgery to provide an enhanced view of small or otherwise inaccessible body structures.

Ophthalmic Pertaining to the eye.

Opioid Synthetic substance that has similar properties to opium.

Oral Pertaining to the mouth.

Order of operations Sequence in which certain tasks must be performed; especially important when solving algebraic equations.

Organelle Specialized part of a cell contained within the cytoplasm that has a specific function.

Organic Derived from living organisms.

Orifice Opening, for example, the mouth.

OS Abbreviation of the Latin term *oculus sinister*, meaning left eye.

Os Latin term meaning mouth or mouth-like opening.

Osmolality Measure of concentration of solutes per unit of volume; also called osmolarity.

Osmolarity Measure of concentration of solutes per unit of volume; also called osmolality.

Osmosis Ability of a solution to diffuse through a semipermeable membrane from an area of high concentration to an area of low concentration, thereby equalizing the concentration of the solution on both sides of the membrane.

Osmotic diuretic Type of drug that increases urine excretion by inhibiting reabsorption of water and sodium from the loop of Henle in the kidney, thereby increasing osmolarity (measure of concentration of solutes per liter of solution). Fluid is moved from the cells to the intercellular fluid and plasma, which is especially useful in reducing intraocular and intracranial pressure.

Osmotic pressure Force exerted by the flow of water through a semipermeable membrane separating two solutions with different concentrations of solute; also called oncotic pressure.

Otic Pertaining to the ear (auricular).

ou Abbreviation of the Latin term *oculus utraque*, meaning each eye (both eyes).

Ounce 1. Apothecary system term that represents the equivalent of 8 drams. 2. Household system term that represents the equivalent of an international avoirdupois ounce (most common—28.350 grams or 437.5 grains), an international troy ounce (usually used to weigh precious metals—31.103 grams or 480 grains), or an apothecary ounce (equivalent to a troy ounce). 3. Used to measure weight of a solid (one sixteenth of a pound/28.349 grams) or volume of a liquid (liquid ounce equals 29.573 milliliters).

Overdosage To take or be administered an excessive amount of a drug.

Ovine Pertaining to sheep.

Oxytocic Drug used to induce labor, strengthen uterine contractions during labor, and contract the uterus to control hemorrhage following an abortion or delivery (vaginal or abdominal) of a neonate.

oz Abbreviation that represents the household system term *ounce*.

P

Package insert Printed detailed description of a drug containing in-depth information that is too extensive to fit on the drug label.

Packed cells Blood component therapy consisting blood cells that have been separated from the plasma; sometimes refers only to red blood cells.

Packet Resembles a miniature envelope and typically contains a small amount (single dose) of a sterile product.

Paradoxical Contradictory.

Parasympathetic Portion of the autonomic nervous system that functions in opposition to the sympathetic nervous system to return the body to homeostasis following a sympathetic response.

Parasympatholytic Drug used to block the effects of the parasympathetic nervous system; capable of decreasing production of secretions, decreasing peristalsis of the gastrointestinal tract, dilating the pupils, and decreasing contractibility of the urinary bladder; also called anticholinergic, antimuscarinic, and cholinergic blocker.

Parasympathomimetic Drug used to mimic the effects of the parasympathetic nervous system; capable of slowing of the heart, pupil constriction, increased gastrointestinal peristalsis, increased production of secretions (such as gastric juices, mucous, saliva, and sweat), increased contractibility of the urinary bladder, increased strength of the skeletal muscles, pupil constriction (miosis), and decreased intraocular pressure; also called cholinergic and muscarinic.

Parenteral Other than enteral (usually by injection).

Partial agonist Type of agonist that produces a weak effect even though all of the available receptors are occupied by the drug.

Passive transport Drug molecules (in solution) move from an area of high concentration across a semipermeable membrane to an area of low concentration by osmosis (diffusion) until the concentration on both sides of the membrane is equal. No energy is expended during passive transport.

Patent (adjective) Open or unobstructed passageway (may pertain to a duct, bodily passage, catheter, tube, or drain).

Patent (noun) Issued by the United States Patent and Trademark Office. Prevents another manufacturer from producing a product for the length of the patent (usually 20 years).

Pathogen Substance capable of causing disease such as a bacteria or a virus.

Pathology Study of disease processes (origin, nature, and course).

Pathophysiology Changes in function related to a disease.

pc Abbreviation of the Latin term *post cibum*, meaning after meals.

Peak effect Time that elapses when the drug is most effective.

PEMDAS Acronym that represents the terms *parenthesis, exponents, multiplication, division, addition,* and *subtraction*; serves as a reminder to employ the order of operations when solving an algebraic problem. Perform the operations inside the parenthesis first, then the exponents, next multiplication and division (from left to right), and finally addition and subtraction (also from left to right).

Penicillin Drug in the beta-lactam group of antiinfective agents; originate from *Penicillium* molds, which are commonly found on the skin of citrus fruits; further divided into four classifications.

per Latin term meaning by/through.

Percent Parts per hundred.

Percutaneously Through the skin.

Pericardium Membrane that surrounds the heart.

Peripheral Superficial; away from the central area.

Peripheral blood vessels Veins and arteries that are located away from the core of the body.

Peripheral nervous system Division of the nervous system comprised of all nerves, ganglia, receptors, and effectors.

Peripheral vein Small vein that is located farther from the heart than a central vein. Examples of peripheral veins include veins of the arms, lower legs, and the scalp.

Peristalsis Wavelike contraction and relaxation of muscles that propels contents through a muscular tube such as the gastrointestinal tract or the ureters.

Peritoneal Pertaining to the abdominal cavity.

Peritoneal fluid Liquid produced within the abdominal cavity that serves to lubricate the internal surfaces.

Per os Latin term meaning by mouth.

Peta- Metric system prefix meaning quadrillion; abbreviated as P.

pH Potential of hydrogen (to gain or lose ions).

Pharmaceutical Pertains to a drug that is prepared commercially or in a pharmacy and/or dispensed by a retail or hospital pharmacist.

Pharmacist An individual licensed by the appropriate State Board of Pharmacy who is educated to prepare and dispense drugs in that state.

Pharmacodynamics Interaction of the drug molecule with the target (receptor, membrane, cell, tissue, organ, or whole body).

Pharmacokinetics Movement of the drug within the body. The four main processes involved in pharmacokinetics are absorption, distribution, biotransformation (metabolism), and excretion.

Pharmacologist One who has knowledge of drugs (origin, composition, action, uses, toxic effects, etc.) and the science of drug preparation. A pharmacologist usually works in a research setting.

Pharmacology The study of drugs; pertains to the composition, properties, and uses of the drug especially those that make it medically effective, and the effects or characteristics of the drug.

Pharmacopeia Reference book that is published by a recognized authority (such as the federal government) sets the legal standards for drug quality, strength, and purity.

Pharmacy Designated location for storage, preparation, and dispensing drugs. The term *pharmacy* may also be used to describe the practice of drug preparation and dispensation as well as other services such as providing the consumer with information concerning the prescribed medication(s) and other clinical services.

Phases of surgical case management Surgical case management is divided into three phases: preoperative, intraoperative, and postoperative. Each phase has components that relate to the patient, operating room, instruments, equipment, supplies, medications, and the surgical team members.

pH scale Measures hydrogen ion concentration. The pH scale ranges from 1 to 14 and represents the difference between the amount of H⁺ (hydrogen) ions and OH⁻ (hydroxide) ions. A pH of less than 7 represents an acid and a pH of greater than 7 represents a base. A pH of 7 is considered neutral. Deionized (distilled) water is neutral because it is neither an acid nor a base because it has no ions to donate and is incapable of accepting any ions.

Photochemical reaction A change in the properties of a substance due to exposure to light.

Physiological Pertaining to the function of an organism. May refer to function of a single cell or the whole body.

Physiological antagonism Type of antagonism that occurs when two drugs are given that cancel the effects of one another.

Physiology Study of the function of the body.

Pico- Metric system prefix meaning trillionth; abbreviated as p.

Pinocytosis A small amount of fluid containing the drug molecule(s) called a vesicle is formed. The entire vesicle is drawn through the membrane. Pinocytosis is a form of active transport that is used in very specific circumstances such as absorption of fat-soluble vitamins.

Pint 1. Apothecary system term that represents the equivalent of 16 fluid ounces. 2. Household system term that represents the equivalent of 2 cups/32 ounces.

Plain Term sometimes used in pharmacology to indicate that an additive has not been combined with a medication.

Plant alkaloid Drug that interrupts various stages of cell division (mitosis) according to the type of drug; also called mitotic inhibitor.

Plasma 1. Liquid portion of the blood (without the formed elements). 2. Liquids found within a cell known as cytoplasm and nucleoplasm.

Plasmalemma Double phospholipid membrane that surrounds the plasma (cytoplasm/protoplasm) of a cell; also known as plasma membrane and cell membrane.

Plasma membrane Double phospholipid membrane that surrounds the plasma (cytoplasm/protoplasm) of a cell; also known as cell membrane and plasmalemma.

Plasma protein binding Ability of some drugs to bind to plasma proteins (such as albumin) to allow for transport and to protect them from being metabolized by various enzymes. Unfortunately, the bound portion of the drug is not available to the target cells, leaving only the free molecules to be delivered to the target cells to accomplish the desired action.

Platelet Cell fragment found in the blood that is part of the blood-clotting sequence; also called thrombocyte.

Platelet aggregation Part of the blood-clotting sequence in which platelets clump together to form the foundation of a thrombus.

Platelet concentrate Blood component consisting primarily of platelets (thrombocytes), which are essential to normal blood clotting.

PM Acronym that represents the Latin term *post meridiem*.

po Abbreviation of the Latin term *per os*, meaning by mouth.

Policy Document containing a plan of action sanctioned by an entity such as a health care facility.

Polymyxin Drug in the polypeptide group that is produced by the organism *Bacillus polymyxa*, which is a Gram-positive bacterium; binds to the bacterial cell membrane disrupting the cell's ability to release toxins; primarily effective against most Gram-negative bacteria.

Polypeptide Amino acid chain linked with peptide bonds; includes the polymyxin group of antiinfective agents.

Porcine Pertaining to swine.

Positive contrast media Radiopaque material used during radiographic studies to enhance visualization by differentiating body structures; examples include ionic and non-ionic iodinated substances and barium; shows as white or light gray on the x-ray image.

Posology Study of dosages of drugs.

Post cibum Latin term meaning after meals.

Post meridiem (PM) Latin term meaning after midday/noon.

Postoperative phase of surgical case management All activities following completion of the surgical procedure (includes the patient's recovery and care of the operating room, instruments, equipment, and supplies).

Potassium-channel blocker Drug that slows electrical impulses as they move through the heart and increases the time between heart beats; reduces the number of potassium ions available to conduct the impulse, slowing movement of the impulse.

Potency Strength.

Pound 1. Apothecary system term that represents the equivalent of 12 ounces. 2. Household system term that represents the equivalent of 16 ounces.

Precipitate Chemical reaction during which a dissolved substance separates from the solution and appears as fine particles suspended in the solution.

Preference card In the operating room, the surgeon preference card is the tool utilized to prepare for the surgical procedure. The preference card is a form of standing orders. The preference card contains all of the pertinent information concerning a specific surgeon's requests for a specific surgical procedure including medication orders.

Preoperative phase of surgical case management All preparatory activities leading up to initiation of the surgical procedure.

Prescription An order written by a physician (or other licensed health care provider) that is required prior to preparing and dispensing certain medications or administering a treatment.

Primary effect Intended drug action; therapeutic effect.

Principles of asepsis Principles related to the practice of sterile technique that include creating a sterile field for each surgical procedure, entry of the sterile team members into the sterile field, and maintenance of the sterile field. The goal of the principles of asepsis is to keep the microbial count to an irreducible minimum.

prn Abbreviation of the Latin term *pro re nata*, meaning according to the circumstances/as needed.

Procedure Description of the manner in which a plan of action (policy) is carried out.

Procoagulant Drug or other substance used to promote blood clotting, maintain a blood clot, or otherwise act to slow or stop bleeding; also called coagulant and hemostatic agent.

Product Result of multiplication.

Proper fraction Numerator is smaller than the denominator.

Properties Distinctive element such as characteristics or traits.

Prophylaxis Term used to describe preventive measures.

Proportion Comparison of two ratios that are equal.

Proprietary name Name that the manufacturer assigns to a drug for marketing purposes; also known as trade name and brand name.

Pro re nata Latin term meaning according to the circumstances/as needed.

Prostaglandins Hormone-like chemical messengers that are secreted by many types of cells in the body and act on nearby tissues; responsible for initiation of the inflammatory response, which results in fever and pain.

Prostatectomy Removal of the prostate.

Protein Essential component of living cells composed of chains of amino acids. Proteins are necessary for tissue repair and growth and are obtained in the diet by eating meat, fish, dairy products, and legumes.

Protein channel Opening formed by a protein through a membrane to allow passage of a substance such as a drug.

Protocol A detailed plan designed to carry out an experiment or a medical treatment.

Proton Positively charged portion of an atom.

Prototype Generalization about the characteristics of the drugs in that classification.

Pseudocholinesterase Enzyme found in the blood plasma responsible for biotransformation of certain drugs (amino esters and the depolarizing neuromuscular blocking agent succinylcholine).

Psychological Pertaining to or influencing the mind or the emotions.

pt 1. Abbreviation that represents the apothecary system term *pint*. 2. Abbreviation that represents the household system term *pint*.

Pulmonary aspiration Entry of food, fluid, stomach contents, or a foreign body into the lower respiratory tract (trachea, bronchi, lungs) by inhalation or mechanical ventilation.

Q

q Abbreviation of the Latin term *quaque*, meaning every.

qd Abbreviation of the Latin term *quaque die*, meaning once every day.

qh/q3h (any number may be substituted, as prescribed) Abbreviation of the Latin term *quaque hora/quaque 3 hora*, meaning every hour/every 3 hours.

qid Abbreviation of the Latin term *quarter in die*, meaning four times per day.

qt 1. Abbreviation that represents the apothecary system term *quart*. 2. Abbreviation that represents the household system term *quart*.

Quaque Latin term meaning every.

Quaque die Latin term meaning once every day.

Quaque hora Latin term meaning every hour.

Quart 1. Apothecary system term that represents the equivalent of 2 pints. 2. Household system term that represents the equivalent of 2 pints/4 cups/32 ounces.

Quarter in die Latin term meaning four times per day.

Quotient Result of division.

R

Radioactive isotope Chemical element that emits gamma radiation, which is used as contrast media to identify tumors, infections, congenital abnormalities, and the function of various tissues; the isotope is given intravenously and a scintillation camera is used to create an image that allows visualization of the area of concern; also called radionuclide.

Radiographic Pertaining to an x-ray.

Radiolucent Substance that allows penetration of x-rays providing contrast of various tissues.

Radionuclide Chemical element that emits gamma radiation, which is used as contrast media to identify tumors, infections, congenital abnormalities, and the function of various tissues; the isotope is given intravenously and a scintillation camera is used to create an image that allows visualization of the area of concern; also called radioactive isotope.

Radiopaque Substance that slows or does not allow penetration of x-rays, providing contrast of various tissues.

Rankine temperature scale Temperature scale commonly used in industrial settings that is based on absolute zero; no number on the scale can be less than zero.

Ratio Expression of a relationship between two numbers or components by comparing them to one another.

Receptor Sensory nerve ending that receives a stimuli and sends information to the central nervous system for processing and a response.

Reciprocal Number that when multiplied by a given number or quantity results in a product of one; synonymous with the term *multiplicative inverse*.

Recombinant To combine segments of DNA from more than one source.

Reconstitute To add a liquid to a dried or concentrated substance to return it to its former condition and/or strength.

Rectal Pertaining to the rectum.

Recurrent 1. Event that happens repeatedly. 2. Turn back; to go in the opposite direction; refers to body structures (nerves, blood vessels, etc.).

Reduced responsiveness Drug tolerance that occurs when the number of receptors that bind to the drug are decreased; also known as cellular tolerance or downregulation.

Reduce to lowest terms Cancellation of all common terms (factors) in the numerator and denominator of a fraction until no common terms remain; synonymous with the term *simplify*.

Relative bioavailability Used to compare the availability of the same drug that has been manufactured differently such as the brand name drug versus the generic version of the same drug.

Remainder Portion that is left after the mathematic process is complete.

Respiratory acidosis High level of acid in the blood (acidemia) and body fluids due to inadequate elimination of carbon dioxide from the lungs; causes include lung disease such as emphysema or pneumonia and administration of medications that suppress respiration such as general anesthetic agents.

Respiratory stimulant Drug that stimulates the central nervous system to increase the urge to breathe, the rate of respirations, and the tidal volume.

Rh factor Antigen found on the surface of red blood cells of some individuals; individuals with the antigen are said to be Rh+ (positive) and individuals lacking the antigen are said to be Rh– (negative).

Rho (D) immune globulin Contains antibodies that suppress the Rh– maternal immune system from attacking Rh+ blood cells from a fetus that may enter maternal circulation during a first pregnancy, thereby preventing hemolytic disease of the newborn in subsequent pregnancies.

Ring syringe Syringe that employs three finger rings instead of flanges. Two of the rings are attached to the barrel and one is attached to the plunger. The rings provide increased stability (control) of the syringe in the hand of the user and allow additional pressure to be applied to eject the contents if resistance occurs. Also called a control syringe.

Roman numeral system System of numbering that uses letters (upper or lower case) to represent numbers but does not include a symbol to represent zero; includes a separate system to denote fractions.

Route of administration Method used to convey a drug into the body.

S

sc Abbreviation that represents the term *subcutaneous*.

Scintillation camera Device similar to a Geiger counter that is capable of detecting gamma radiation emitted from radioisotopes; also called a gamma camera.

Scored Scratch or notch in the neck of an ampule to allow the glass to break at the desired location.

Scruple Apothecary system term that represents the equivalent of 20 grains.

Secondary effect(s) Known side effect of a drug that prompts use of the drug for additional purposes.

Sedative Minor tranquilizer used to produce a state of calm and reduce anxiety; also called anxiolytic.

Seizure Change in consciousness, emotion, sensation, vision, taste, and muscle tone (including loss of muscle control or muscle twitching and tightening that cause spasmodic movement) that result from abnormal electrical activity in the brain.

Semi-critical item Medical device, such as an airway maintenance device, that will come in contact with non-intact skin or a mucous membrane; must be disinfected with at least an intermediate-level agent.

Semipermeable membrane Membrane that allows some molecules to pass through, but not all.

Semisolid Of a consistency that is between a solid and a liquid. Creams, foams, gels, lotions, suppositories, and unguents (ointments) are examples of semisolids.

Sex hormones 1. Hormones of the adrenal cortex that promote development of secondary sex characteristics. 2. Hormones secreted from the ovaries in the female (estrogens and progesterone) and from the testes in the male (testosterone) that are activated at the time of puberty under the control of other hormones that originate in the pituitary gland.

Shelf life Length of time that a product may be stored and remain suitable for use.

SI Abbreviation representing the term Systeme International d'Unites.

Side effects Expected but undesirable, generally mild, and often tolerable or manageable effects of a drug that are not therapeutic. Examples of side effects include, but are not limited to, skin irritation, nausea, vomiting, constipation, diarrhea, dry mouth, dizziness, and drowsiness.

sig Abbreviation of the Latin term *signa*, meaning write (usually an indication to the pharmacist that the directions that follow should be translated and written on the label for the patient).

Signa Latin term meaning to write.

Simple fraction Contains only one numerator and one denominator.

Simplify Cancellation of all common terms in the numerator and denominator of a fraction until no common terms remain; synonymous with reduce to lowest terms.

Six rights Model used to ensure that a drug is handled and administered correctly. The six rights are the right patient, right drug, right dose, right route of administration, right time and frequency, and right documentation/labeling.

Slip tip Tapered syringe tip designed to fit inside of a needle hub and secure the needle via friction.

Small bulb syringe Syringe for irrigation and aspiration of small wounds or natural body openings that is constructed as a single unit of soft plastic that has a bulb on one end and a tapered opening on the other end; also known as ear syringe, nasal syringe, and ulcer syringe.

Sodium-channel blocker Drug that lengthens the amount of time needed for an electrical impulse to move from the sinoatrial node, through the heart, to the Purkinje fibers and stimulate the ventricles to contract or increase the amount of time between heart beats; reduces the number of sodium ions available to conduct the impulse, thereby slowing movement of the impulse.

Solid The particulate form of matter.

soln Abbreviation that represents the term *solution*.

Solute Substance of a mixture in the larger amount. Typically the liquid portion of a mixture.

Solution Mixture of two or more substances that combine easily. Solutions are homogenous.

Solution bag Glass or polyvinyl chloride container that can range in size from 50 milliliters to 5 liters. More than 200 commercially prepared solutions are available. A solution bag is used in conjunction with an administration set or a transfer device to deliver the solution to the patient or to the sterile field. Also called an IV bag.

Solvent Substance of a mixture in the smaller amount. May be another liquid or a solid that is dissolved by the solvent.

Soporific Central nervous system depressant classified as a narcotic; used to induce sleep; also called hypnotic.

Sorbitol Nonelectrolyte solution used for bladder irrigation because it does not conduct electricity or harm the blood cells and is not sticky. Sorbitol is also used as a sweetener and a non-stimulant laxative.

sq Abbreviation of the term *subcutaneous*.

Square root A divisor of a number that when squared results in the same number. For example, the square roots of 9 are 3 and 3 because $3 \times 3 = 9$.

Stain Pigment used to color tissue; used when coloration is needed permanently or for long duration; not easily removed or absorbed.

Standard time Time-keeping system that uses a 12-hour clock in which the 12 numbers repeat; designations of AM and PM are used to represent morning and afternoon; synonymous with civilian time.

Standing orders Pre-established set of orders for patients with similar conditions.

Staphylococci Characteristic arrangement of round bacterial cells that form in clusters.

Stat Abbreviation of the Latin term *statum*, meaning immediately.

Statum Latin term meaning immediately.

Sterilant Chemical or physical agent that kills all microorganisms including bacterial spores.

Sterile technique Rules and practices related to maintaining the principles of asepsis.

Streptococci Characteristic arrangement of round bacterial cells that form in chains.

Strong agonist Type of agonist that produces the greatest effect even though only a small percentage of the available receptors on the plasmalemma may be occupied by the drug.

Subacute Disease or medical condition that is not as severe as acute but not as long-lasting as chronic.

Subconjunctival Pertaining to the tissue beneath the conjunctiva.

Subcutaneous Beneath the skin; pertaining to the adipose tissue.

Sublingual Under the tongue.

Subtraction Calculation of the difference between two numbers.

Subtrahend Number to be subtracted from another (minuend).

Sulfa drug Synthetic antiinfective agent that works by disrupting synthesis of folic acid, thereby negatively impacting production of deoxyribonucleic acid (DNA) and purine; primarily effective against many Gram-positive and Gram-negative bacteria; sometimes called sulfonamide.

Sulfonamide Synthetic antiinfective agent that works by disrupting synthesis of folic acid, thereby negatively impacting production of deoxyribonucleic acid (DNA) and purine; primarily effective against many Gram-positive and Gram-negative bacteria; sometimes called sulfa drugs.

Sum Result of addition.

Superficial Near the surface.

Suppository Medication that is in a solid or semisolid form that has been shaped cylindrically for insertion into the rectum, urethra, or vagina.

susp Abbreviation that represents the term *suspension*.

Suspension Consists of a liquid and one or more solids that do not dissolve. Suspensions are heterogenous.

Sustained-release Maintains steady liberation of the drug for a prolonged period.

Symbol Character used to represent something else; for example, = is a symbol used to represent the word *equals*.

Sympathetic Portion of the autonomic nervous system that functions in opposition to the parasympathetic nervous system; allows for the fight-or-flight response to stress, anger, or an emergency situation.

Sympatholytic Drug that inhibits the effects of the sympathetic nervous system; also called adrenergic antagonist and adrenergic blocker.

Sympathomimetic Drug that mimics the effects of the sympathetic nervous system; also called adrenergic or adrenergic agonist.

Synapse A small gap where nerve impulses pass with the aid of a neurotransmitter.

Synergist A drug that works together with one or more other drugs to produce an enhanced effect, making the cumulative effect of the combined drugs greater than the effect of each drug individually.

Synthesis Formation of a complex substance from simpler elements that is reliable and reproducible in a laboratory setting.

Synthetic Substance produced in a laboratory (artificially) rather than naturally.

Syringe A cylindrical device with either a plunger or a bulb attachment that is used to inject fluids into or withdraw fluids from the body. Syringes may be manufactured from glass, metal, plastic, and/or rubber.

Syrup An aqueous solution that has been sweetened with sugar to enhance the taste.

Systeme International d'Unites (SI) Official name of the metric system; French version.

T

T Abbreviation that represents the household system term *tablespoon/tablespoons*; the abbreviation Tbsp may also be used.

t Abbreviation that represents the household system term *teaspoon/teaspoons*; the abbreviation tsp may also be used.

tab Abbreviation that represents the term *tablet*.

Tablespoon Household system term that represents the equivalent of 3 teaspoons.

Tablet Medicated powder that has been compressed to form a small pellet.

Tamponade 1. Use of a plug of cotton, bone wax, or other material inserted into an orifice or wound for the purpose of absorbing blood or applying pressure to slow or stop bleeding. 2. Condition in which the heart is compressed and unable to function correctly due to accumulation of fluid in the pericardium.

Tank Tubular (cylindrical) pressurized metal container that is typically used to store a gas. Medical gases, such as oxygen and nitrous oxide, are often stored in a large tank in a central location and piped to the point of use and delivered via an outlet; or a smaller portable cylinder may be employed; also known as a cylinder.

Tbsp Abbreviation that represents the household system term *tablespoon/tablespoons*; the abbreviation T may also be used.

Teaspoon Household system term that represents the equivalent of 60 drops.

Tensile strength Ability of a substance to resist rupture when force (tension) is applied.

Tera- Metric system prefix meaning trillion; abbreviated as T.

Teratogenic effects Drug effects that cause malformations that affect an embryo or a fetus, resulting in a congenital defect.

Ter in die Latin term meaning three times per day.

Tetracycline Antiinfective agent that disrupts protein synthesis of the cell, rendering the cell incapable of reproduction; effective against a wide variety of Gram-negative and Gram-positive bacteria.

Therapeutic effect Intended drug action; primary effect.

Three verification process Safe medication practice that involves checking each medication (name, strength, expiration date, and any other pertinent facts) three times.

Thrombocyte Cell fragment found in the blood that is part of the blood-clotting sequence; also called platelet.

Thrombolytic Drug that destroys fibrin, which is a major component of a blood clot (thrombus); also called fibrinolytic.

Thrombus Blood clot; primarily made of fibrin.

tid Abbreviation for the Latin term *ter in die*, meaning three times per day.

Tidal volume Amount of air moved in and out of the lungs with each breath.

tinc Abbreviation for the term *tincture*.

tinct Abbreviation for the term *tincture*.

Tincture An alcohol-based solution.

Tissue binding Administered drug has an affinity for a certain type of tissue such as muscle or fat where it is bound, making a portion of the drug unavailable to the target cells. However, when the drug is released from the tissue, a lingering effect of the drug may be noted; also known as depot storage.

Tocolytic Drug used to suppress uterine contractions and arrest premature labor.

Tolerance A result of a decreased response to the same dose of a particular drug over an extended period of time. As a result, the dosage must be increased to produce the desired response. Tolerance may be physiological or psychological and is usually seen with narcotic analgesics, alcohol, and benzodiazepine as well as other psychotropic drugs. Tolerance is described in three categories: metabolic, cellular, and behavioral.

Toomey syringe Specialty syringe typically used during urologic procedures. Syringe consists of a transparent barrel with markings to indicate the capacity and a plunger. The plunger has a rubber stopper on the barrel end and a large thumb ring that allows the user to draw in the desired contents or eject the contents under pressure while maintaining control of the syringe on the opposite end. The interchangeable tip of the syringe is designed to be attached to standard urology instruments or to a Foley catheter. Also called a piston syringe.

Topical Pertaining to a surface. Topical drugs are applied to a surface (may pertain to the skin, mucous membrane, or an exposed surface within the body).

Toxic Having a poisonous effect.

Toxic effects Poisonous effects of a drug that are capable of causing injury or death and are usually related to overdosing; however, a toxic effect may also be seen when metabolism or excretion of the drug is impeded.

Toxicology Study of the poisonous effects of a substance.

Toxin Poison; includes the bacterial (tetanus, diphtheria, etc.), plant (ricin), and animal toxins (snake venom).

tr Abbreviation for the term *tincture*.

Trademark Issued by the United States Patent and Trademark Office; a word, phrase, symbol, design, or combination thereof that identifies and distinguishes an item; usually pertains to the trade/brand name of a product.

Trade name Name that the manufacturer assigns to a drug for marketing purposes; also known as the proprietary name and the brand name.

Tranquilizer Drug used in the treatment of psychoses, neuroses, to relieve nausea and vomiting, as a synergist of an analgesics, and to treat anxiety, stress, and irritability; also known as a neuroleptic.

Transcutaneous Through the skin.

Transdermal Through the skin.

Transfer device Rigid spout attached to a solution bag that allows the solution to be transferred (poured) into a container on the sterile field.

Transfusion Transfer of blood or blood components from a donor to a recipient; donor and recipient may be the same individual (autotransfusion).

Transmucosal Through a mucous membrane.

Transport To move or cause movement from one area to another.

Transporters Substances such as proteins bind with the drug molecules to allow distribution of the drug to the target cells and excretion of the drug. Without transporters some drugs would be rendered useless.

Transurethral Through the urethra.

tsp Abbreviation that represents the household system term *teaspoon/teaspoons*; the abbreviation t may also be used.

Tube 1. Small flexible metal or plastic container that is sealed at one end and has a capped opening at the other from which a semisolid substance (such as a cream, gel, or ointment) may be squeezed. 2. Hollow cylindrical device inserted into a body cavity, duct, or vessel to decompress the structure, create negative pressure, maintain patency of a lumen, or administer fluids or gasses.

Turbidity Murky or cloudy in appearance.

Twist tip Threaded syringe tip option that allows a needle to be twisted (screwed) securely in place. Also called Luer-lok® tip.

Type and cross match Test performed on blood from both the donor and the recipient to identify the blood type, Rh factor, and the presence of antibodies in the donor blood that could be harmful to the recipient.

U

U Abbreviation that represents the term *unit*.

Ulcer syringe Syringe for irrigation and aspiration of small wounds or natural body openings that is constructed as a single unit of soft plastic that has a bulb on one end and a tapered opening on the other end; also known as small bulb syringe, nasal syringe, and ear syringe.

ung Abbreviation of the Latin term *unguentum*, meaning ointment.

Unguent Latin term meaning ointment.

Unguentum Latin term meaning ointment.

Uniform Resource Locator (URL) Sequence of characters used to reference an internet source.

Unit Type of measurement that has a standard physical quality (such as quantity, size, and weight).

United States customary units Measurement system primarily used in the United States to determine length, weight, and volume; also referred to as the household system.

Universal blood donor Individuals with the blood type O–.

Universal blood recipient Individuals with the blood type AB+.

Ureters Passageway that connects the kidneys to the urinary bladder.

Urethra Passageway that connects the urinary bladder to the exterior of the body; allows for excretion of urine.

Urethral Pertaining to the urethra.

URL (Uniform Resource Locator) Sequence of characters used to reference an internet source.

Urologic Pertaining to the study of the urinary tract. The urinary tract consists of the kidneys, ureters, bladder, and urethra.

Urticaria Hives.

ut dict Abbreviation of the Latin term *ut dictum*, meaning as directed.

ut dictum Latin term meaning as directed.

V

V Roman numeral symbol that represents the number five.

Vaccine Preparation administered to provide immunity to a specific pathogen.

Vagal blocker Drugs such as H_2 receptor blockers (H_2 antagonists) and cholinergic blockers (anticholinergics/parasympatholytics/antimuscarinics) that are used to block the effects of the vagus nerve.

Vaginal Pertaining to the vagina.

Vapor Volatile liquids that vaporize or evaporate easily.

Vasoconstrictor Drug that tightens (constricts) the smooth muscle of the wall of a blood vessel, decreases the diameter of the lumen of the vessel, and increases resistance to blood flow, raising the blood pressure; also called vasopressor.

Vasodilator Drug that relaxes (dilates) the smooth muscle of the wall of a blood vessel, thereby increasing the diameter of the lumen of the vessel, decreasing resistance to blood flow, and lowering the blood pressure.

Vasopressor Drug that tightens (constricts) the smooth muscle of the wall of a blood vessel, thereby decreasing the diameter of the lumen of the vessel and increasing resistance to blood flow, raising the blood pressure; also called vasoconstrictor.

Vaughan-Williams classification system Method for classifying antidysrhythmic drugs and some miscellaneous drugs used to treat dysrhythmias; consists of four main classifications.

Ventilator A mechanical device that delivers artificial respiration.

Ventricle Cavities or chambers found within an organ such as the heart or the brain.

Verification Method/process used to confirm accuracy.

Vesicle Small sac that usually contains fluid.

Vial Small plastic or glass bottle that contains a sterile medication that may be in either solution or powder form. A vial is sealed with a sterile rubber stopper that is held in place with an aluminum seal. Additionally, a plastic cap is attached to the aluminum seal to protect the sterility of and to allow easy access to the rubber stopper.

Virus Group of pathogens that are smaller than bacteria and are capable of multiplication only within living cells.

Viscoelastic Substance that possesses both viscous (thick, gelatinous consistency) and elastic (flexible, but capable of maintaining original shape) properties.

Viscosity The thickness of a liquid or a semisolid.

Vital signs Provide an overview of an individual's general condition; vital signs include temperature, pulse, respirations, and blood pressure. Each vital sign has an assigned range of normal values.

Vitamin Organic compounds essential to homeostasis. Vitamins are classified as fat soluble (vitamins A, D, E, and K because they are stored in body fat and in the liver) and water soluble (vitamin B complex and vitamin C because they are not stored in the body and are excreted in the urine). Some vitamins are naturally acquired in the diet from plant and animal consumption and others are manufactured within the body.

Volatile liquid A liquid that vaporizes or evaporates easily.

Vomiting Regurgitation; ejection of the stomach contents through the mouth; reverse peristalsis; also called emesis.

von Willebrand's disease Blood clotting disorder related to a deficiency of von Willebrand factor (vWF), which is a protein that is required for platelet aggregation.

W

w With.

w/o Without.

Water soluble Capable of being dissolved or liquefied in water.

Weak agonist Type of agonist that produces approximately the same effect as a strong agonist, but must occupy a greater percentage of the cell's receptors.

Whole blood Donated blood product for transfusion that does not have any portion removed, although an anticoagulant may be added.

Withdrawal Occurs when an individual who is addicted to a drug discontinues use of the drug. Withdrawal may occur suddenly or gradually. Physical and psychological manifestations of withdrawal can vary in intensity and severity from very mild to extremely serious, and in some situations may be deadly. Symptoms of withdrawal can last from as little as a few hours to as long as several weeks. Examples of withdrawal symptoms include nausea, vomiting, diarrhea, constipation, sweating, and tremors. Some individuals experience a rebound effect in which the problem for which the drug was initially administered returns in a seemingly more severe fashion until homeostasis is reestablished; also known as detoxification.

Wound Area of damaged tissue, as from a surgical incision or traumatic injury.

X

X Roman numeral symbol that represents the number ten.

X-ray Image obtained with the use of a form of electromagnetic radiation that is recorded on film or digitally.

Y

Yard Household system term that represents the equivalent of 3 feet/36 inches.

yd Abbreviation that represents the household system term *yard/yards*.

Yeast Type of single-celled fungus that reproduces by budding.

Yocto- Metric system prefix meaning septillionth; abbreviated as y.

Yotta- Metric system prefix meaning septillion; abbreviated as Y.

Z

Zepto- Metric system prefix meaning sextillionth; abbreviated as z.

Zetta- Metric system prefix meaning sextillion; abbreviated as Z.

Zonule of Zinn Ring of fibrous tissue that connects the crystalline lens of the eye with the ciliary body.

Zonulysis Use of an enzyme to dissolve the zonule of Zinn to facilitate removal of a cataract.

Zoologic Term typically used to distinguish lower animals from humans, but a few drugs classified as having an animal origin are derived from human sources.

INDEX